W9-BYH-933

The Mental Health Practitioner and the Law
///

The
Mental Health
Practitioner
and the Law

A Comprehensive Handbook

///

Edited by
Lawrence E. Lifson, M.D.
and Robert I. Simon, M.D.

Harvard University Press
Cambridge, Massachusetts
London, England
1998

Copyright © 1998 by the President and Fellows of Harvard College
All rights reserved
Printed in the United States of America

Library of Congress Cataloging-in-Publication Data

The mental health practitioner and the law : a comprehensive handbook
  / edited by Lawrence E. Lifson and Robert I. Simon.
     p.   cm.
  Includes bibliographical references and index.
  ISBN 0-674-69721-9 (alk. paper)
  1. Psychiatrists—Malpractice—United States.
  2. Psychologists—Malpractice—United States.
  I. Lifson, Lawrence E. II. Simon, Robert I.
  KF2910.P753M46 1998
  344.73′044—dc21   97-41510

With loving appreciation to our wives

Marcie G. Lifson and Patricia A. Simon

and to our children

Deborah and Jennifer Lifson

and

Robert, Patrick, and Brett Simon

///CONTENTS

Introduction   1
Lawrence E. Lifson, M.D., and Robert I. Simon, M.D.

LIABILITY PREVENTION

 1. The Harvard Medical Practice Study   7
    Troyen Brennan, M.D., J.D., MPH

 2. Informed Consent   23
    Marilyn Berner, J.D., LICSW

 3. Liability Issues with Managed Care   44
    James Hilliard, J.D.

 4. Write Smarter, Not Longer   54
    Marilyn Berner, J.D., LICSW

 5. Child and Adolescent Therapy   72
    Renee Tankenoff Brant, M.D., and Hon. Jonathan Brant

 6. The Perspective of the Insurer   89
    Peggy Berry Martin, M.Ed., A.R.M.

 7. What Your Licensing Board Expects of You   101
    Richard Waring, J.D.

MALPRACTICE MINEFIELDS

 8. Litigation Hot Spots in Clinical Practice   117
    Robert I. Simon, M.D.

 9. Supervisor, Supervisee, and Medical Backup   140
    Thomas G. Gutheil, M.D.

10. The Violent Patient   153
    James Beck, M.D., Ph.D., and Prudence Baxter, M.D.

11. The Suicidal Patient   166
    Robert I. Simon, M.D.

12. Pitfalls of Prescribing Medications   187
   James Hilliard, J.D.

13. Boundary Violations in Psychotherapy   195
   Robert I. Simon, M.D.

14. Termination of Treatment with Troublesome Patients   216
   James Hilliard, J.D.

THE CLINICIAN IN COURT

15. Witnesses, Depositions, and Trials   225
   Thomas G. Gutheil, M.D.

16. Patients Who Sue and Clinicians Who Get Sued in the
   Managed Care Era   237
   Harold J. Bursztajn, M.D., and Archie Brodsky, B.A.

17. The Wellsprings of Litigation   250
   Thomas G. Gutheil, M.D.

18. Ethical and Effective Testimony after *Daubert*   262
   Harold J. Bursztajn, M.D., and Archie Brodsky, B.A.

19. Suggestions for Expert Witnesses   281
   Larry H. Strasburger, M.D.

20. Narrative Truth, Historical Truth, and Forensic Truth   299
   Alan W. Scheflin, J.D., L.L.M.

21. The Perspective of the Plaintiff's Attorney   329
   Clyde D. Bergstresser, J.D.

22. Listen to Your Lawyer   344
   David Gould, J.D.

23. A View from the Bench   357
   Hon. Kermit V. Lipez

Epilogue   371
Glen O. Gabbard, M.D.

Contributors   385

Index   387

The Mental Health Practitioner and the Law
///

Introduction

Lawrence E. Lifson, M.D.
Robert I. Simon, M.D.

Clinical practice without undue fear of legal liability is fundamental to the practitioner's peace of mind. In fact, the fear of being sued can lead to unduly defensive reactions that may interfere with the appropriate treatment of the patient. The patient's welfare should be the clinician's unfettered concern. When the clinician focuses on providing good clinical care, employs sound risk management techniques, and carries adequate malpractice insurance, the fear of a malpractice claim should dissipate. The concept of clinical risk management emphasized throughout this book is a means for achieving such equanimity.

Clinical risk management is defined as the combining of professional expertise and knowledge of the patient with a clinically useful understanding of legal issues governing mental health practice in order to provide optimal care of the patient and, only secondarily, to reduce the risk of legal liability. A working knowledge of the legal regulation of clinical practice is essential. Such knowledge helps dispel unduly defensive reactions that may inhibit the clinician from utilizing a wide spectrum of effective treatments.

This book presents the major risk management areas and legal pitfalls encountered in current clinical practice. It focuses on practical knowledge and skills designed to decrease the practitioner's likelihood of being sued, and to increase the likelihood of prevailing if sued. This book also emphasizes the practitioner's professional, ethical, and moral duty to provide competent care to each and every patient.

/ / /

There are three basic spheres of influence that affect the working lives of mental health professionals: the therapist's duty to provide competent care to patients; the patient's right of self-determination to receive or reject such care; and the decisions and directives of courts, legislatures, and non-governmental agencies that regulate professional practice. Effective mental health treatment must encompass the tension between clinical practice and legal requirements.

For example, the imposition of the *Tarasoff* duty upon therapists to warn endangered third parties was viewed with much alarm. Because of the liability consequences, many therapists resisted accepting this as a professional duty. They viewed it as an unwarranted intrusion by the law into their professional lives. Thus, the moral principles underlying the duty to protect potential victims from violence by mental patients were often overlooked. Few psychotherapists would disagree with the need to protect an endangered third person from a patient who intends to do physical harm. What initially appears to be a conflict between the therapist's duty to maintain the confidentiality of patients and the law's requirements to safeguard the public can be viewed with less rancor when the commonality of underlying moral concern for the safety of another person is appreciated by both the law and the therapists. In the final analysis moral and ethical considerations are always an integral part of good clinical care.

We have witnessed an explosion of liability suits against health professionals with an attendant flood of anxiety on the part of clinicians. This has had a negative impact on patient care, partly by encouraging the practice of defensive medicine. Malpractice insurance premiums have soared, and some clinicians have even stopped seeing patients. Ironically, and sometimes painfully, unduly defensive practices have often subjected clinicians to even greater liability.

In an attempt to deal with this increased risk of liability, the Harvard Medical School Department of Continuing Education, in conjunction with the Harvard Risk Management Foundation, instituted an annual conference on liability prevention for mental health clinicians. Initially these conferences focused on new developments in malpractice prevention. It soon became apparent that we needed to place greater emphasis on the appearance of the practicing clinician in the courtroom. We thus added a second conference addressing the ever-increasing involvement of the clinician in court, be it as defendant, treating clinician, fact witness, or expert witness.

Our conferences were attended by many clinicians from outside the mental health field. In response, we introduced two additional annual conferences for medical and surgical practitioners: one on liability prevention and one on how to survive in a court setting.

This book is an outgrowth of our experience regarding risk management for the practicing clinician. Unlike most books in the field of risk management, this book is clinically based, responding to the needs of the practitioner upon entering the twenty-first century. It is both clinical and practical in approach and is organized into three sections.

The first section addresses the basic issues important for liability prevention. As in all sections, the contributing authors include both clinicians and attorneys. Troyen Brennan begins the book with a description of the seminal Harvard Medical Practice Study and its implications for malpractice prevention. This section also includes discussion of issues of informed consent and managed care liability in chapters written by James Hilliard and Marilyn Berner. Ms. Berner also presents a "documentation workshop," challenging the clinician's need to be overinclusive in documenting clinical care by her "write smarter not longer" strategy. The chapter by Renee Tankenoff Brant and Jonathan Brant covers unique aspects of risk management of child and adolescent treatment. Peggy Martin then offers a view from the perspective of the malpractice insurance carrier. This section concludes with a chapter by Richard Waring, who details what state licensing boards expect of practitioners.

The second section identifies the malpractice minefields, or high-risk areas for lawsuits. Robert I. Simon discusses current and future hot spots in legal liability, highlighting two of the most common high-risk areas confronting mental health clinicians—the management of the suicidal patient and the violation of treatment boundaries, particularly in the so-called gray areas. Thomas G. Gutheil deals with the poorly understood legal implications facing both the supervisor of clinical care and the physician who provides medical backup for other clinicians, be they medical students or senior nonphysician clinicians. James Beck and Prudence Baxter write about how to minimize risk in treating the violent patient. And James Hilliard advises about how to cope with two of the fastest-increasing threats of lawsuit: the pitfalls of prescribing medication and of terminating treatment with difficult patients.

The final section offers a survival guide for clinicians whose testimony is required in court, whether as defendant, treating clinician, fact witness, or expert witness. This section provides an introduction to courtroom demeanor and trial techniques for clinicians involved with the courts. Thomas G. Gutheil guides us through the various roles the clinician may play in court, and identifies the ingredients of clinician-patient relationships that are most likely to result in lawsuits. Harold Bursztajn and Archie Brodsky make it clear that the likelihood of a lawsuit has more to do with the personalities and interaction of particular patients with particular clinicians than with particular outcomes, and offer practical pointers for clinicians on the witness stand. Larry Strasburger discusses how to be most effective in testifying as an expert witness. Alan Scheflin delineates the differences between narrative truth, historical truth, and forensic truth and the implications of these differences for mental health clinicians in court. The section concludes with the perspectives of the plaintiff's attorney, the defense attorney, and the judge. Clyde Bergstresser warns clinicians of potential situations and circumstances that would encourage him, as a plaintiff's attorney, to bring suit. David Gould advises clinicians on how best to defend against that suit. Judge Kermit Lipez presents an invaluable perspective from the bench and offers practical suggestions on what a clinician should do in order to prevail when sued. Finally, in the book's epilogue, Glen O. Gabbard focuses on the psychology of the clinician and how fear of liability may impair the clinician's capacity to provide competent treatment.

The distinguished contributors to the book not only address the major areas of risk management and legal pitfalls encountered in clinical practice but also instruct clinicians about the legal process and the courtroom situation. This knowledge will enable clinicians to minimize the chance of being sued while enhancing the chance of successfully defending against such suit. Most important, the contributors present clinical risk management in a clear, concise manner that not only limits the risk of legal liability but betters patient care.

Liability
Prevention

/ / /

1

The Harvard Medical Practice Study

Troyen Brennan, M.D., J.D., MPH

There is very little empirical information regarding the manner in which accident law compensates individuals who have suffered injury, or prevents the activities that led to such injuries. Few major studies detail the levels of compensation available to those injured in accidents.[1] Even less is known about the deterrent effect of tort litigation. Much of the information that is available focuses on no-fault automobile insurance and rates of fatal accidents,[2] particularly in the province of Quebec.[3] Even data as simple as the numbers of claims brought in common law courts are generally unavailable.

An exception to this rule of scant empirical evidence regarding torts is found in the area of medical malpractice. Perhaps because there is so much research in other areas of health policy, social scientists have long been interested in medical malpractice. Hence there is comparatively a great deal of information about suits of providers and hospitals by patients. Much of this information has been generated in the last decade, partially in response to tremendous variations in claims rates over that time. There have been a number of studies analyzing the impact of tort reform on medical malpractice claims rates.[4] Specific case studies have clarified the manner in which changes in tort doctrine can diminish the number of claims brought by plaintiffs.[5]

Students of medical malpractice have also begun to gather thorough information on longitudinal cohorts of claims. For instance, Sloan and colleagues have compiled the results of jury verdicts in several jurisdictions and have begun to analyze the variation in outcomes,[6] building on some earlier work by Danzon.[7] Other investigators have turned their attention to the experience of defendants, particularly physicians, to identify the characteristics that may lead to more frequent actions by plaintiffs.[8] Still others have focused on what kinds of medical interactions lead to suits.[9] Perhaps the most thorough effort to understand the dynamics of malpractice litigation is Thomas Metzloff's study of several hundred claims over a three-year period in North Carolina.[10]

Questions of efficient litigant behavior, and of the impact of statutory reforms of personal injury law, have been the central focus of empiricists, but more wide-ranging institutional analyses have begun to appear. For example, the accuracy of malpractice insurance pricing[11] and the validity of settlements by insurers are among the concerns now being assessed by researchers.[12]

But while the intensity and depth of research into medical malpractice liability have grown tremendously in the last five to ten years, we must acknowledge that the most important work in this field is now over ten years old. If one wants to analyze the foundations of accident law, it is vital to compare the universe of accidents to the universe of litigation. Perhaps the only place where this has been done in tort law is with regard to medical malpractice. In 1975 Don Harper Mills and colleagues undertook the California Medical Association's Medical Insurance Feasibility study.[13] They reviewed records from more than thirty hospitals in the state of California in order to estimate a statewide medical injury rate, and the subset due to negligence. Using this data, Patricia Danzon undertook a parallel analysis of malpractice litigation,[14] and demonstrated that there was significant underclaiming by injured victims.

The availability of such thorough and fundamental research allows us to pinpoint unanswered questions. First, the CMA's analysis of medical records did not involve a random sample. Hence it was impossible to develop population estimates of injuries. Nor could Danzon estimate the relative claims rates by injured and uninjured plaintiffs. Moreover, the research has not totted up the costs of accidents and the relative adequacy of tort law's compensation function.

To address these and other issues, a group of investigators from the Harvard School of Public Health, Harvard Medical School, and Harvard Law School began a collaborative study of malpractice litigation and hospital-based medical injury. First, we used state-of-the-art research methodology to estimate the number of adverse events, and the percentage of all adverse events that were due to negligent or substandard care, in a random sample of New York hospitals in 1984. Next we compared the results of our hospital records analysis with those of a comprehensive analysis of all litigation records from New York medical professional liability insurers. Third, we completed surveys of injured individuals as well as uninjured controls to understand the costs of injury suffered by patients. Much of this research has now been published in technical medical journals. Herein I describe many of the results of this multifaceted study in a less technical manner.

Little of this empirical research relates to psychiatry. In fact, the Harvard study omitted psychiatric hospitalizations and psychiatric hospitals. However, this general overview is likely to have implications for mental health clinicians and their practice.

The Epidemiology of Medical Injuries in Hospitals

A review of medical records to develop an accurate estimate of the incidence of medical injury in hospitals was the cornerstone of the Medical Practice Study. As noted above, tort litigation is intended at least in part to reduce the occurrence of poor outcomes. Thus an accurate estimate of the numbers of patients injured and the extent of resulting disability is central to evaluating the efficacy of tort litigation.

Defining medical injury is conceptually challenging. Since patients are in hospitals because they are sick or in a state of ill-health, the further injury or illness caused by medical practice is not always readily disentangled from the original disease process, making judgments about causation difficult. Moreover, causation is just a threshold finding. From the viewpoint of tort law, only those disabilities caused by substandard care are compensable. Thus, in addition to the medical causation issue, we had to judge the presence of negligence.

An "adverse event" is a medical injury, defined as an incapacity that is the result of medical care, not of the disease for which the patient was hospitalized, that either prolongs the hospitalization or leads to disability at the time of discharge. A "negligent adverse event" is one caused by care that fails to reach the standard of the average medical practitioner. In addition to the critical "causation" and "negligence" judgments, we also asked our record reviewers to characterize the disability associated with adverse events.

In the more than 31,000 medical records reviewed, we uncovered a total of 1,133 adverse events that occurred as a result of medical management in the hospitalization under investigation or required hospitalization for treatment of an injury suffered elsewhere. Of this number, 280 were the products of negligent care. We estimated the incidence of adverse events in New York in 1984 to be 3.7 percent. Among the adverse events, 27.6 percent were due to negligence, that is, 1 percent of all hospital discharges had a negligent adverse event.

These figures are quite similar to those compiled in California a decade earlier. While the California Medical Association's negligence rate was somewhat lower and the rate of potentially compensable events somewhat higher, these differences are probably not statistically significant. Overall, the resonance between the two estimates suggests that approximately 4 percent of all hospitalizations result in adverse events and more than one-quarter of these are due to substandard care. Thus, the risk of injury for hospitalized patients is quite high.

"Weighting" these figures up to population estimates provides perhaps more helpful information regarding the epidemiology of medical injury and deficient care. Among the 2.6 million hospital discharges in New York in 1984, 56,000 involved adverse events that gave rise to minimal impairment from which individuals recovered within one month. Another 13,500 led to moderate impairment but with recovery in less than six months. Therefore more than 70 percent of adverse events led to short-term disability. There were also large numbers of patients who suffered more serious injuries: 3,800 adverse events produced permanent impairment causing a disability of 1–50 percent; more than 2,500 led to permanent total disabilities; and 13,400 adverse events caused death.

Similar to the CMA study, the percentage of adverse events due to negligence varied according to the seriousness of the injury. Only 23 percent of adverse events causing impairments that lasted less than six months were the result of negligence. However, 34 percent of the adverse events that led to permanent total disability and 51 percent of deaths from adverse events were due to substandard care.

These numbers are quite striking when compared to other important sources of accidents in this country. This is especially true of the fatality rate. Extrapolating the number of adverse event–related deaths to the United States at large, we estimate there are 180,000 iatrogenic deaths annually, and that more than 90,000 of these are due to negligence. Medical injury thus dwarfs the mortality associated with motor vehicle accidents (40,000 deaths per year), and occupation-related mishaps (6,000 deaths per year).

Moreover, the 2,500 permanent total disabilities in New York extrapolate to approximately 35,000 permanently disabled individuals on a national basis. These cases represent enormous personal suffering as well as huge costs for social benefit programs. Thus the burden of morbidity and mortality caused by medical care is substantial.

The information we have gathered on individual hospitals is likely to be more closely related to quality. Negligence rates in institutions can provide very useful insight into the kind of care rendered. The hospitals with higher proportions of substandard care are probably not providing superior medical treatment. On the other hand, adverse events in themselves do not signal poor quality, but rather may reflect the severity of the illnesses of the patients admitted to a particular institution.

Our results revealed striking differences in adverse event rates and negligence. We found a nearly sixteenfold variation between hospitals in rates of adverse events. After standardization for differences in clinical severity and elimination of those hospitals in which we reviewed fewer than 900 records, there was still a twelvefold variation. The percentage of adverse events due to negligence ranged from 0 to 70. Such variations are enormous from a statistical point of view. We must conclude that the rate of medical injury, and the quality of care, varies substantially from hospital to hospital.

Survey of Litigation Records

The review of medical records was only the first step in our research. The second step concerned a study of malpractice litigation in New York in the 1980s, focusing especially on 1984. We intended to calculate the overall annual rate of malpractice litigation, and to compare this with the annual rate of negligent adverse events, which we had already calculated to be approximately 27,000 of the 2.6 million discharges from New York hospitals in 1984. We also wished to match the litigation survey with the medical record survey so as to understand what sort of cases produced litigation. The result, we hoped, would provide us with a comprehensive comparison of medical care with medical malpractice litigation.

In theory, every episode of a medical injury that results from substandard care could give rise to successful litigation. Indeed, this would be an optimal outcome in a functional analysis of the tort system. The more negligent adverse events that produce lawsuits, the greater is the deterrent effect and the more adequate is compensation for injury. On the other hand, suits that arise out of medical injuries that are not caused by substandard care, or that arise in cases in which no injury from medical treatment has occurred, frustrate the goals of malpractice litigation. Such suits induce dissonance in the deterrent signals for providers of health care, and any compensation they produce increases unnecessarily the costs of the common law approach.[15]

As noted earlier, Patricia Danzon has explored these issues in some detail.[16] After reviewing the California Medical Association Study, Danzon used information available from the National Association of Insurance Commissioners (NAIC) to estimate the ratio of negligent adverse events to claims. She concluded that there were ten instances of injury caused by substandard practice for each malpractice claim. Moreover, based on the less than 50 percent probability that any claimant would obtain a settlement or award from a defendant, Danzon concluded that only one patient receives compensation per 25 instances of injury from negligent care.

After the completion of her original work, claims rates increased a good deal, especially in the early to mid 1980s. Accordingly, Danzon revised her estimates, stating in 1988 that the negligent injury to claims ratio had probably fallen from ten to five.[17] These estimates are the best available for any area of tort litigation regarding the number of potential to actual legal actions by plaintiffs. Moreover, in light of this information, most commentators have concluded that the huge gap between potential and actual suits will frustrate any effort to provide no-fault compensation, in which all injuries, not just negligent injuries, would be eligible for money awards. No-fault simply appears to be too expensive.

Danzon could only comment on the comparison of the overall litigation rates with medical injury rates. It was not possible to link the NAIC data to the information from the CMA hospital record review. Thus Danzon could not generate information on rates of litigation within the subset of cases involving negligent adverse events. It may have been that many of the claims in California arose from cases in which substandard care injured patients. But it is equally possible that the lion's share of suits or requests for payment arose from cases in which there was no injury or no negligence. Thus Danzon's study is silent concerning the accuracy of tort litigation.

The questions raised by the landmark studies of the CMA and Danzon, more than anything else, motivated the design of our study. In the record review, we were determined to develop a random sample with reliable and valid review procedures, thus attempting to surpass the original California study. So too we were committed to completing a comprehensive review of litigation records and to matching those litigation records with the sample of hospital records, allowing us to address the issue of tort litigation's efficiency.

The first step was to compile comprehensive and accurate information on suits and requests for payment in New York for the 1980s, especially 1984. Since the enactment of malpractice reform legislation in New York in 1975, professional liability insurers have faced stringent reporting requirements. A central repository is located at the Office of Professional Medical Conduct of the Department of Health.

Using several estimation procedures, we calculated that there were 3,500–3,800 patient claims in 1984. Comparing this with the over 27,000 negligent adverse events we uncovered, we conclude that there are 7.2 adverse events due to negligence for each patient claim. Assuming that only half of these result in payment, it appears there are 14.4 negligent adverse events for every paid claim. Looking at patient claims opened in 1985 and 1986, we developed quite similar estimates.

To go beyond information provided by Danzon and others, and to estimate the overall efficiency of tort litigation, we next matched the claims data base to the record review results. During the record review, we had noted important identifying information on each patient. The same sort of information was available from insurance company data. To match, we undertook exhaustive computer and manual techniques. First the computer used a phonetic program to find patient names common to both data sets. Any potential pairs were then studied using additional descriptive information from the record sample and claims records.

In this way we identified 98 persons in our record sample who had filed claims against 151 health care providers. Using the description provided by the insurers as well as the data from the hospital charts, we attempted to discern whether or not the accidents that gave rise to the malpractice claim arose out of the medical management provided during the hospitalization. For 48 of the 98 individuals, we concluded that it was more likely than not that the care in the sample hospitalization led to the claim. One of these claims did not fit the criteria for the incidence estimates. Thus there were 47 claims/sample matches.

The juxtaposition of the medical record review with the claims information generated striking results. Among the 47 matches, only 8 concern cases in which there was a negligent adverse event. Using population-based figures, this suggests that less than 2 percent of negligent adverse events resulted in claims. The remainder of suits and requests for payment arose out of cases in which we judged there was no negligent adverse event. Ten occurred in hospitalizations that led to adverse events but no negligence. Another three hospitalizations contained some evidence for a medical injury, but did not reach the required threshold. Finally, 26 of the claims arose out of medical care in which there was no evidence of an adverse event. The result is that large numbers of claims followed hospitalizations in which our review process uncovered no injury and/or no negligence;

on the other hand, the true odds of a claim following an actual negligent adverse event is much closer to 1:50 than 1:8.

It is perhaps understandable that there are claims from cases in which there is no negligent injury. First of all, attorneys must often go through a sifting process before determining whether or not there is a valid suit. Therefore a certain number of exploratory suits are to be expected in medical malpractice litigation. Many of the "false positive" cases we have identified may be explained by such sifting. Over the course of time, we should be able to identify the suits that lead to payment, providing a better idea of the efficiency of the tort system. Other studies have suggested that the problem with frivolous claims is not so great.[18]

Nonetheless, our primary finding, that there exists a huge gap between negligent adverse events and claims, still stands. Even if we interpret the matching results as conservatively as possible, the conclusion we are left with is that less than one out of twenty-five injuries from substandard care produces litigation or request for payment. Of course, this means that there is potential for a great deal more malpractice litigation than we now experience. Indeed, given the cyclical nature of tort litigation, especially in the malpractice area, there is every reason to believe there could be another crisis of malpractice litigation in the near future.

Economic Costs of Patient Injury

In the review of medical records we asked physicians to assess the physical impairments suffered by patients as a result of adverse events. These estimates obviously could not be completely accurate, as not all dimensions of patient losses are defined in hospital charts. Nor is it possible to gauge with complete accuracy the ability of individuals to recover from injuries. Finally, similarly injured individuals may ultimately suffer very different levels of disability.

A record review is also inadequate for developing precise information about sources of compensation available for the injured. A number of social welfare programs replace lost income for severely handicapped individuals.[19] Indeed, in 1984, tort provided $39 billion, only one-tenth of the total paid for injury and illness by loss-shifting programs.[20] Medical care costs of injuries to patients can be covered by a variety of governmental programs, but especially Medicare and Medicaid.[21] Given the existence of this partial social safety net, one cannot assume that patients bear all the costs of medical injury. Therefore, to assess the compensation task of tort law, it is important to define the economic extent of medical injury and the collateral sources of compensation available to patients who are injured.

The survey of patients was designed to assess not only the cost of negligent injury but that of all injury-based adverse events. As discussed in the previous section, a compensation gap exists between negligent adverse events and litigation. There is a further gap between all adverse events and litigation. Previous studies, especially that by Danzon, suggested that given the discontinuity between medical injuries and litigation and the known costs of medical malpractice litigation, it would not be possible to move to any no-fault alternative. The point of our patient survey was to provide accurate information on the size of this gap, accounting for the costs of accidents compensated through other sources.

We designed a method for assessing the cost of patient injury based on telephone surveys. After culling hospital charts for information, we turned names and telephone numbers over to a private survey research firm. The patient lists included all individuals who had suffered adverse events. This firm located the patients, and for those willing to participate, gathered a broad array of socioeconomic data. Interviewers did not ask any questions about tort litigation and were unaware of the overall hypothesis of the study.

With the gross information on economic costs, we next assessed the *net* economic costs of medical injuries. This required a micro-analysis of each injury associated with an adverse event. Two of us judged the overall impact of the injury on work, household production, and health care costs by studying the results of the survey as well as the information from the medical records review. Using the population weights for each case, we could calculate the total costs for all losses attributable to adverse events in New York in 1984. This figure could then be readily compared to the actual costs of medical malpractice litigation in New York.

As noted, we assumed that any kind of no-fault alternative for compensation of patient injury would pay only for the net cost of injury, after application of other collateral sources. This is a defensible policy position, and is in keeping with developments in the reform of tort law itself. However, some third-party payers of medical care costs, especially the federal government, refuse to take a first position for payment if another source is available.[22] In later analyses of our data we intend to define the overall costs should some programs refuse to act as collateral sources.

We also excluded pain and suffering from our calculation of costs. Most no-fault compensation claims are indeed restricted to economic costs. However, a good case can be made for compensation for pain and suffering, even under administrative no-fault plans. The comprehensiveness of our survey methods allowed us to develop many permutations of different costs, and to tailor the mock programs to different political constraints.

To estimate the size of a hypothetical no-fault plan, we first calculated the gross costs of underlying illnesses and adverse events. The 98,000 individuals who suffered adverse events lost over $20 billion in 1984. The bulk of the total was medical care expenditures ($14.5 billion). Lost wages accounted for $2.5 billion. Recall that these large figures included all costs of underlying illness and adverse events, not just those attributable to adverse events.

We then reduced these net costs by attributing costs to adverse events as opposed to the underlying illness. The isolation of costs due to the adverse event from the universe of costs of all illness produced substantial reductions. For instance, for workers who had suffered adverse events, the net wage loss decreased from $2.5 billion to $467 million. Household production losses dropped from $3.4 billion to $1.5 billion. Health care costs decreased to $1.8 billion.

This is not surprising. Many adverse events are suffered by chronically ill individuals. Their u. derlying illnesses cause long-term disability. Therefore, disentangling the disability due to adverse events from that caused by preexisting disease is quite important to any no-fault program.

From the overall total, we then subtracted the reimbursement available under other compensation plans, as well as income tax and consumption deductions. This reduced the bill a good deal further. For instance, the attributed wage losses for workers were $467 million. However, after deduction for income tax and consumption deduction, the net direct wage losses were only $235 million. Attributed medical care costs were $1.8 billion. However, injured individuals were compensated $1.56 billion through third-party insurers. Thus the total net medical costs were only $240 million.

The information on the sources and extent of compensation from collateral sources within the hypothetical no-fault plan was quite illuminating. On the one hand, insurance benefits for medical care reimbursed more than 85 percent of the doctor and hospital bills. On the other hand, compensation from all sources for wage losses for workers covered less than 20 percent of the total net wage loss. Furthermore, no plan existed for shifting the costs associated with household production. This suggests that the most important gap to be covered by tort awards or other alternatives is the long-term disability of injured individuals.

Combining the amounts for all the various subgroups of the population, discounting appropriately, and then developing present-value figures for 1989 dollars, we estimated the overall costs of the hypothetical no-fault plan to be $1,024 million. Lost wages and lost household production represented more than 70 percent of this total.

The final sum is considerably less than the $1.2 billion expended in New York State for medical liability insurance in 1992. This information suggests, for the first time, that a no-fault program for medical injury could be an affordable alternative to tort litigation. Of course, several caveats attend this conclusion. First, we are comparing the estimates of compensable losses suffered by patients injured in 1984 to malpractice costs estimated by insurers for patients injured in 1988. This is a reasonable assumption, however, if one grants that the injury rate for individuals is likely to be quite stable (as is suggested by comparison of the New York data with California data from ten years ago). Moreover, our present-value estimates include an adjustment of 1984 losses into 1989 dollars, accounting for most of the inflation during the four-year period.

It is also true that our estimate does not include any administrative costs. Similar costs associated with a tort system are greater than 50 percent of the total. It is doubtful that a no-fault compensation scheme for medical injury would involve such high costs. Indeed the best-known analogy, workers' compensation, has administrative expenses of about 20 percent.[23] Nonetheless, we believe that a patient injury no-fault program may be somewhat more difficult to operate than the workers' compensation system, especially because of the problems of disentangling injury from disease. Thus adding a 20 percent administrative allowance to our compensable figure would yield a lower limit on the total program costs. The Swedish no-fault compensation scheme for medical injuries has administrative costs of 25 percent.

Finally, and perhaps most important, we do not include the costs of psychiatric malpractice, which can range between 3 and 10 percent of total liability costs for large channeling programs.

In any case, our research demonstrates how there can be both a huge tort, let alone no-fault, gap in claims brought for iatrogenic injury, and yet little or no gap in costs between the present tort system and a hypothetical no-fault plan. First, the program we envision takes into account the actual size of economic losses, not just the fact of physical impairment. The second reason there is little or no cost gap is that negligent injuries are likely to be the most severe, both in physical and economic terms. Therefore, the present system is dealing with some of the most severe injuries. Third, we reduced the no-fault costs, using the assumption that collateral sources would take the first position for payment. Fourth, there is little doubt that the tort system puts a great deal of resources into administrative costs, and generously compensates pain and suffering. Spending less on administration, and nothing on pain and suffering, reduces the cost differences between tort and no-fault considerably.

One must consider other benefits of moving to the no-fault plan. For instance, the dollars spent on defensive medicine might drop considerably.[24] In addition, fairness may argue for a no-fault system. In our present fault-based system, two individuals may be similarly harmed by medical care. However, if one's injury is the result of substandard care and the other's is not, only the former escapes the burden of the accident. The latter party may properly ask, why do we allow the costs of faultless accidents to lie where they fall?

In summary, the data from our survey of injured individuals suggests for the first time that the no-fault alternative to medical malpractice litigation might be affordable. Further analyses of the data and new estimates of costs will better define the affordability issue. But compensation is only half of the functional analysis of torts.

/ / /

Empirical analysis can be very valuable as one studies policy options. Eventually, however, the policymaker must rely on values and beliefs to fill in the gaps left by researchers. On that note, I offer the following thoughts about reform of malpractice law, realizing that others might move in a different direction while viewing the same facts.

First, it is clear that there are many injuries caused by medical management in American hospitals, a substantial minority of which are presumably preventable. This must represent a challenge for providers, especially physicians, to study cost-effective means to prevent them. It is folly to suggest that it would be efficient to prevent all injuries. But the fact that some hospitals have much lower rates of injury, yet remain competitive, suggests there are some low-cost prevention strategies available.

Second, it is difficult to support further conventional tort reform as an answer to the "malpractice problem." Tort reform decreases numbers of claims, which is the aim of chronic defendants. But this research shows that there is startling underclaiming by injured individuals. Tremendous numbers of injured patients are not compensated, and their potential deterrent signals go unsent. If we are to rely heavily on tort litigation for deterrence, further efforts to make it more difficult to sue are not warranted.

Third, a no-fault alternative to our present approach appears affordable. Several countries have such schemes in place, compensating all medical injuries through an administrative system rather than litigation of only those caused by fault.[25] We have shown that a program similar to that in Sweden, if supplemented by mandatory collateral-source offsets, would cost New York approximately $1 billion per year. This is roughly equivalent to the amount now paid by New York physicians and hospitals in malpractice insurance premiums. This estimate of a no-fault system's cost does not include any administrative expenses. Administrative costs could range as high as 40–50 percent, depending on how the system is constructed.

Further, such policy conjecturing is beyond the scope of this chapter, which is intended to provide an even-handed overview of recently developed empirical information on the functioning of medical malpractice in one state. We hope this data, plus that recently developed elsewhere, will raise the policy discussion to a new level of sophistication and provide background for efforts to prevent medical injuries.

With regard to the specific problem of psychiatric malpractice, we will need to gather more data. The large studies of medical injury and malpractice litigation presently available do not address psychiatric diagnoses. Future research should aim at this target.

Notes

This chapter is reprinted in part from Troyen A. Brennan, "An Empirical Analysis of Accidents and Accident Law: The Case of Medical Malpractice Law," *St. Louis University Law Journal* 36, no. 4 (1992): 823–878.

1. D. Harris et al., *Compensation and Support for Illness and Injury* (Oxford: Oxford University Press, 1984).
2. See J. Landes, "Insurance Liability and Accidents: A Theoretical and Empirical Investigation Effect of No-Fault Accidents," *Journal of Law and Economics* 25 (1982): 49; A. Zador and M. Lund, "Reanalysis of the Effects of No-Fault Auto Insurance on Fatal Crashes," *Journal of Risk and Insurance* 53 (1986): 226; J. Kochanoowski and E. L. Young, "Deterrent Aspects of No-Fault Automobile Insurance: Some Empirical Findings," *Journal of Risk and Insurance* 52 (1985): 269.
3. R. A. Devlin, "Some Welfare Implications of No-Fault Automobile Insurance," *International Review of Law and Economics* 10 (1990): 193.
4. See E. K. Adams and S. Zuckerman, "Variations in the Growth and Incidence of Medical Malpractice Claims," *Journal of Health Politics Policy and Law* 9 (1984): 475; P. Danzon, "The Frequency and Severity of Medical Malpractice

Claims: New Evidence," *Law and Contemporary Problems* 49 (1986): 57; F. A. Sloan, "State Response to the Malpractice Insurance Crisis of the 1970s: An Empirical Assessment," *Journal of Health Politics Policy and Law* 9 (1985): 629; J. Coyte, D. Dewees, and M. Triebilcock, "Canadian Medical Malpractice Liability: An Empirical Analysis of Recent Trends," *Journal of Health Economics* 10 (1991): 143; F. A. Sloan, M. Mergenhagen, and R. Bovbjerg, "Effects of Tort Reforms on the Value of Closed Medical Malpractice Claims: A Microanalysis," *Journal of Health Politics Policy and Law* 14 (1989): 663.

5. An especially thorough study of the reforms in Indiana, including a cap on economic damages, can be found in several articles by Eleanor Kinney. See E. Kinney and R. Gronfein, "Indiana's Malpractice System: No-Fault by Accident?" *Law and Contemporary Problems* 54 (1991): 169; R. Gronfein and E. Kinney, "Controlling Large Malpractice Claims: The Unexpected Impact of Damage Caps," *Journal of Health Politics Policy and Law* 16 (1991): 441.

6. See R. Bovbjerg et al., "Juries and Justice: Are Malpractice and Other Personal Injuries Created Equal?" *Law and Contemporary Problems* 54 (1991): 5; F. A. Sloan and J. Hsieh, "Variability in Medical Malpractice Payments: Is the Compensation Fair?" *Law and Society Review* 24 (1990): 601.

7. See P. Danzon and R. E. Lillard, "Settlement Out of Court: The Disposition of Medical Malpractice Claims," *Journal of Legal Studies* 12 (1983): 345.

8. See F. A. Sloan et al., "Medical Malpractice Experience of Physicians: Predictable or Haphazard?" *JAMA* 262 (1989): 3291; R. Kravitz, E. Rolph, and T. McGuigan, "Malpractice Claims Data as a Quality Improvement Tool: 1. Epidemiology of Error of Four Specialties," *JAMA* 262 (1991): 2087; E. Rolph, R. Kravitz, and T. McGuigan, "Malpractice Claims Data as a Quality Improvement Tool: 2. Is Targeting Effective?" *JAMA* 262 (1991): 2093.

9. See R. May and C. Stengel, "Who Sues Their Doctors? How Patients Handle Medical Grievances," *Law and Society Review* 24 (1990): 105; T. Kellett, "Healing Angry Wounds: The Role of Apology and Mediation in Disputes between Physicians and Patients," *Journal of Dispute Resolutions* (1987): 111.

10. See T. Metzloff, "Resolving Malpractice Disputes: Imaging the Jury's Shadow," *Law and Contemporary Problems* 54 (1991): 43.

11. See F. A. Sloan and A. Hassan, "Equity and Accuracy in Medical Malpractice Insurance Pricing," *Journal of Health Economics* 9 (1990): 289.

12. See R. C. Cheney et al., "Standard of Care in Anesthesia Liability," *JAMA* 261 (1989): 1599.

13. See California Medical Association, *Medical Insurance Feasibility Study* (Sacramento: Sutter, 1977).

14. See P. M. Danzon, *Medical Malpractice: Theory, Evidence and Public Policy* (Cambridge, Mass.: Harvard University Press, 1985).

15. Randy Bovbjerg and collaborators have compared jury verdicts in malpractice cases with other torts. See Bovbjerg et al., "Juries and Justice," p. 10. The authors cite extensively to other literature in this rich field.

16. See esp. Danzon, *Medical Malpractice*.

17. See P. M. Danzon, "Medical Malpractice Liability," in R. E. Litan and R. W. Clifford, eds., *Liability Perspectives and Policy* (Washington: Brookings Institution, 1988).

18. See, e.g., R. C. Cheney et al., "Standard of Care in Anesthesia Liability." These investigators found that a large percentage of cases (42 percent) were paid that were not actually the result of negligence. However, many of the amounts paid by the insurers were small, indicating that insurers were willing to pay to eliminate nuisance claims.

19. For example, the OASDHI program provides $33 billion for spouses and children of deceased workers. See U.S. Department of Health and Human Services, Social Security Administration, *Social Security Insurance: Annual Statistical Supplement* (1988). Private pension plans provide another source of compensation for survivors. See A. Munnell, *The Economics of Private Pensions* (Cambridge, Mass.: Harvard University Press, 1982). The Social Security Disability Program and the Social Security Income Program (SSI) also provide disabled individuals with income support.

20. See J. O'Connell and A. Guinivan, "An Irrational Combination: Relative Expansion of Liability Insurance and Contraction of Loss Insurance," *Ohio State Law Journal* 49 (1988): 757.

21. Medicare provides health insurance for all individuals who are eligible for social security, old age, or disability insurance programs. See 42 U.S.C. Section 1395(c), 1395(0) (1982) supp. 3 1985. See generally E. Kinney, "National Coverage under the Medicare Program: Problems and Proposals for Change," *St. Louis University Law Journal* 32 (1988): 872. Medicaid coverage is a more complicated issue, as it is tied to SSI and Aid to Families with Dependent Children (AFDC) eligibility. See generally R. Blendon and T. Moloney, eds., *New Approaches to the Medicaid Crisis* (Washington: Urban Institute, 1982).

22. See Department of Health and Human Services, Health Care Financing Administration, "Medicare Is Secondary Payer in Medicare Recovery against Third Parties," proposed rule, 53 Fed. Reg. 22335, 6-15-1988. See also *Abrams v. Heckler*, 582 F. Supp. 1155 (S.D. N.Y. 1984); *Rubin v. Sullivan*, F. Supp. (D. Hawaii, 1989).

23. See G. Priest, "The Current Insurance Crisis and Modern Tort Law," *Yale Law Journal* 96 (1987): 1521, 1560.

24. See R. A. Reynolds, J. A. Rizzo, and M. L. Gonzales, "The Costs of Medical Professional Liability," *JAMA* 257 (1987): 2776 (suggesting the overall costs of defensive medicine are $10.6 billion); G. Hershey, "The Defensive Practice of Medicine: Myth or Reality?" *Milbank Memorial Fund Quarterly* (1973): 131; L. Tancredi and J. Barondess, "The Problem with Defensive Medicine," *Science* 200 (1978): 879.

25. This is an issue we intend to study in Sweden and New Zealand, where no-fault systems for compensation of medical injury are already in place. See

M. M. Rosenthal, *Dealing with Medical Malpractice: The British and Swedish Experience* (Durham, N.C.: Duke University Press, 1988); J. Hellner, "Compensation for Personal Injury: The Swedish Alternative," *American Journal of Comparative Law* 36 (1986): 613–633; C. Oldertz, "Security Insurance, Patient Insurance and Pharmaceutical Insurance in Sweden," *American Journal of Comparative Law* 34 (1986): 635. On New Zealand see A. Gellhorn, "Medical Malpractice Litigation (U.S.)—Medical Mishap Compensation (N.Z.)," *Cornell Law Review* 73 (1988): 170.

2

Informed Consent

Marilyn Berner, J.D., LICSW

Informed consent is the cornerstone of the contemporary clinician's ability to treat and the linchpin of the patient's right to accept or reject clinical care. 'Twas not always thus: the concept that patients have a right to full disclosure of a proposed treatment, including an assessment of risks and benefits, as well as a discussion of possible side effects and unintended, but possible, sequelae, is a relatively modern invention. The refinement of this invention roughly parallels the development of an attention to personal, in addition to property, rights in American jurisprudence.

As early as 1914 Justice Cardozo articulated this principle, saying, "Every human being of adult years and sound mind has a right to determine what shall be done with his own body; and a surgeon who performs an operation without his patient's consent commits an assault, for which he is liable in damages" (*Schloendorff v. Society of New York Hospital,* 1914). Most of the issues which have subsequently arisen to plague clinicians, patients, attorneys, and courts alike germinate from this deceptively simple statement. The issues coiled within it, waiting only for the right conditions to begin to sprout, include such questions as these:

1. Who is a human being?
2. Who is an adult?
3. What does sound mind mean?
4. What constitutes an operation?
5. Are there exceptions to the rule, or to parts of the rule?
6. Is assault and battery the only theory under which a patient may recover damages, or is the law flexible enough to accommodate the emerging body of negligence law?

Intentional Torts versus Negligence

As any first-year law student knows, a battery consists simply of a touching which has not been consented to. (Although Justice Cardozo refers to it as an assault, it is, technically speaking, a battery; the assault is the moment which precedes the battery and includes the surgeon's intent, as well as her apparent capability at that moment, to commit the touching.) The early cases dealt with discomfiting medical events such as consenting to have one's diseased left leg removed, and waking to find oneself missing additional parts as well.

These situations were relatively straightforward and could be fitted easily into the law of assault and battery. It was not until the early 1960s that a troubling question began to reach the courts: Was consent a mere technicality, or was there some substance to it? A number of state courts, primarily in the midwest, found that patients were entitled to "adequate" information about proposed treatments, including the risks of the proposed therapy, and information about alternative treatments, if they were to be able to give a meaningful consent. In this way a new legal doctrine emerged, that of informed consent. Like many ideas which sprang up in the 1960s, this one and its descendants remain with us today. What concerns us here is how this concept has changed clinical practice by imposing obligations on both clinicians and patients in ways that were unforeseen by Justice Cardozo.

The new cases, which involved nondisclosure of the possible adverse effects of electroconvulsive and insulin shock therapy, established that "a reasonable medical practitioner, under some circumstances, would make full disclosure of all risks which had any reasonable likelihood of occurring, but in others the facts and circumstances would dictate a guarded or limited disclosure" (*Aiken v. Clary*, 1965). The careful, rather vague wording, which defers in large part to clinical discretion, represents the characteristic hesitation of courts in promulgating a new rule. (In a fascinating socioclinical footnote to history, the defendant doctor testified that his justification for making less than full disclosure to Mr. Aiken, who was diagnosed as suffering from "process schizophrenia," of the hazards of insulin shock therapy, was that Mr. Aiken was "real shook." This vernacular formulation of Mr. Aiken's mental status presumably influenced the court to issue its own rather guarded pronouncement.)

This rule had the effect, by expanding the concept of consent to require disclosure by the clinician, of removing a whole class of cases from the exclusive jurisdiction of the theory of battery, an intentional tort, and allowing it to move into the burgeoning field of negligence law. In addition to raising the issue of what constitutes the reasonable and appropriate scope of disclosure, this development gives rise to a number of practical consequences for clinicians. In some jurisdictions plaintiffs can sue under both assault and battery and negligence theories, at least theoretically increasing exposure for clinicians. In addition, negligence actions are in general governed by a longer statute of limitations than intentional tort actions, again increasing exposure for clinicians. The scales of justice are somewhat balanced by the fact that most negligence actions require expert testimony in order for the plaintiff to meet his burden of proof. The measure of damages is also affected by the theory the plaintiff uses. Under an intentional tort theory, the plaintiff can recover nominal damages without showing an actual injury, and in addition may recover punitive damages if she can show an element of malice. Under a negligence theory, a plaintiff may recover only for the harm he actually suffers. Last, and perhaps most important, many malpractice policies exclude coverage for intentional torts, which again, at least theoretically, increases the clinician's exposure.

Disclosure: How Much Is Enough?

So, you may ask yourself, how much disclosure is enough? One standard is defined above; some states have adopted a somewhat more stringent rule, reasoning that the *Aiken v. Clary* rule grants unlimited discretion to clinicians, and in effect guts the requirement altogether. The more stringent rule, articulated in the case of *Canterbury v. Spence* (1972) has been characterized as defining "the breadth of disclosure to include any risk which either singly or in combination with other risks would be deemed significant by the average patient in deciding whether to accept or forgo the therapy" (Reisner and Slobogin, 1990, p. 186). This rule has in turn been criticized for leaving the therapist open to unknown risks of liability, since it leaves it to the plaintiff to decide if whether what the therapist said or did not say was material to her decision. It does not require expert testimony and may rely solely on the plaintiff's own testimony. The conflict between these two standards remains very much alive, and which rule controls varies according to jurisdiction.

Reasonable Disclosure

A closer look at the court's opinion in *Canterbury v. Spence* is illuminating. Mr. Canterbury sued Dr. Spence for his alleged negligence in the performance of a laminectomy and for his failure to inform him beforehand of the risk involved. The court found that Dr. Spence did in fact have a duty to inform Mr. Canterbury of the risks involved in the operation in order for him to make a considered decision. It said:

> The context in which the duty of risk-disclosure arises is invariably the occasion for decision as to whether a particular treatment procedure is to be undertaken. To the physician, whose training enables a self-satisfying evaluation, the answer may seem clear, but it is the prerogative of the patient, not the physician, to determine for himself the direction in which his interests seem to lie. To enable the patient to chart his course understandably, some familiarity with the therapeutic alternatives and their hazards becomes essential.
>
> We now find, as a part of the physician's overall obligation to the patient, a similar duty of reasonable disclosure of the choices with respect to proposed therapy and the dangers inherently and potentially involved. (*Canterbury v. Spence,* 1972)

The experienced reader of legal writing will recognize the highly elastic adjectival standard of "reasonableness" used to modify the noun "disclosure." The experienced clinical reader of legal writing will know that "reasonable" is to legal discourse what "appropriate" is to clinical discourse. "Reasonable" and "appropriate" are, like obscenity, harder to define in the abstract than to recognize in the concrete here and now. Sensitive perhaps to such perceived criticism of the promulgation of a vague standard, or, more likely, responding to similar arguments in the defendant-appellee's briefs, the *Canterbury* court provides a lengthy footnote filling in some of the blanks of what constitutes "reasonable" disclosure:

> Some doubt has been expressed as to ability of physicians to suitably communicate their evaluations of risks and the advantages of optional treatment, and as to the lay patient's ability to understand what the physician tells him. We do not share these apprehensions. The discussion need not be a disquisition, and surely the physician is not compelled to give his patient a short medical education; the disclosure rule summons the physician only to a reasonable explanation. That means generally informing the patient in nontechnical terms as to what is at stake: the therapy alternatives open to him, the goals expectably to be achieved, and the risks that may ensue from particular treatment and no treatment. So informing the patient hardly taxes the physician, and it must be the exceptional patient who cannot comprehend such an explanation at least in a rough way. (*Canterbury v. Spence,* 1972)

These cases establish the information component of informed consent: what lawyers refer to as one of the "elements" of informed consent. They set out the two-part standard regarding the information necessary to satisfy the reasonableness requirement imposed by the courts. The two components consist of what is known as the *professional standard* and the *materiality standard*. The professional standard is that information which the reasonable average clinician would provide to a patient under similar circumstances. The materiality standard views the situation from the patient's perspective, looking at the amount of information which the average patient would consider significant in deciding whether to accept or reject the therapy proposed. "Significant" translates into "material" in legal parlance; hence "materiality standard": that information which the reasonable average patient would require to make an informed decision under similar circumstances. This standard has come in for criticism similar to the criticism of the *Aiken v. Clary* standard, which was felt to be flawed in that it appeared to allow for unfettered discretion on the part of the clinician, to the extent that commentators feared that the basic rule would disappear. The materiality standard, complained critics, because it permits factfinders in the litigation process to decide in a given case whether a fact was material based solely on the plaintiff's testimony, tips the scales unfairly in favor of plaintiffs. It does so by making it possible for a plaintiff to establish a prima facie case solely on lay testimony, without any expert testimony required. As one commentator asks, rhetorically, we presume, "To what extent does this approach invite intentional or unintentional fabrication by the plaintiff?" (Reisner and Slobogin, 1990, p. 186).

Hypothetical Scenarios

How do these rules translate into the everyday work of treating patients? *Aiken v. Clary,* and *Canterbury v. Spence,* and the cases which follow them establish some general requirements which need to be included in the provision of information by clinicians in order for patients to give informed consent to treatment.

1. *The nature of the patient's condition (his diagnosis, in nontechnical terms) and the proposed treatment, or treatments, must be disclosed.* For example:

> Mr. Jones, you have an illness which makes it difficult to separate reality from your own thoughts. I have found that treatment with a medication known

as Clozaril is useful in treating some of the particular problems that you have been having, particularly the voices inside your head.

Ms. Smith, the films from XYZ Clinic show an increased density in the outer left quadrant of your left breast. I recommend some additional views of that breast here at ABC Clinic.

Mr. Beck, based on our interview and your depression scale score, I think you are suffering from depression. I recommend a ten-week course of cognitive therapy.

2. *A second requirement is disclosure of the nature and probability of the material risks involved.* This recalls the materiality standard, and includes both infrequently occurring risks with more significant possibility of harm and more frequently occurring risks which pose less significant risk of harm to the patient. For example:

Mr. Jones, there have been some reported cases of blood disease as a result of taking Clozaril, so we will need to get blood samples from you on a regular basis if you decide to take this medication.

Ms. Smith, this is not an emergency, but the risk is there that while the films may simply represent a difference in technique between the two clinics, there may in fact be something which needs to be treated. I think you should come in within the next few weeks.

Mr. Beck, cognitive therapy poses no risks to you that I am aware of.

3. *Information regarding the reasonably expected benefits must also be conveyed to the patient.* For example:

Mr. Jones, if you take the Clozaril the way I've prescribed it, and your blood work is okay, I think you can expect not to be bothered so much by the voices and to feel much more like getting back into your other activities, like going back to work.

Ms. Smith, if you come in for more views of your left breast, we will be better able to tell whether we're actually seeing something in your breast, or whether what we see is simply a matter of different techniques, and then we won't need to be concerned any longer.

Mr. Beck, I expect you'll find that as we have an opportunity to think together about how you're feeling and how to change it, you'll begin to feel better.

4. *At the same time, you, the clinician, need to be clear about your inability to predict results with certainty.* For example:

Mr. Jones, I can't say for sure that you won't develop problems with your blood, or that you'll definitely feel better. What I can say is that when other patients with problems like yours have tried Clozaril, they've felt better and done better, and most of them have had no blood problems.

Ms. Smith, I can't say for sure that what looks like an area of increased density is or isn't just that. What I can say is that, without additional views, we'll continue to have this question and no answer.

Mr. Beck, I can't guarantee you a positive result; what I can tell you is that the research and my own experience show that most people feel less depressed after a ten-week course of therapy and find that it is very useful in helping them to cope with things that come up in their lives.

5. *If the procedure or treatment you are proposing is irreversible, you must inform your patient of that fact.* For example:

Mr. Jones, I must tell you that if you continue to take Trilafon, there is a risk that you will develop a condition known as t.d., or tardive dyskinesia. This condition causes involuntary movements of the mouth, tongue, and face, and if it occurs, it's irreversible; we can't give you anything to change it.

Mr. Canterbury, I want to be sure you're aware that once I perform the surgery to fuse the vertebrae in your spine, I won't be able to undo it; it's an irreversible operation.

Mr. Morosa, as far as we know, any side effects you experience as a result of the antidepressant medication will be reversible; that is to say, they will stop once you discontinue the medication.

6. *Finally, you must explain to your patient the expectable result of no treatment and alternative treatments, along with the risks and benefits of each.* For example:

Mr. Jones, you know that your condition, schizophrenia, doesn't get better by itself. While we can't cure it, we can treat it. If you decide to take the Clozaril, I think there's a good chance you'll feel better and things will improve in your life. We will need to monitor your blood, but there's only a small chance of developing a problem there. If you take Thorazine, or Trilafon, as you have in the past, there's a greater chance as time goes on that you'll develop t.d., and as I've said, there's nothing we'll be able to do about that. The worst thing to do, in my opinion, would be to do nothing; to have no treatment at all. We can pretty much guarantee that if you follow that course, you'll feel worse, and your behavior and living conditions will deteriorate. You'll probably wind up in the hospital again.

Ms. Smith, I sense that you're reluctant to come in for more views of your left breast. The alternative would be to come in again a year from now, on your regular once-a-year schedule, which is recommended for women over 50. The risk there is that if this area of greater density isn't a result of different techniques at the two clinics, we may miss a potential mass in your breast which would be much more amenable to treatment now than a year from now.

Yes, Mr. Beck, it is possible that you may begin to feel less depressed if you do nothing at all. It sometimes happens. The risk is that you may continue to be more vulnerable to depression again in the future if you forgo the opportunity to learn ways to cope differently with troubling events in your life. And yes, there are alternative forms of treatment for depression. I would certainly recommend that you have an evaluation for a course of antidepressant medication, as well. Often the combination of medication and psychotherapy is the most effective treatment. And yes, psychoanalysis is an alternative, and may very well provide a deeper insight into the roots of your depression. The drawbacks are that it could be quite a while before you see results, and that it will probably be quite expensive, and not covered by your insurance plan.

Knowledge of Assent

You might think that we had exhausted the topic of disclosure, if not informed consent, at this point. Not so. There are a number of issues we have not addressed. For instance, how do you know that the patient has consented? And was the consent voluntary?

Since the law has moved from the assented-to touching as a defense to assault and battery into negligence law and the requirement of informed consent, necessitating the presence of the dual ingredients of awareness and assent, there have been relatively few cases raising the issue of patient awareness. However, in any malpractice case involving an informed consent issue, the factfinder must judge whether the patient-plaintiff intended, by the totality of his verbal and nonverbal expression, to consent to the treatment. The factfinder makes this determination according to an objective standard, the ''reasonable person'' standard. (By now this should sound familiar to the alert reader of legal materials.) This means, in brief, that the plaintiff must establish, as part of meeting his burden of proof, the rather difficult proposition that a reasonable average therapist would not have concluded, in similar circumstances, that the patient-plaintiff was not aware of the risks that had been communicated, and that he had also not indicated in any way, ambiguous or definite, that he was willing to undertake the proposed treatment.

As Reisner and Slobogin point out, when informed consent cases are litigated they turn, at least in part, on issues of credibility. The patient and the therapist may have substantially different recollections of what was disclosed. The patient will contend that disclosure was not sufficient to make him aware of the risks involved, while the therapist will maintain that she made full disclosure of all the risks, that the plaintiff was aware of them and knowingly consented to the treatment. For this and other reasons, it is a good idea to keep written notes of this conversation (see Chapter 4). What merits some discussion here is the situations—medical, surgical, and psychiatric—in which the presence of the patient's informed consent is, for various operational reasons, put at issue. For example, when Dr. Surgeon discusses the risks and benefits of the proposed surgical procedure with his patient, but neglects to have his patient sign the informed consent form required by his hospital, he sets the stage for later trouble in the event of litigation. This may occur when he has the patient sign the form after the administration of the preoperative Demerol when the patient is recumbent on a gurney in the corridor outside the operating room.

A similar situation obtains in the psychiatric arena in the case of electroconvulsive treatment. Likewise, in the practice of psychotherapy, when a psychotherapist proposes, for example, an open-ended course of psychodynamic treatment for depression, and the patient fails to experience a subjective sense of improved well-being, or his life situation deteriorates. The stage is again set for trouble when the transference intensifies in a negative way and the patient feels the therapist is to blame for the lack of improvement. Whose recollection regarding the discussion, or lack of it, of the risks and benefits of a medication evaluation and a possible course of antidepressant medication in addition to the talk therapy will be most reliable?

Voluntariness

We turn now to the issue of voluntariness and its mirror image, coercion. Was the patient's consent voluntary or was it coerced in some way? How is the clinician to know? Without voluntariness, or in the presence of coercion, there can be no informed consent. At this point in our journey, the informed clinical reader realizes he should be asking some version of the question, What must the reasonable average clinician provide to, and hear from, the patient in order to assure herself that the patient's consent is truly voluntary?

The law provides some guidance: consent is presumed to be voluntary. This means that a patient, later a plaintiff, who asserts that his consent was not voluntary, but coerced, has the burden of proof on that element, as on all elements, of his prima facie case. (The prima facie case consists of a "list" of the items which compose the skeleton of the plaintiff's complaint. For instance, the prima facie case of assault and battery requires proof of each of the following:

1. The defendant
2. intended
3. and had the apparent present ability to touch
4. and did touch
5. the plaintiff
6. without his consent
7. and the plaintiff suffered harm as a result.

If the plaintiff provides sufficient proof for all seven items, he has established his prima facie case. The issue for the factfinder (judge or jury) on the issue of consent, then, is whether the plaintiff has convinced it that "a particular set of circumstances was sufficiently coercive as to lead to the conclusion that but for such pressure, consent would have been withheld" (Reisner and Slobogin, 1990, p. 204).

It's easy to see that a decision reached as someone holds a gun to a person's head or a knife to her throat is involuntary or coerced. But what about subtle forms of coercion? What about the example given earlier in which the patient has been medicated and is already on his way to the operating room? Even assuming that there was a valid informed consent at a prior office consultation which Dr. Surgeon neglected to document, does the post-medication, in-the-corridor form signing allow room for the resolution of the patient's ambivalence? Does it take into account the possibility that the patient may have changed his mind? Or is the situation one that the courts would consider "inherently coercive"?

Institutionalized Populations

In practice, the cases which reach the courts on this issue arise in institutional settings, which raises the question of whether the institutional milieu itself exercises so much control over a person's life that voluntary choice is impossible. In these situations, courts have found that consent was coerced, rather than voluntary, not because an individual did not have the opportunity to make an effective choice, but because the basic "bargain" was unfair, as a result of the individual's vulnerability. In these circumstances, even the threat to withhold some privilege or the promise of a benefit has been held to be coercive. The traditional risk-benefit analysis is overridden by a moral judgment about the overall vulnerability of the presumed-to-be-consenting individual, whether he is an inmate or a patient. For instance, an agreement by prisoners to donate blood in return for reasonable remuneration has been upheld by the courts ("blood time" is the colloquial expression for credit toward an early release earned by the donation of blood). It has been criticized by those who argue that voluntary consent to any medical procedure that is without any direct therapeutic benefit to the inmate is impossible.

Courts have so far declined to follow this absolutist position on behalf of inmates, preferring to decide each case on its own facts rather than to establish a rule of law. Nevertheless, this issue remains alive for those clinicians who work in institutional settings and who must grapple on a daily basis with the questions of whether voluntary informed consent exists or is necessary under the circumstances. These questions themselves raise a plethora of issues which we will address shortly, but it is worthwhile to pause here for a moment and consider briefly the issues raised in the area of experimental or research procedures carried out on institutionalized patients. This topic serves in some ways to place the issue of informed consent under a microscope for close inspection.

Only one existing case directly addresses the issue of whether institutionalized patients have the capacity to give informed consent to intrusive experimental treatment, and it is not an appellate opinion, merely a trial court ruling, and therefore without precedental value. *Kaimowitz v. Department of Mental Health of Michigan* (1973) held that a patient committed involuntarily under the then-existing criminal sexual psychopath law could not provide informed consent for experimental psychosurgery. The *Kaimowitz* court went on to say that "involuntarily confined mental patients live in an inherently coercive institutional environment," and that "they are not able to voluntarily give informed consent because of the inherent inequality in their position." Furthermore, the court added, "The keystone to any intrusion upon the body of a person must be full, adequate and informed consent. The integrity of the individual must be protected from invasion into his body and personality not voluntarily agreed to . . . Consent is not an idle or symbolic act; it is a fundamental requirement for the protection of the individual's integrity."

While no commentator has disagreed with the *Kaimowitz* court regarding the necessary importance of voluntary informed consent, there have been numerous criticisms of the decision on policy grounds, on the grounds of empirical evidence, and on the grounds that the decision itself is internally illogical. There are later cases which hold differently, but in these cases, the institutionalized population consists of prisoners, not involuntarily committed psychiatric patients or developmentally disabled individuals. It is certainly conceivable that courts see these populations as inherently different, accustomed as they are to hearing repeatedly the testimony which leads them to transform defendants into prisoners deserving punishment, a group readily distinguishable in judicial eyes from patients deserving treatment.

The second variable which distinguishes *Kaimowitz* from other situations is that it involved experimental treatment. While it would seem a matter of common knowledge that much, if not most, psychiatric research, especially that involving medication, is carried out on institutionalized patients, drug trials appear not to raise the same level of alarm that experimental surgery raised in 1973, and would presumably raise today. This is perhaps a reflection of the societal expectation that drug trials will be carefully monitored, and therefore do not have the irreversible potential of surgery. Remember, for instance, the *Canterbury* court's emphasis on the irreversibility of Mr. Canterbury's laminectomy. Finally, we can only speculate regarding the almost universal unconscious narcissistic investment in an intact body and psyche which may also have influenced the revulsion of the writer of the *Kaimowitz* opinion at the intrusion and potentially irreversible loss represented by the experimental psychosurgery proposed in *Kaimowitz*.

Competence as an Element of Informed Consent

We have yet to consider a crucial issue which has been present in all of the situations we have discussed thus far, and which has been addressed in the cases. This issue is competence. Competence is a legal conclusion which attempts to define and describe the elastic and ever-changing set of circumstances within which a person is considered to be able or unable to manage any one or more of life's tasks. It is best understood as a process, rather than as an event or a thing. In this way, we can more readily understand how a person can be competent to perform one task but not another.

Correspondingly, we can see how a person may be competent to perform a task at 9 A.M., but incompetent at 3 P.M., or vice versa. Competence can be influenced by emotion, such as depression, mania, or grief; or by physiological changes, such as hypoglycemia, Alzheimer's, or high fever; or by cognitive ability.

If we think back to our discussion of coercion and voluntary assent, and to the example of the patient who signs the consent form after medication and on his way to the operating room, we can see immediately that there is an additional issue to consider: Was this patient competent to assent to the imminent surgery? Or did the administration of the preoperative Demerol and its attendant feeling of devil-may-care euphoria effectively destroy the patient's competence to assess the risks which might lie ahead? We can see more clearly in this hypothetical example how it is useful to conceptualize competence as a process. The patient in this situation was probably competent to consent to treatment at the time of the discussion in Dr. Surgeon's office. However, in the corridor after the Demerol, he probably was not. Similarly, people who suffer from a variety of psychiatric and medical conditions experience fluctuations in competence, which often mirror the fluctuations in their physiological status as well as in their mental status.

Courts are concerned with competence in a broad array of situations, both civil and criminal. Historically, the criminal process has been concerned with whether a person is competent to stand trial for the offense with which he is charged, and whether at the time of the alleged offense he was competent to form the required specific intent which the law requires to convict someone of a crime. More recently, the criminal justice system has addressed the issue of whether a person convicted of a crime and facing a death sentence is competent to be executed. In the civil system, courts are concerned with whether a person is competent to be a witness (known as testimonial capacity), whether a person is competent to direct the disposition of her property after her death (known as testamentary capacity, and generally felt to be the least demanding standard), the capacity to manage one's own financial and personal affairs (people who cannot perform these functions may be subject to broad or limited conservatorships or guardianships), and, finally, the capacity to give, or refuse, informed consent to medical treatment.

The general rule of law regarding competence is quite simple. All adults are presumed to be competent and must be treated as such unless and until a court has found them incompetent. This includes persons diagnosed as having major mental illness, or developmental disabilities, whether institutionalized or living in the community. This rule stems from the preference in this society, and reflected in its laws, for autonomy—the freedom to make and act upon one's own decisions. While the rule itself is simple, its application can be complicated, and of course there are exceptions, which we will examine shortly. For the moment, let us consider competence specifically as it relates to the issue of informed consent.

Four Elements of Competence

Competence is another essential "element" of informed consent, like voluntariness and disclosure of adequate information. It includes four basic and interrelated sub-elements, the first of which is that the person in question have a factual understanding of the situation, which includes the relevant needs and alternatives. For example, in order to establish an essential element of competence, a thirty-year-old woman with bipolar disorder and cervical cancer must understand what the cervix is, and the role it plays in her reproductive life.

The second sub-element requires an appreciation of the seriousness of the condition and the consequences of accepting or rejecting treatment. Appreciation includes an affective as well as a cognitive component, and in our example, would appear to call for some expression of trepidation or apprehension, rather than *la belle indifférence,* regarding the possible inability to bear children if treatment is accepted, or the possibility of death if treatment is rejected.

The third sub-element is the requirement that the patient express a preference. This preference does not have to be consistent with the clinician's preference, or with what she thinks would be in her patient's best interest. In our example, the patient may express a preference to preserve her reproductive capacity even at the risk to her own life, or she may say that preserving her own life is paramount. Both are indications of competence. If, however, she simply said that she didn't care, or couldn't decide, or said "It's up to you, Doc, whatever you say," or "Go away, don't bother me," concerns would be raised regarding her competence.

The fourth and final sub-element of competence demands that the patient be capable of working with the information disclosed by the clinician in a rational fashion. In our example, that means being able to keep the information reality-grounded and separate from whatever delusional material or psychotic thinking which may be present at various times as a result of the bipolar disorder. For clinicians who treat comparatively less disordered, private practice outpatients, issues regarding competence may arise seldom, if ever. While the clinician whose patient steadfastly refuses a trial of antidepressant medication may experience worry and frustration, he may very well never question the patient's competence to make that decision. For those clinicians who work in inpatient or outpatient settings with seriously or chronically mentally ill patients, or with a developmentally disabled population, the issue of competence is always present. This leads us to contemplate two additional issues: how to think about competence in chronically ill patients, and the right to refuse treatment.

Competence and the Chronically Ill

The difficulties here stem from confusion about what competence means, and from reliance on old ways of thinking about competence as a thing, or as an event which happens once and once only. As anyone with experience in working with inpatient populations can tell us, some of the most seriously ill patients can experience lucid intervals. Is such a patient competent during those intervals? This question is easier to contemplate if we remember to think of competence as a process. First we need to remind ourselves of the basic legal presumption of competence. If the patient is not subject to guardianship, we must assume his competence.

Then we need to ask another question: Competent to do what? Since this is a chapter on informed consent, let us skip testamentary and testimonial capacities and the capacity to manage one's own legal, financial, and other affairs, and confine ourselves to the matter at hand. Suppose that you, as the patient's psychiatrist, are recommending a change in medication. Your patient is not subject to guardianship, although he suffers from a serious and chronic mental illness. As you discuss the proposed medication change with him, you keep in mind the four sub-elements of competence, along with the requirements of reasonable disclosure and voluntariness of assent. You have explained what you think the advantages of the new medication are—a decrease in persecutory voices, and an increased ability to participate in the activities of daily life. What next? You must have a conversation with your patient which allows you to ascertain, first, whether he understands the facts of the situation. Does he know that continuing to take his current medication may increase his already present, but mild, tardive dyskinesia? Does he understand that there is a relationship between taking medication and the presence and severity of his voices? Does he understand the relationship between his ability to manage his daily activities and the restoration of grounds privileges?

Second—and often difficult in this situation—does your patient appreciate the seriousness of worsening tardive dyskinesia symptoms? Does he appreciate the importance of complying with staff requests to draw blood regularly to monitor his progress? Does he realize that things are likely to get worse for him if nothing is changed? This often overlaps with the third criterion: Does he express a preference? For patients who manifest the "negative symptoms" of schizophrenia, for example, or who are profoundly depressed, it is often hard to get a clear expression of preference.

Finally, can he use the information you provide in a rational fashion, or does it get incorporated into his existing delusional system? Is he too paranoid, or too preoccupied in dealing with his persecutory voices, to be able to take in this information and understand how it applies to him? Answers in the negative to questions about his ability to use the information rationally raise the issue of competence, but must always be considered in the context of the totality of the situation.

The Right to Refuse Treatment

The requirement of informed consent brings with it a close relative, the right to refuse treatment. This right is based on the preference for autonomy embedded in our legal and social systems, and on certain constitutional principles. It parallels the basic law of competence in its simplicity: all competent adults have the right to make basic decisions concerning their own bodies, and therefore their own medical treatment, even though their decisions may be at odds with what their physician might choose, or even with what a majority of other patients might choose under similar circumstances. This means that competent adults are free to refuse any and all treatment. Moreover, it means that incompetent adults have the same right, although someone else, usually a guardian, may be required to exercise that right on their behalf.

In practice, when someone refuses medical treatment which caregivers feel is necessary, the result is often resort to the legal system, since family members and even guardians are commonly thought not to possess the necessary objectivity. The court then usually appoints a *guardian ad litem,* someone who acts on the patient's behalf only for the duration of the litigation concerning the proposed treatment. The guardian ad litem arranges for a competence examination, interviews the patient, family members, and others involved in caring for the patient. The court considers all the evidence presented (and may ask for additional evidence) and makes a judgment as to whether the patient is or is not competent to refuse the proposed treatment.

Involuntary Commitment Is Not Necessarily Incompetence

Even involuntarily committed competent patients have an absolute right to refuse not only medical treatment but treatment with antipsychotic medications. This is an important point which is often a source of confusion to clinicians. The reason for the confusion is a blurring of the distinction between competence, which, as you remember, is presumed of any adult, and the standard for involuntary commitment, which is always some variation of inability to care for oneself, or danger to oneself or others. Involuntary commitment does not negate the presumption of competence. This is in part because the standard for involuntary commitment is more of a "snapshot" of a moment in time, while competence is a dynamic process.

In many jurisdictions, initial involuntary commitment does not require judicial intervention; in all jurisdictions, a judgment of incompetence, whether narrowly or broadly defined, requires a judicial proceeding. In addition, all jurisdictions require a judicial proceeding in order to continue an involuntary commitment beyond its initial stages. Even if granted, this long-term involuntary commitment does not negate the presumption of competence or constitute the equivalent of a competency proceeding, which mandates a separate request to the court for a judgment of incompetence and appointment of a guardian.

When an involuntarily committed patient is found by a court to be incompetent to decide whether or not to consent to treatment with antipsychotic medication, a number of states require a judge to make a decision after a full adversarial hearing. The judge is required in most jurisdictions to reach her decision by using what is referred to as a substituted judgment analysis. This means that the judge must figure out what the patient would want if he were competent and in the same situation. She must not substitute her own judgment for that of the patient, or make a judgment which she considers to be in the patient's best interest. The same procedure, and the same standards, are used in most jurisdictions to make medical decisions for persons who have been found incompetent to make those decisions for themselves. All of the elements of informed consent apply to the judge, who then adds the substituted judgment element to her decisionmaking process.

Exceptions to the Rules

EMERGENCY

The rule that competent adults must give informed consent to medical treatment is suspended in emergency situations. When a person arrives unconscious at the emergency room lifesaving measures are begun without waiting for consent. The analogous psychiatric situation is presented by the out-of-behavioral-control psychotic patient in a psychiatric hospital. In these circumstances, the requirement of judicial intervention to authorize unconsented-to antipsychotic medication is lifted. The rationale is that this situation presents the equivalent life-threatening danger to the patient or to others that the emergency-room arrival does. Both situations are felt to be time-limited, and require the return to informed consent procedure as soon as possible.

THERAPEUTIC PRIVILEGE

The doctrine of therapeutic privilege, alluded to in *Canterbury v. Spence,* is becoming increasingly rare. It allows a physician to withhold full disclosure of the risks associated with a treatment if disclosure might cause serious physical or psychological detriment to the patient. It is not recognized in many states because of its uncertain parameters and the difficulty of justifying it in operational terms, since it cannot be used solely to overcome the patient's refusal to follow the physician's treatment agenda. It cannot be used with third-party authorizers such as guardians.

WAIVER

Another relatively rare exception is waiver. This occurs when a competent patient requests not to be informed regarding a proposed treatment or procedure. Although upheld by some courts, it is definitely a minority view and arises infrequently in litigation.

PROXY

An additional exception, also fading from legal view, is that of proxy, or good faith, consent, usually obtained from family members on behalf of a patient who has not been adjudicated incompetent. This principle has no basis or support in the law, and would almost certainly not be sufficient to overcome a competent patient's right to refuse treatment. It arises more frequently in the medical/surgical arena than in the psychiatric, where it continues to operate in an informal, often oblique manner. This often takes the form of corridor conversations between clinicians and spouses, siblings, or adult children of patients who the clinician or family suspect are not competent or whom they fear to upset.

TREATMENT REVIEW BOARDS

Treatment review boards are most often involved in research projects; their role is not necessarily to substitute consent but to ensure that researchers follow relevant informed consent procedures. Statutes in a few jurisdictions may allow spouses to substitute consent in certain circumstances. Courts themselves in some states follow a doctrine of making a decision on a patient's behalf based on what they consider to be the patient's best interest, rather than following the substituted judgment (what an incompetent patient would do in the same circumstances if he were competent) analysis.

ADVANCE DIRECTIVES

A last exception to the requirement of informed consent occurs in the case of advance directives. This includes devices such as the living will, the health care proxy, and the durable power of attorney. These and other similar arrangements allow a competent person to authorize another to make decisions on her behalf when and if she is no longer able to make them for herself. They exist in every jurisdiction, and are most commonly used in medical/surgical situations. There is no reason why a competent psychiatric patient may not avail himself—and his treatment providers—of the same opportunity to engage in advance planning. An often-cited example is the situation of the patient with bipolar illness, who, when competent, executes an advance directive to the effect that, should he become manic and/or psychotic in the future, he is to be medicated even if he objects vigorously when the episode occurs. Although there are no reported cases on this subject, there is no reason to expect that such a directive would not survive a legal challenge providing there was adduced sufficient proof of competence at the time of signing the document.

Children

The requirement of informed consent is also somewhat differently formulated in the case of children. Contrary to the general rule for adults, children are presumed to be incompetent to consent to treatment; their parents exercise those rights for them. This doctrine is known as substituted consent, and its rationale is twofold: to protect children from their own immaturity, and to protect the interests of their parents who are financially responsible for them. This exception has its own exceptions, as well as its own complications. The law realizes that in certain situations the interests of parents and children may not coincide. Most states have statutes which authorize courts to substitute their own consent for parental consent in the children's best interest. These cases usually involve young children and arise where parents have religious beliefs which prohibit certain medical procedures such as blood transfusions or surgery or medication.

Parents' and children's interests may also not coincide in the case of older children and adolescents. These cases are more likely to involve consent to testing for pregnancy and venereal disease, and for contraception, abortion, and treatment for drug dependence. The law recognizes that, without freedom from parental knowledge, minors might be reluctant to seek testing or treatment. In addition, some states have enacted statutes which permit minors to receive mental health treatment without parental consent (Reisner and Slobogin, 1990).

There are two other legal doctrines which permit courts to allow minors to make their own informed consent decisions. The first is the doctrine of the *emancipated minor,* which applies to children who are no longer receiving parental guidance or financial support. Children can achieve this status through marriage, enlistment in the armed forces, failure of their parents to support them, or judicial decree based on a wide variety of fact patterns. A similar doctrine is that of the *mature minor,* which allows minors of sufficient maturity and intelligence to make their own medical and treatment decisions. As Reisner and Slobogin point out, these are essentially subjective judgments which in some cases may leave clinicians open to liability, and in which parental involvement, if at all possible, may be the safer course.

No discussion of informed consent involving children would be complete without some mention of children whose parents are separated or divorced. The parents of children from intact families have equal rights to substitute consent for their children. Separated or divorced parents may have the same equal rights either under state law or pursuant to a court order. It is increasingly rare for one parent to have the entire right and the other parent to have none, but the laws vary from state to state, and it is always a good idea to be clear about this. Many separated or divorced parents are able to put aside their differences in medical situations involving their children, but many are also unable to keep their children's health and treatment needs from becoming entangled in their own feelings and behavior. These situations can be extremely trying for all concerned, including clinicians, and legal advice and even judicial intervention are sometimes necessary to obtain a clear mandate for treatment. Unless a clear emergency situation presents itself, examination and treatment should not proceed without the consent of a parent or a judicial order.

References

Aiken v. Clary, 396 S.W. 2d 668 (1965).

Appelbaum, P., and T. Gutheil (1994). *Clinical Handbook of Psychiatry and the Law.* 2nd ed. Baltimore: Williams and Wilkins.

Bursztajn, H. B., et al. (1991). "Beyond Cognition: The Role of Disordered Affective States in Impairing Competence to Consent to Treatment." *Bulletin of the American Academy of Psychiatry and the Law* 19, no. 4, 1991.

Canterbury v. Spence, 464 F. 2d 772 (1972).

Kaimowitz v. Department of Mental Health for the State of Michigan, Circuit Court for Wayne County, Civil Action no. 73-19434-AW, 1973.

Reisner, R., and C. Slobogin (1990). *Law and the Mental Health System.* St. Paul: West Publishing.

Schloendorff v. Society of New York Hospital, 211 N.Y. 125 (1914).

Simon, R. (1992). *Clinical Psychiatry and the Law.* 2nd ed. Washington: American Psychiatric Press.

3

Liability Issues with Managed Care

James Hilliard, J.D.

The term "managed care" generally refers to the management of the cost of health care services chiefly by the imposition of restrictions on access to and reimbursement of those services. Fee-for-service payment was traditional in the United States up to the time of the advent of managed care in the mid to late 1970s. Managed care has become the predominant method of doing business in a rapidly changing health care industry.

The term "managed care" is derivative of the manner by which services are rendered. Insurance companies, employers, and other parties who are responsible for paying for health care services (the payors) (1) *manage* health care services by negotiating for health care contracts, medical supplies, and medical devices; (2) offer financial incentives to encourage employees (enrollees) to utilize such health care providers, who, in turn, agree to treat the enrollees on a discounted basis; and (3) impose certain restrictions on access to health care services. The change in the means by which services are delivered under a managed care system has created additional liability not only for the managed care organization but also for the direct provider of the services.

Managed care's necessary focus on cost containment is often in conflict with standards of care that physicians have traditionally applied. This inherent conflict is particularly strong in the arena of treatment for the mentally ill. The incentives that a managed care system may impose to underrecognize, underdiagnose, and undertreat patients do not easily mesh with the comprehensive and long-term treatment that is required for patients with severe mental illness.

Third-Party Contractual Liability

Contracts between providers and managed care companies usually contain provisions which broadly govern various aspects of the relationships between the two. Such contracts typically include provisions relating to the timeliness, nature, and quality of services that the provider agrees to render to the patient. Specific provisions range from the creation of an obligation on the part of the provider to see the patient immediately in the event of an emergency to the delineation of the standard of care that is expected of the provider. Provisions regulating the standard of care may be tailored to fit the particular specialty that is practiced by the particular contracting provider.

Although these agreements are between the provider and the managed care organization, the patient may be the intended "beneficiary" of the promises contained within. Accordingly, if the provider violates a provision intended to benefit the patient and the violation results in harm to the patient, the patient may have a cause of action in *contract* against the provider for damages relating to the provider's breach of the agreement. This is not an action for negligent malpractice; it takes the form of a contract action and, therefore, is not covered by medical malpractice insurance.

In a recent Massachusetts case, *St. Charles v. Kender,*[1] a patient, who was a member of an HMO, called her primary care physician when she started experiencing discomfort during the early stages of her pregnancy and prior to having seen her physician. The physician was unavailable and the patient left a message. The primary care physician did not respond to the patient's call for two days despite the fact that the message clearly termed the situation as an emergency. Finally, with continuing discomfort, the patient took herself to a hospital, where she miscarried. The contract between the provider and the managed care company required that the provider respond to patient emergencies within one to two hours. The patient filed suit against the doctor in contract, alleging that she was the third-party beneficiary to the contract between the doctor and the managed care company. The trial court found that the doctor was not contractually liable to the patient, but upon further review, the appellate court held that a subscriber to a managed care contract is an intended third-party beneficiary of those provisions of the contract which describe the nature of the medical services that physicians are to provide to their patients. Breach of those provisions gives rise to a cause of action in contract to the patient.

Physicians/providers need to be aware of those clauses in their provider contracts and manuals concerning standards and quality of care expected to be provided to their patients under the plan. Failure to abide by the agreements as stipulated in the contract will expose the provider to liability that may be uninsured.

Provider Lawsuits Resulting from the Actions of the Managed Care Organization

One of the major aspects of the managed care concept is the review and preapproval of services. Utilization reviewers are employed in all facets of managed care to communicate their opinions concerning services requested, by either the patients or primary care providers, to such primary care providers and/or other specialists who are approved by the managed care companies to provide services. The request for services does not always result in approval, especially in light of the emergence of aggressive management by managed care companies of services, and therein lies a contentious issue that has spurred a great deal of controversy and litigation.

DUTY TO TREAT

An issue to keep in the forefront is that doctors are always liable to their patients for failure to treat within the established standard of care, and that it is the treating physician's ultimate responsibility to determine what is medically necessary. It is sometimes difficult to reconcile these two concepts with a managed care environment where the primary concern is often cost containment. It goes without saying that a managed care's financial dictates may, at times, affect the level of care. Indeed, those financial dictates may lead to decisions that are contrary to the provider's opinion not only about the standard of care but also about the medical necessity for the care. It is this refusal on the part of the managed care company to authorize treatments which the provider believes are medically necessary that gives rise to the conflict between the provider, managed care company, and the patient.

In the seminal case *Wickline v. California*,[2] a participant in a state-funded managed care program sued the state, contending that the negligent administration of its prospective utilization review procedures had caused her premature discharge from the hospital. After the patient had undergone complicated surgery to correct a vascular problem in her leg, her physicians requested approval from the state's payor system for an eight-day extension of her hospital stay. In review of the patient's case, the state's consultant only authorized payment for a four-day extension, after which the treating physicians discharged the patient. After the discharge, the patient allegedly suffered an exacerbation of her medical problems which led to her rehospitalization and the eventual amputation of her leg. Suit was filed against the state carrier, and a jury returned a verdict for the patient based on its finding that the patient had suffered harm as a result of "the negligent administration of the state's cost control system."

The holding of the case was reversed by the appellate court, which found that the state's payor system was not liable to the patient and that the utilization-review decision was not the proximate cause of the patient's injury. The appellate court further reasoned that the treating physician, who was not a defendant, was ultimately responsible for the patient's treatment because he had made the decision to discharge her. The court noted that the treating physician could have sought additional extensions from the state's program if he believed the patient needed to remain in the hospital. The court further found that "the physician who complies without protest with the limitation imposed by a third-party payor when his medical judgment dictates otherwise cannot avoid his ultimate responsibility for his patient's care." However, in view of the facts of the case, the court found that although the physician did not protest the state's discharge decision, he did not violate the appropriate standard of care in authorizing the discharge of the patient.

While the court did not directly address the issue of the physician's liability, it did indicate that a managed care company may be held liable when medically inappropriate decisions result from defects in the administration or design of cost-containment features. For example, the court noted that liability may be imposed on a managed care organization when an appeal made on a patient's behalf is not given fair treatment or "when requests for medical care are arbitrarily ignored or unreasonably rejected."

The *Wickline* case raises several issues for providers., What roles should providers be playing with respect to advocating for their patients? Furthermore, if providers do advocate on behalf of their patients, to what degree must they combat a decision by a managed care company that, in their opinion, will negatively impact the patient? It is clear only that if a provider blindly complies with a decision made by a managed care company that the provider does not agree with on a medical basis, the doctor may be liable for any consequential injuries suffered by the patient.

While refusals, approvals, and other dictates of managed care companies or agencies may affect the shape of the treatment that is provided, this does not redefine the standard of care. Rather, the payors' focus on cost containment has created a line of decisionmaking that is often separate and distinct from the standard of care that a providing physician must apply. When these two methodologies are at odds with one another, the managed care decision may put pressure on a physician to provide the lesser level of care that is prescribed by the payor. This unfortunate byproduct of managed care is not be confused with the standard of care that has been carefully honed as a result of the continued evolution and technological advancement of medical services.

In cases where allegedly substandard care causes injury to a patient, litigation becomes the forum not only to allocate the liabilities of the provider and the payor but also to reaffirm what is the actual standard of care that a physician must apply. In such an action the opinions of the managed care company regarding the allowable level of treatment are merely evidentiary in the definition of the standard of care that physicians are bound to apply. Other evidence is gathered though the record as well as the testimony of expert witnesses who possess either demonstrable insight to the type of medical services at issue or familiarity with the actual facts being debated in the courtroom.

Such litigation has the important functions of both redefining the standard of care and reaffirming that the standard of care supersedes the decision of a managed care company in the event that the two do not coincide. Often, such cases result in legislative codification of the standard of care, as was the case where the threshold hospital stays for mothers following birth were increased from the managed care industry standard of twenty-four hours to the current legislative mandate of forty-eight hours.

In order to shield themselves from liability, physicians should take certain affirmative steps:

APPEAL RIGHTS

Physicians should take affirmative steps to ensure that their patients are informed that they have a right to appeal when a managed care company denies services that the physician believes are medically necessary. Not only should physicians advise their patients of their rights to appeal a denial of services, they should also be careful to record that they have so advised. Often, merely telling the patients of their right is not enough. Providing them with documentation of the right to appeal, if requested, is important, and copies of other consultants' reports that would aid the patients in their appeals should also be provided. Furthermore, in *Sarchett v. Blue Cross of California*,[3] the court held that the mere existence of a documented right to appeal denials of coverage does not operate to discharge liability, especially where it is evident that the patient does not understand the right to appeal.

Equally important is that physicians understand the grievance procedure and appeal rights as related to themselves. When providers are allowed to appeal denial of services by a managed care company, they should make every effort to take advantage of appeal and grievance procedures on behalf of their patients. Whatever appeal processes are available should be disclosed to the patient and exhausted by the physician so that, ultimately, if harm comes to the patient as a result of a decision by the managed care company, it cannot be attributed to the negligent care of the provider.

THE DECISION TO TREAT OR TRANSFER

During the period of appeal, the physician is faced with a dilemma—the dilemma of whether to treat without payment or to transfer the patient. Physicians should take caution not to abandon patients despite an HMO's refusal to pay. Often, physicians can continue to treat with an arrangement with the patient for direct payment or reduced payment (physicians should always refer to their contract if they are going to charge the patient directly) or, in some cases, the provider may have to continue to treat even though no payment is available. Referrals may be a source of continuing treatment for the patient, but precipitous termination and/or an attempt at a referral where no real alternative service is available can be viewed as abandonment. It is important to document all steps taken when attempting to resolve a patient's need for treatment when the managed care company has refused to authorize such treatment.

The Indemnification Clause

Most contracts between providers and managed care companies contain a so-called indemnification/hold harmless clause that contains wording similar to this: "Provider agrees to indemnify and hold harmless the HMO for all losses, costs, including reasonable attorneys' fees resulting from any claims, actions, causes of actions, or lawsuits against the HMO as a result of provider's provision of services under this agreement."

This clause that most providers unknowingly are bound to as a result of the cursory signing of the contract states that, if the managed care company is sued for any reason whatsoever with respect to the provider's treatment of the patient, any loss then sustained by the managed care company, including reasonable attorneys' fees, is to be paid by the provider to the managed care company. Usually there is no stipulation in the indemnification clauses that the duty to indemnify the managed care company turns on an adjudication of the provider's negligence. Indemnification clauses are not covered under malpractice insurance policies, as they are contractual and do not arise out of negligent behavior. Accordingly, if a managed care organization lays claim against a provider under the terms of the indemnification clause, the provider will be personally responsible for such losses.

Providers should read their managed care contract before they sign it, or have their attorney review all its terms. If they have already signed a contract with an indemnification clause, additional insurance may be available to cover the indemnification clause. If the contract is to be renewed and has yet to be signed, it is recommended that the physician or the physician's attorney contact the managed care organization and advise them that the indemnification clause should be stricken from the contract. In some cases, managed care organizations will strike the clause. In the event that they refuse to strike the clause, the second line of defense should be that the clause should apply but only to the extent that the provider is insured for third-party indemnification agreements. Such an amendment to the clause may appear somewhat illusory if the provider does not carry the insurance. However, it is protection nevertheless. The third line of defense should be that the clause should be amended to require that any losses sustained by the managed care company that are attributed to the provider will be effective only as a result of an adjudication, including all appeals, by a court of competent jurisdiction wherein it is found that the provider was the negligent party and what percentage of such negligence was attributed to the provider.

Confidentiality of Records

A managed care company's right to access a patient's records held by a provider has been an issue of controversy within the terms of the provider's agreement. Most contracts with providers require the provider to allow the managed care company full access to all patient records made by the provider. Paradoxically, there are also clauses in the same contracts that require the provider to protect the patient's confidentiality to the fullest extent of the law.

Providers should keep in mind that as a general rule the confidentiality of psychiatric records belongs to the patient and the "duty" to maintain the confidentiality belongs to the provider. The managed care company is *not* a party to the patient's record unless the patient agrees to make it a party and approves access by signing a full or limited release. Of course, there may be statutory provisions that give insurance companies limited access to patient records as a payor of health services. However, the patient is the one who ultimately decides whether the managed care company may have access to his or her confidential record. The patient's refusal may result in the insurer's refusing payment and canceling the insurance altogether, but this is an issue for the patient to resolve. Releasing the record to the managed care company in reliance on the terms of the provider agreement may violate the patient's right to confidentiality. Such a right, unless waived, supersedes the contractual duty to release confidential records.

Providers should discuss the issue of access to records with their patients at the early stages of treatment to avoid problems later and to determine early on the process of records access by the managed care company.

Besides routine access for billing and utilization review, there are other areas of records confidentiality that a provider must be aware of: patient access, court order, subpoena, mandatory reporting, and consultations.

PATIENT ACCESS

As a general rule and in most states, patients have a right to access all or at least a summary of their outpatient records. Because of the generally more serious nature of the illnesses afflicting inpatients, and the concurrent risk of the exacerbation of such illnesses, there are more restrictions placed on patients' access to their *inpatient* psychiatric records than to their outpatient records. These restrictions are usually found in the statutes and licensing board regulations. Providers should check to see what their states' laws or regulations allow. The patient must be competent in order to request and sign for such release. In those cases where the patient is not competent by reason of age or mental infirmity, either a parent or a guardian should sign the request.

COURT ORDER

Psychiatric records are treated differently in most states from medical records in that they enjoy a "privilege" from being subpoenaed for certain reasons during litigation. That privilege usually belongs to the patient, and it may be waived in order to have the record released, or it may be invoked to preclude the provider from releasing the records to the subpoenaing party (this is usually done with a motion to quash or a protective order). Most privileged communication statutes also contain exception clauses when under certain circumstances a privilege would not apply. For example, in the case of adoption or child abuse or when patients place their "state of mind" into evidence in a personal injury case, most states will *not* recognize the patient's privilege and will require the record to be released.

A court order usually results from a due process hearing on whether or not the record is subject to the privilege. Court orders will override the privilege and require the provider to release the records either in their totality or for the purposes of a limited or "in camera" review. Providers need to seek legal consultation in cases where there is any doubt about the process of obtaining records under court order.

SUBPOENA

Subpoenas differ from court orders in that they are usually issued by attorneys in the process of discovery in lawsuits. Subpoenas are not always appropriate to access psychiatric records or testimony. When a subpoena is accompanied by a valid court order *or* a signed release from the competent patient, the provider may release the patient's records. When there is a question concerning the validity of a release or subpoena, legal counsel should be sought.

MANDATORY REPORTING

Mandatory reporting is usually a creature of statute and contains the following elements:

1. The provider (who must come within the reporting class) is mandated to inform a state or federal agency or other designated individual based upon the reasonable belief that certain facts are present.
2. The provider's failure to report subjects him or her to either criminal (fine) or civil penalty.
3. The provider is vested with civil immunity from an action by the patient for reporting under such a statute.

The most common mandatory reporting statutes arise in the following contexts: child abuse, duty to warn or protect, elder abuse, disabled abuse, gunshot/knife wounds.

Mandatory reporters experience the most difficulty when they hesitate to report an incident because of their concern for the impact it will have on the patient, family, or victim. The purpose of most mandatory reporting statutes is to obviate the reporter's discretion to decide whether certain acts will result in physical or emotional or sexual abuse, neglect, or harm. Usually a reasonable basis to believe that certain events occurred *or* that a communication has been made to the mandated reporter is all that is necessary to trigger the statute. Mandated reporters must understand that the decision not to report on a situation that at first glance appears to fall within the requirement for reporting may result in a retributory action against them. Therefore, providers should document their reasons for believing that the statutory or mandatory threshold has not been met and a report is not warranted. This will provide some protection in the event that an action is brought for failing to report.

CONSULTATIONS

Often a consultation on a difficult issue is in keeping with the standard of care. Therapists do not have to reveal the identity of their patient in order to seek a consultation. Under these circumstances, no breach of confidentiality occurs. When it is necessary to reveal the identity of a patient for a consultation, the patient's permission is necessary. A note in the patient's chart that permission was granted is usually sufficient. In all cases, whether the patient's identity is or is not revealed, a note of the consultation should be made.

/ / /

While the pitfalls in the ever burgeoning arena of managed care can generally be avoided though the application of the tried and tested standards of medical practice that were pervasive before the advent of managed care, some of the basic paradigms have been shifted. A physician's duty to a patient can no longer be viewed in a vacuum. The potential for liability, though basically still rooted in the duty that a physician owes a patient, can arise in a variety of contexts, and can expose a physician to a level of responsibility that could not have been perceived before the advent of managed care. From liability arising out of contract theory to the wrongful disclosure of a patient's records, the risks of exposure to a provider are daunting and ever-increasing.

While a provider's diligence toward a patient's needs, rights, and records, as well as careful scrutiny of his or her relationship with the managed care payor, may absolve that provider from some of the risks chronicled herein, liability in the managed care context is anything but settled. Managed care is still a relatively new phenomenon, and the courts are likely to see and enforce a variety of new claims against managed care companies and the providers employed by them.

Notes

1. 38 Mass. App. Ct. 155, 646 N.E.2d 411 (1995).
2. 228 Cal. Rptr. 661 (Cal. App. 2 Dist. 1986).
3. 43 Cal.3d 1, 233 Cal. Rptr. 76, 729 P.2d 267 (1987).

4

Write Smarter, Not Longer

Marilyn Berner, J.D., LICSW

It is not sufficient to practice your profession to the best of your ability. You must also document, and keep records sufficient to convince a neutral factfinder that you have done so. The practical realities of how to do that are what this chapter is about. We will examine inpatient, outpatient, medical/surgical, and psychotherapeutic situations. There are some basic rules which apply to all situations. The rules which are most basic, and which apply to all settings and situations, are these:

1. Write smarter, not longer.
2. If you didn't write it down, it didn't happen.
3. Never, ever change a record.

Writing Smarter

Writing smarter means being succinct. It means doing what you were taught to do all those many years ago during your training. It means assessing the information presented to you by a patient, and collateral sources, if relevant, and documenting that assessment. Further, it means making a response to that information, a response in which you exercise your clinical judgment at various decision points. Finally, it means documenting that response and exercise of clinical judgment. In the exercise of clinical judgment, you are essentially conducting a risk-benefit analysis, and it is helpful to use a decision-tree model, which orders your thinking and offers a flexible obsessionality to fit varying levels of anxiety. Consider this hypothetical situation:

You have a female patient who presents as depressed, with suicidal thoughts and a history of suicide attempts, a recent miscarriage, and a supportive husband. You will be here for two weeks, then away for three weeks. Your analysis of the risks and benefits of various treatment approaches follows the branches of the decision tree. You need to assess the risks and benefits of medication versus no medication, and hospitalization versus no hospitalization, and to document your assessment, your response, and your rationale for your decisions. You also need to document the weight you give to her history and to the current presence of a supportive spouse. You must also document that you have considered your time-limited availability and its effect on your decision. Is this a new patient in a clinic? In a private practice? In a hospital emergency room? You must indicate that the presence or absence of a treatment alliance, and the availability of backup coverage, figured in your treatment rationale and how those facts figured into your decision. Finally, you must document the patient's competence to participate in the treatment planning process.

COMPETENCE

Patient competence is the element most often omitted from notes. (An exception seems to occur in the case of state-funded systems of care. This may be a function of the population served, with its preponderance of clients with major mental illness, which forces people in the system to think about competence in a different way. See Chapter 2.) It may be that a partial explanation of the failure to document the patient's competence is that we take it for granted. In fact, clinicians are assessing competence all the way through the assessment interview, in the same way we are assessing mental status. When we get to naming the last five presidents, or counting backward from one hundred by sevens, we are looking for confirmation of what we think we already know. It is the surprise, or the unexpected break in the pattern, that gets our attention.

Documentation of competence should be explicit, and should include consideration of affect, cognition, and the treatment alliance. In our hypothetical situation, what is the effect of the patient's affective state on her competence? Can she reliably agree to follow a plan that the two of you develop together? Can she plan with you at all? Does she need her husband to be included in the planning? Does she need him to be kept out? Can you and she rely on her husband's support? If they are on the verge of separating, does that change her affective state, and therefore her competence to participate? How intelligent is she? Does her depression limit her access to her cognitive resources?

Finally, there is the treatment alliance to consider. Is she a long-time patient of yours? A patient you have never seen before? Is she a patient of a colleague who has provided you with some background? Does she have a connection to the hospital or clinic with which you are affiliated? Is she your first referral from a new managed care plan? All of these questions (and more important, their answers) affect your assessment of the patient's competence, and therefore, your decisions. They all deserve some weight in your response.

What might the note documenting this clinical encounter look like?

2/3/96. Saw Joan F., 28 y.o.m.f. Here with husband. Seemed depressed; chief complaint: suicidal thoughts. Not psychotic. Hx: 2 suicide attempts, miscarriage x2 wks, prev. hx prozac, norpramin, psychotherapy with gd. effect. Doesn't want hospital. Plan: Prozac 10 mg q AM x4d, then 20 mg q AM., see again Fri. Refer for psychotherapy.

A smarter note might look like this:

2/3/96. Saw Joan F., a 28 y.o. m.w.f. who came in with her husband. Ms. F. states she is experiencing suicidal thoughts after suffering a miscarriage two weeks ago. No plan. Mood and affect depressed. Poor eye contact; dress casual to sloppy; grooming adequate; slumped posture. Reports trouble falling asleep, early A.M. awakening. No appetite. Feels sad, "not interested in anything." Spoke with husband, who corroborates this and appears anxious and concerned.

No psychotic symptoms. Fund of knowledge good. Has hx of 2 prior suicide attempts, 1 after end of previous relationship, 1 after previous miscarriage. (See old chart.) States she does not want to be hospitalized again; wants to manage at home. Has done well in past on both prozac and norpramin. Last seen in this practice 18 months ago by C.B., LICSW, with whom she had a good relationship, but who is no longer here. Agreed to have husband join us; slightly more animated in his presence. Says they "have no secrets." Husband states he will "do whatever she needs," and that family will help out.

Plan:

1. Start Ms. F. on Prozac 10 mg q AM x 4d, then Prozac 20 mg qd.

2. Daily telephone check-in with Ms. F. and husband until Friday.

3. Ms. F. to spend afternoons and evenings with mother or mother-in-law while Mr. F. at work.

4. See both Mr. and Ms. F. again on Friday; introduce them to R.S.,

LICSW, who will set up therapy appointment, and to L.T., M.D., who will cover while I am away. Reassess at that time and formulate new plan.

5. Ms. F. appears competent to engage in this planning and to carry out plan. Agrees to call immediately if she feels worse, and if she begins to think about a plan. Understands my obligation to hospitalize her if necessary even if she objects.

Writing smarter also means remembering the essentials of grammar. Now, as in seventh grade, the misplaced modifier is not your friend. The following two real-life examples could have been avoided, or corrected, if the clinicians had either paid more attention while writing the notes or reread them before signing them. This example is from a 1987 discharge summary from a hospital in the Northeast:

> History: This is a 30 year old white female who was brought in to YYY Hospital Emergency Room on the morning of 10-31 with a self-inflicted stab wound of the abdomen. She was found to be hypotensive. She was taken to the Operating Room by Dr. ZZZ, where she sustained a self-inflicted laceration of the left lobe of the liver.

A jury could be forgiven for having some questions about whether operating room procedures at YYY Hospital met accepted standards of care. The next example is also from a facility in the Northeast:

> Identifying data: the patient is a 22 year old male admitted to Great Big Medical Center on 5-9-89 with a history of psychotic behavior, evaluated at Neighborhood Clinic earlier and seen by a Social Worker there with a chemically induced psychosis.

The question of whether this social worker's behavior met accepted standards of care would never get to a jury, since if this note were an accurate reflection of events at the clinic, the insurer would settle the case before trial.

As most of you are no doubt aware, there are financial as well as risk management incentives to write smarter, not longer. To quote an insurer who is most concise on this subject: "In essence, notes should state who rendered what service; why, when, and to whom. The notes must be legible and signed by the person providing the service. The unreadable will be unread, thereby making benefit determination impossible" (Blue Cross/Blue Shield, date unknown.)

Payors of all stripes want documentation of progress. They want to know whether they, and their insureds, are getting what they are paying for.

They do not want intimate details of the therapy process. The various Blue Cross/Blue Shield organizations periodically issue documentation guidelines which are quite clear. Most managed care organizations do the same; some provide clinicians with their own organizational forms which indicate what information is required.

In November of 1994 the *Medicare B Newsletter* published guidelines for documentation which were developed jointly by the American Medical Association and the Health Care Financing Administration. Unlike the Blue Cross guidelines, which were intended specifically for mental health providers, the Medicare B guidelines are intended for all providers. These guidelines are clear and unambiguous, and manage to be quite extensive, without lapsing into obsessional bureaucratese.

PROGRESS VERSUS PROCESS

The payor focus on progress leads us to a consideration of the difference between progress notes and process notes. Table 4.1 outlines the distinctions.

Let us look at an example:

4/3/91. Mr. Smith is beginning to realize that his oedipal longings for his cold and distant mother, complicated by the years of sexual abuse by his seductively intimidating uncle, now Archbishop Jones, contribute to his confused sexual boundaries, drug selling, cocaine abuse, pimping, and manipulative behavior. The crucible for this is, of course, his increasingly eroticized

Table 4.1. PROGRESS NOTES VERSUS PROCESS NOTES

	Progress notes	*Process notes*
Location	"Front," "ward," "clinic," or "public" chart	Therapist's private notes
Content	Facts, observations, tests, procedures, treatments, services, lab results, medications *only*	"Anything that comes to mind"; conscious or unconscious, fact or fantasy
Viewpoint	Operational/descriptive	Therapeutic/investigative
Purpose	Treatment planning, recording, documentation, and utilization review	Understanding total patient for treatment
Language	Austere, factual, descriptive, clear and legible, showing follow-up of problems; may be problem-oriented format	May be quotations from doctor or patient, may use private shorthand or abbreviations, etc.

transference to me. His increased need for me as a primitive selfobject manifests itself as a disintegration product in increased antisocial behavior, such as slashing the tires of my colleagues' cars, and threatening their children as they return from school, and then blatantly and provocatively lying to me and forcing me to cancel several appointments with him.

Is this a progress note? Let us examine it against the criteria in Table 4.1. First, *location*. Is this a note that belongs in a "public" chart? Or does it read more like some therapist's private notes? Second, *content*. Does it document observable or measurable progress, lab results, medications? Or does it read more like the therapist's own stream-of-consciousness musings? Third, *viewpoint*. Is the perspective operational or descriptive? While some of it is descriptive, it is highly subjective and laden with theoretical jargon. Fourth, what is the *purpose* of this note? Does it assist accrediting bodies, utilization reviewers, supervisors, or treatment teams in the performance of their tasks? Or does it appear to reflect the therapist's idiosyncratic attempt to understand the total patient for treatment? Last, *language*. While this note does not use quotations from the patient or the clinician, or private shorthand, it would be a stretch to describe it as austere. It certainly does not follow a problem-oriented format (let alone a solution-oriented one, as favored by many managed care organizations). Most damaging, there is in this lengthy, but not too smart, note no evidence of follow-up of any of the several serious problem behaviors referred to. There is some assessment, but the only response is in the theoretical realm, and none in the behavioral arena of the real world. As a progress note, it gets an F.

When I talk with clinicians about documentation and recordkeeping, someone usually asks, at about this point, some variation of the question: "You keep telling us to write smarter, not longer, but there is all this information that has to be documented. Can't I just use some kind of form?" Translated into the legal question it is, this question asks: "Is there a form I can use that will capture all of the relevant information, take little of my time, and still protect me from liability?" The answer to this question, like the answer to all legal questions, is "It depends." If you can get the necessary relevant information onto a form, then it is fine. There is no case law or statute that says you cannot use a form. Probably the best alternative is a form that allows for a checkoff, plus some space to write a narrative note. I have seen some computer-generated forms which consist of a monthly calendar with a numeral for the date in each box, and a place to check off Y or N in response to four questions: Depressed? Suicidal? Psychotic? Medication? A narrow band of space for notes runs under each week's boxes, not really big enough for much more than a reference to another location in order to document a response to a "yes" answer to any of the four questions.

If you are designing a form, you must be sure the form allows you to document your assessment and your response and your patient's competence in sufficient detail to satisfy neutral factfinders. Further, you must decide whether to rely on the economy version, as in the previous paragraph, or to upgrade to a form that allows you a cushion of protection. Until a neutral factfinder considers the question, and an appellate court either upholds or reverses that decision, we are left to make our best judgment on the information we have available. The traditional SOAP format (Subjective: what the patient said; Objective: what the clinician observed or learned from collateral sources; Assessment: how the clinician tied the first two together and arrived at a conclusion; Plan: the clinician's recommendations for treatment) and its variations are adequate to contain the necessary information. The November 1994 *Medicare B Newsletter* suggests a somewhat similar seven-point format for capturing the essential information.

The second question which often arises at this point in the discussion goes as follows: "This all seems to apply to hospitals and clinics; what about my solo practice, half of which consists of self-pay patients who do not use their insurance?" This is an excellent question, with complicated answers which are different for every fact situation. It is true that without some institutional oversight there is technically no need for progress notes. Several questions remain, however. How are you and your patient going to keep track of his progress? How are you going to define progress? Are you able to keep track of all the therapies you are engaged in without notes? Most important, we need to acknowledge that some therapies go badly, that some patients are unhappy with their therapists, and that unhappiness sometimes leads to litigation.

In the event of litigation, if you have no progress notes, you are likely to be in trouble. It will be your (former) patient's word against yours. (And perhaps she will have been keeping written records.)

If You Didn't Write It Down, It Didn't Happen

Because the practice of clinical recordkeeping is of such long standing, and because courts in particular understand that the reason for clinical documentation is, in fact, not for the convenience of attorneys and judges, but to further the goal of good patient care, "everyone" expects that clinicians will keep records. "Everyone" means your patients, your professional society's ethics board, your professional discipline's licensing board, the newspapers, the general public, and perhaps most relevant for us in this chapter, the courts. Courts know what everyone else knows, and courts expect clinicians to keep records documenting their work. Here is a paraphrase of what one court had to say on the subject: "Dr. (X) in his testimony states that various of these steps, such as talking to (patient) were taken but not recorded in notes. I cannot give full credit to this testimony. Even if it were true that steps were taken and daily visits occurred, the failure to record them was in itself a breach of hospital rules and a serious departure from reasonable medical practice."

To paraphrase Cassandra, there is even worse news to come. Namely, if you neglected to make progress notes, but you did keep personal "process" notes to remind you of your associations, countertransference reactions, and theories about the treatment, these notes may not be private at all, but may be "discoverable" in the event of litigation involving your patient, or between you and your patient. "Discoverable" in legal terms refers to documents or other information which, in the event of a lawsuit brought against you by a former patient (or in the context of any litigation), will be available to other parties in the litigation. If you are muttering to yourself, "I thought this stuff was confidential," it is clearly time for a brief review of the basics of confidentiality and privilege.

CONFIDENTIALITY AND PRIVILEGE

It is still quite true that the basic rule is that communications between doctor and patient, and in virtually all jurisdictions, between psychotherapists and patients, are confidential and privileged. As in all discussions of legal principles, it is the definitions and the exceptions that provide the trouble. First, the distinction between confidentiality and privilege. Confidentiality refers to the broad right, established by ethical tradition and recognized by the law, to keep communications with physicians, lawyers, psychotherapists, and clergy private, and not available to third parties. Privilege is a narrower offshoot of confidentiality, more accurately referred to as "testimonial privilege," and refers to the right of all persons to refuse to testify, or to prevent other persons from testifying, in court regarding matters which are considered confidential. (A useful mnemonic device for distinguishing between the two is as follows: COnfidentiality is the Clinician's Obligation; PRivilege is the Patient's Right.)

The patient's right not to testify, and to prevent you from testifying, regarding the therapy, springs from your obligation to keep the fact, as well as the substance, of the therapy confidential. This is a very real obligation; if you violate this obligation, you may be liable in tort for malpractice and invasion of privacy, for breach of contract, for ethical violations, and for violation of your licensing statute. To make matters worse, if such a lawsuit does not allege malpractice or another form of negligence, but relies, for instance, on a breach of contract theory, your malpractice insurer may decline to defend you. In the event that your patient sues you, she is considered to have waived her privilege by calling into question the issue of her mental health. (The reverse is also true; if she does not pay her bill, and you sue her, her privilege is waived. However, the intimate details of her psychotherapy would most probably be excluded from testimony on grounds of irrelevance, unless you could show that she had sought help for a long history of failing to pay her bills.)

The exceptions to this rule, like the exceptions to all rules of law, serve to define it. The law attempts to balance a variety of competing interests, among them the right to have treatment for any condition be a private matter between a citizen and his treater; the rights of litigants to present their cases in court to secure justice; the rights of insurers to ensure competent and equitable treatment and to prevent fraud; to make sure that people are able to get treatment in emergency situations; and the right of all citizens to enjoy a high degree of personal liberty and privacy versus the right of other citizens, and society in general, to be protected against violence.

In practical terms, the absolute right to confidentiality has been substantially eroded. When I do trainings on this subject, I find that I must devote ninety percent of my time to the ever-expanding list of exceptions to the general rule. For example, in Massachusetts, the exceptions, in addition to the two already mentioned, include these:

1. *Tarasoff* situations.
2. The need for involuntary hospitalization.
3. If a court decides that a therapist has relevant information related to parental fitness in a custody or adoption case.
4. If a therapist believes that a child, elderly person, or handicapped person in the patient's care is suffering abuse or neglect.
5. If the patient introduces the issue of mental or emotional condition in any litigation (not only litigation between patient and therapist), including litigation after the patient's death where this is an issue, such as a will contest.

6. If a court issues an order authorizing access to records to defense counsel in a case where the patient has alleged sexual assault, as well as in some other criminal cases.
7. To provide information regarding diagnosis, prognosis, and course of treatment to an insurance company or government agency paying for treatment.

Not surprisingly, many clinicians, as well as many consumers and advocacy groups, consider the exceptions to have swallowed the rule already, and indeed, many clinicians regularly issue caveats warning that they cannot guarantee confidentiality to patients who use insurance. As this book is being written, public debate on this issue centers on proposed new federal legislation whose supporters assert that it will protect patient confidentiality, and whose opponents argue equally vigorously that it will undermine it. In the judicial branch, the Supreme Court has recently decided that the patient-psychotherapist privilege recognized in most states will protect patients who litigate in federal court. Some jurisdictions have enacted "consumer protection" legislation designed to inform patients at the outset of treatment of possible exceptions to their expectations of confidentiality.

While no one wants to argue that patients should not be informed, many clinicians express concern that presenting this information in the initial sessions will have a chilling effect on people's willingness to seek help when they need it and to be candid if they do. This is particularly true in situations where lawyers advise their clinician clients that in order to conform their behavior to the requirements of these laws, they must provide their patients with a written statement of these exceptions to confidentiality in order to obtain a valid informed consent to treatment.

This presents a dilemma for clinicians and lawyers alike. As lawyers are well aware, too much documentation in the area of informed consent can boomerang. Five-page, single-spaced forms setting out all the possible sequelae to a proposed treatment, from hangnail to death, and presented to the already anxious patient, are routinely found by judges and juries not to be worth the trees they felled, if an actual meeting of the minds between practitioner and patient did not occur. This is as true in medical and surgical cases as it is in psychiatry. On the one hand, the clinician can breathe easier if she has written documentation of her effort to comply with the law. On the other hand, she may have introduced into the therapy some issues of distrust which may retard the development of a working treatment alliance, or in some instances, prevent its development entirely. From the patient's perspective, he is now forewarned, but the issue of whether his forearming will ultimately be to his therapeutic benefit is less clear.

CONFIDENTIALITY SCENARIOS

It may be useful at this point to consider some hypothetical scenarios.

First scenario: Your patient is a twenty-two-year-old college senior whose parents are paying for his therapy. His parent calls with a routine request having to do with the form of your bill to the insurance company. After a brief conversation, the parent inquires how your patient is doing in therapy, asks what you think of his prognosis, and wonders how his parents ought to be responding to what they consider his outrageous behavior. You cannot discuss the treatment or the prognosis without your patient's consent, since he is an adult. You can diplomatically understand the parental concern, but you must explain that without an explicit consent from your patient you are extremely limited in what you can say, although you will be happy to listen to what they have to say. You must then discuss with your patient what his limits are regarding communication with his family. The final agreement, if there is to be any disclosure, should be in writing so that it is clear to both of you what you are agreeing to. A note in the chart that your patient competently authorized a release of information may be adequate, but if there is later disagreement between you and your patient, whether or not there is litigation, a note in the chart will simply be your word against his. A written disclosure agreement, signed by both of you, and enunciating the issues agreed to, narrows the field of disagreement (and perhaps your liability) considerably.

Second scenario: You have the same patient and family situation—but it is an emergency. The same rules apply, but it is harder to follow them, because your anxiety, and perhaps your anger and narcissistic injury, which may already be causing you to second-guess your clinical judgment, get in your way. What you need to do is to provide practical information on how family members should respond to the emergency, as well as information on what role you will play. You need to help contain the family's emotions and preserve your patient's confidentiality so that the treatment can continue when the emergency is over. In the unhappy event that your patient has succeeded in taking his own life, you must continue to preserve his confidentiality for the moment. In many jurisdictions, the legal rule has been that "the privilege [of confidentiality] died with the patient." This is no longer clearly the case in many states, so it is a good idea to get legal advice before disclosing any information to the patient's family. This does not preclude your meeting with the family at some point, sooner rather than later, to offer whatever consolation you can, and to help the family begin to manage their feelings about their loss. In addition to being careful not to reveal confidential information, of course, you must avoid being defensive, or expecting the family to console you. This is not only a decent human thing to do, but is a good risk management technique, as discussed elsewhere in this book.

Third scenario: Your patient is a child. You will, if the child is from an intact family, have some communication with the parents, who presumably not only are paying for the treatment but are responsible for, and invested in, the child's welfare. While it is not always clear what privacy rights children actually enjoy under the law, good clinical practice requires that you work out some rules or guidelines which protect the child's confidences and the integrity of the therapy, while allowing the parents to remain appropriately involved. If the child's family is not intact, the situation offers a rich potential for complication, as discussed in Chapter 2. Joint legal custody, which gives both parents the same rights to be involved in and informed about their children's treatment, is increasingly the trend. This can be changed by judicial order, and if the situation is acrimonious it may be necessary to obtain, through the parents' attorneys, copies of the orders or agreements which spell out the rights and obligations of all concerned.

Fourth scenario: You are an inpatient therapist treating the same twenty-two-year-old college senior. The rules for communicating with his family are the same: you may not discuss his care with them unless he agrees. You may discuss the case with other members of his treatment team, and with your supervisor. They are within what the forensic psychiatrist Thomas Gutheil has referred to as the "circle of confidentiality," which encompasses the direct caregivers, the larger treatment team, and the supervisors of those people. The treatment team may not meet with the patient's family without the patient's permission, nor may any member of the treatment team discuss the case with the patient's former or subsequent therapists without his consent.

A Return to Writing Smarter, Not Longer

Another way to write smarter, not longer, is to keep your notes clinical and patient-centered. For example, do not write "Patient irrational and threatening to sue me," but write "Patient's apparent dissatisfaction and threat of litigation may lead to difficulty following medical advice."

This brings us to the issue of treatment team disagreement. Such disagreement provides an occasion when writing smarter is even more challenging than when writing an individual note. The disagreement should take place in the team meeting, not in the chart. What appears in the chart should be the documentation of the process of arriving at a team decision. An impasse on the treatment team requires the team to obtain a consultation, which must also be documented. In the chart, on the record, dissenting opinions are not allowed; the treatment team is not the Supreme Court. A good note might read: "After much discussion of the risks and benefit of treatment plan X vs. treatment plan Y, the team sought and obtained consultation from Dr. Expert on Z date. Subsequent to the consultation, the team developed the following treatment plan, for the following reasons." The language of the last sentence of this note is important: it is the treatment team's plan, not Dr. Expert's. Formulation of a plan is the team's responsibility, and the liability, if any, is also theirs. The team, like any individual therapist, cannot hide behind the consultant's opinion. Similarly, the team is not required to follow the consultant's advice. It is advisable to document why you sought the advice, what the advice was, and why you decided to follow, or not to follow, it.

The final topic to consider under the general rubric of writing smarter concerns institutional incident reports. Two factors—timing and affect—increase the difficulty of keeping the report clinical and patient-centered. All institutions have procedural rules requiring incident reports to be written close in time to the actual occurrence of the incident. This is an aid to recall, but also emphasizes the role of affect. If an incident is serious enough to require a report, the chances are high that the writer will bring some affect to the writing of it. This may very well influence the writer's ability to maintain a clinical perspective, which, in the spirit of progress notes, should be operational, descriptive, factual, clear, and austere. It is usually a good idea to go over it once or twice before you enter it into the record. Report on what you observed; what others said and did; do not attribute feelings or motivations to others or characterize their behavior. Since many incidents which trigger the need for a report involve violence, or the threat of it, maintaining clinical objectivity can be a challenge. Let us consider a pair of hypothetical notes involving an assault and battery on a staff person by a patient.

3/5/96. B.B. refused to go to his day program today, and spent the morning roaming around the house, being obnoxious and provocative to staff, and trying to start a fight with L.L., who had also stayed home today feeling miserable with a cold, earache, sore throat, high fever, and headache. For no apparent reason other than basic meanness, he was taunting L.L. about his cold. When poor L.L. told B.B. to leave him alone, B.B. hauled off and slugged him in his already painful head, pushing him against the cold wall. When I attempted to intervene, he put his hands on me and pushed me into the couch, knowing very well the rule against physical contact between residents and staff.

3/5/96. B.B. refused to go to his day program today, and remained in the residence. During the morning, he was observed to be increasingly agitated, and engaging in verbal hostility with L.L., another resident who had remained in the residence due to illness. When L.L. told B.B. to leave him alone, B.B. punched him in the head, pushing him against the wall. When I attempted to intervene, B.B. put his hands on my shoulders and pushed me into the couch.

It should be clear that the second note is smarter than the first; it does not attribute motivations to B.B., nor does it betray the writer's biased perspective of B.B. as nasty aggressor and L.L. as innocent victim. It is more successful at maintaining a clinical, descriptive viewpoint throughout, including the recounting of the assault and battery on the writer.

Never, Ever Change a Record

The third of our rules, *Never, ever, change a record,* is not the same as Never, ever make a mistake. The issue here is how to correct a mistake in the record without breaking the third commandment of recordkeeping. Corrections should be in real time, contemporaneously labeled, and transparent. This means that you should not attempt to make the record look as if there never had been a mistake in it. When you discover a mistake, you must acknowledge it and then correct it. This what we mean by "real time." "Contemporaneously labeled" means that you must write "error" in the margin of the note, to alert the reader to both the existence of the error and the subsequent correction. "Transparent" means that the correction should refer to the site of the error but not hide it. It means no whiteout and no indelible black magic marker. For instance, if you wrote "Cogentin" but you meant "Benadryl," draw one line through "Cogentin," and write "error" in the margin, with your name, licensed discipline, and the date. The same applies, of course, if you write "dissociated" when you mean "disheveled," or "incoherent" when you mean "incontinent."

What about sins of omission? Suppose you decide to review your recent progress notes. As you read, you notice that in one case you saw the problem, assessed the risks and benefits of several treatment options, discussed them with your competent patient, and then outlined a treatment plan which he agreed to. But for some inexplicable reason, you forgot to document several elements of this process. What to do? Take a fresh progress note, date it today, and write: "As I review my note for (whatever date), I see that I have forgotten to indicate that . . ." It conveys the necessary information to others who may need to read the note, it does not attempt to hide the error, and in the event of subsequent litigation, it will certainly be better than no note at all.

A Return to If You Didn't Write It Down, It Didn't Happen

This brings us back to reconsideration of our second rule. We have already seen that the judicial system expects us to document our clinical activities. Some practitioners hew to the line that if you keep no notes, there is nothing to hang you with. However, as we know, there is more than one way to assure self-destruction, and keeping no notes is one of those ways. It is not an option for clinicians who work in institutional settings or group practices, and it is not wise for solo practitioners.

There are three main problem areas subsumed under this general heading. The first has to do with available information that does not make its way into the chart, often because the oral discussion in treatment team meetings is the primary vehicle of communication, while the chart is relegated to a rather rote "charting" session. This is much more often the case in mental health than in medical-surgical settings, where the chart really is the primary vehicle of communication among the caregivers. It also includes the many discrete and isolated, but important, bits of information that are conveyed orally from one clinician to another in the parking lot, or noticed as you observe, or interact with, a patient at an other-than-scheduled-appointment time.

The second area that sometimes presents a problem is the failure to document that you followed up on something that you noticed. One of the failings of the F-graded progress note earlier in this chapter was that it contained no indication that either of the two very serious, and even criminal, acts of the patient had been followed up on by the therapist. If you noticed something, you must document that you responded to it. Mention of a tremor in a patient on lithium should include a further note documenting what your response was. Here are two examples:

Mr. S. displayed moderate tremor in both hands. After discussion of the tremor, he agreed to continue current dosage level of lithium until lab results are available in two days, since depressive symptoms persist.

Ms. P. reported an increase in dissociative episodes, with a decreased ability to attend to the concrete necessities of her life. I will contact her case manager to find out what day treatment options are available to help her focus better on grounding techniques.

These notes state what the patient reported, and document that you heard it, followed up on it with some response, and that you had a reason for that particular response.

The last reason for not falling into the "if you didn't write it down, it didn't happen" trap is the most important. While we are focused in this book on your liability and how to prevent it, the first and foremost rationale for good documentation and recordkeeping is that it promotes, enables, facilitates, and is essential to good patient care. Relegating charting, or documentation, to a weekly, biweekly, or monthly session does a disservice to you (by increasing your risk of liability), to your ability to stay on top of the treatment, and to your professional development. It does a grave disservice to your patients if you are not on top of the treatment, and may well constitute malpractice. It also presents a potential risk to your patients by what I think of as the runaway bus factor. If you get hit by a runaway bus on the night before your monthly charting session, a whole month of work will be lost for your patients. It will be harder for your grieving colleagues to help your patients if they are hobbled by both lack of information and anger at you.

The final issue which requires a modicum of attention is that of computer records and computerized documentation. To start with our first rule, "Write smarter, not longer," consider this. In a large, comprehensive computerized system, all clinicians have access to the system. What security measures prevent unauthorized persons from calling up your record, just as your physician does? To some extent, fears regarding the confidentiality of computerized record systems reflect our fear of new technology itself. And the technology does bring its own undeniable problems. When popular entertainment inundates us with stories of teenage hackers breaking into the Pentagon, how can we not fear that our medical records are equally vulnerable? The issue is not that computer systems lack security protections. The fear is that for every system there is someone who, for any combination of reasons, sees those protections as a challenge to be overcome. What difference does it make how smart your documentation is if someone else can undo it?

Or consider a different sort of problem: in an effort to maximize efficiency and save space, a computer record system is set up so an individual clinician can access only the last ten encounters. Does this affect the clinician's ability to write smarter rather than longer, or does it require a "longer" summary after every ten encounters? How does it affect continuity of care? Suppose you are new to the case; how can you follow up on something that your predecessor noticed but did not treat eleven encounters ago? What provisions are there for override in emergencies or other situations? Who decides?

The second and third rules present their own interesting issues. How, in a computerized system, can clinicians correct mistakes? How will the system distinguish between unauthorized entry and authorized after-the-fact correction? If there is one central authority through whom corrections must be funneled, how long is the lag time between your noticing the error and the appearance of the correction in the record? How will the reader of the record be able to distinguish between a corrected note and a note that was correct in the first instance, a potentially crucial distinction in some malpractice cases? What is the effect on patient care in the interim? And what are the legal consequences of the lag? If this seems farfetched, consider the current situation in some large noncomputerized systems, where it takes a month for a surgeon's dictated operation note to return to the surgeon for a signature. If you, the surgeon, get a letter from a lawyer in that interval, what is the legal status of your dictated but unsigned note? And if your coverage needs to know what you saw and what you did while you are in Africa and your patient turns up in the emergency room, where will she turn? Questions like these do not yet have answers.

In summary, there are three basic rules which, if followed, will minimize the risk to both you and your patients: (1) Write smarter, not longer. (2) If you didn't write it down, it didn't happen. (3) Never, ever change a record.

References

Appelbaum, P., and T. Gutheil (1991). *Clinical Handbook of Psychiatry and the Law.* 2nd ed. Baltimore: Williams and Wilkins.

Berner, M. (1994). "Responsible Practice, Smart Documentation." *The Psychotherapy Letter*, April. Providence: Manisses Publications.

"Documentation Guidelines for Evaluation and Management Services" (1994).

Medicare B Newsletter, November. Hingham, Mass.: CandS Administrative Services for Medicare.

Gutheil, T. (1980). "Paranoia and Progress Notes." *Hospital and Community Psychiatry* 31, no. 7 (July).

Langman-Dorwart, N. (1995). "Letter to Mental Health Providers with Medical Record Keeping Guidelines." Blue Cross/Blue Shield of Massachusetts, Aug. 7.

Shorter-Fahimi, M. (1995). "Medical Record Documentation in the Age of Managed Care." *Green Spring* 1, no. 2 (Fall).

5

Child and Adolescent Therapy

Renee Tankenoff Brant, M.D.

Hon. Jonathan Brant

Risk management issues in the practice of child and adolescent therapy are substantially similar to those involved in practice with adults but with some additional wrinkles. Therapists working with children must be concerned about consent and confidentiality. However, because the child or adolescent is usually below the legal age for consent to treatment, a number of unique legal issues relating to consent arise. In addition, treatment of children and adolescents usually occurs in a family context. Parents or other family members may be involved in treatment related to the child's treatment. As a result, there are issues related to recordkeeping, confidentiality, and privilege which are unique to child and adolescent psychiatry (Benedek, 1992).

In optimal circumstances the psychological and legal interests of parents and children coincide. Parents seek to nurture and protect their children and promote a child's healthy growth and development. However, the interests of parents and children under stress may diverge. The families of children in treatment may be stressed by separation or divorce, child abuse or domestic violence, or parental mental illness or substance abuse. These family circumstances raise concerns about potential risk of physical or mental harm to the child.

When family circumstances place a child at risk, the child therapist faces unique challenges. Legal requirements designed to protect children and adolescents such as mandatory reporting statutes may intrude upon the normally private conversations between child, parent, and therapist. Where there are protective concerns, the therapist faces a dilemma regarding maintaining therapeutic confidentiality versus breaching confidentiality to fulfill legally mandated reporting requirements (Barnum, 1990; Benedek, 1992). Stressful family circumstances sometimes lead to legal proceedings in which attorneys and judges request or order the participation of a therapist. Child therapists must balance the clinical, legal, and ethical requirements of their therapeutic role with requests that they participate in legal proceedings.

Finally, children and teenagers can become a threat to themselves or others and can become involved in criminal or delinquent activities. A therapist working with children must confront these risk situations in a manner similar to an adult therapist but with additional considerations given the developmental and legal status of the minor child or teenage patient.

This chapter will review the basic issues which are essential to sound clinical risk management for the child and adolescent therapist. We hope that this review will diminish practitioners' anxiety about legal liability and facilitate the excitement and pleasure that should accompany therapeutic work with growing children and their families.

Basic Issues in Risk Management

INFORMED CONSENT

A therapist must obtain consent for providing treatment. With an adult patient this is not a conceptually difficult issue, because a competent adult can consent to treatment. However, with a child or adolescent the situation is more complicated (Benedek, 1992; Koocher and Keith-Spiegel, 1990). Most children and adolescents are younger than the statutory age required for consent to treatment. This age varies from state to state but is usually no younger than sixteen and more commonly eighteen.

In the case of an intact two-parent family, either parent may consent to treatment of a child or adolescent (and thereby incur legal responsibility for paying for the services). A single parent can also obviously consent to treatment for a child. Whenever a therapist sees a child or adolescent whose parents are divorced or legally separated, the therapist must be aware of the legal custodial arrangements concerning the child. The legal custodian generally has the right to give or withhold consent to treatment, and the noncustodial parent has no such right. Because treatment requires informed consent, it is imperative that consent be obtained from the proper party. This becomes even more complicated in the event of joint legal custody of children. In such circumstances, either parent may consent to treatment, but because of shared legal custody, it is preferable that the therapist obtain consent from both parents.

While parents or guardians are legally required to give informed consent for treatment, a child therapist should also try to inform the child or adolescent about the treatment process and enlist the child's cooperation and assent in a manner consistent with developmental and therapeutic considerations (Benedek, 1992). Informed consent should include discussion of the nature and goals of treatment, parental and family involvement, and risks and benefits of treatment. Financial arrangements and cancellation policies should be negotiated with responsible parties. Special consideration must be given to informed consent regarding medication of the child. Parents must be informed about the potential risks and benefits of medication. Children should be included in these discussions in a manner that is developmentally appropriate.

There are a few situations in which a therapist may offer treatment to a child or adolescent without obtaining parental consent. These include emergency treatment and treatment of adolescents who because of marriage, parenthood, or military service are considered "emancipated" or "mature" minors who are permitted to consent for themselves in some states. In addition, some states permit children and adolescents seeking treatment for venereal disease and drug or alcohol abuse to consent to treatment without parental involvement. As a general rule confidentiality should accompany a minor's ability to consent to treatment (Simon, 1992a).

RECORDKEEPING

As with any patient, a therapist seeing a child or adolescent should keep records of that treatment. Such records should, of course, conform to both ethical standards for the profession and to any state laws or regulations.

Recordkeeping with child and adolescent patients becomes complicated because of the likelihood that parents and sometimes other family members are also being seen in therapy. The therapist will probably be hearing what the child has to say about each of the parents and what each of the parents has to say about the child and the other parent. A decision will have to be made whether meetings with the parents or other family members are part of the child's treatment, or whether parental or family treatment is separate from that of the child. The therapist will also have to decide whether records of parent or family meetings are part of the child's record, or whether parental or family therapy records are kept separately.

These details of recordkeeping become salient when the therapist receives a request for release of some or all of the child's therapeutic records. Generally, the minor child's parents have legal authority to see the child's record and to consent to the release of the record to third parties. As a child grows older, a therapist may decide to discuss release of records with the child and obtain the child's consent, although this may not be legally required.

Issues of access to and consent for release of records become more complicated when parents are separated or divorced. The custodial parent, or both parents in a joint custody situation, may well have access to the records of therapy upon request and must consent to release of records to other parties such as schools. The therapist must be careful to record statements made by one family member about another family member in a neutral and accurate manner. The therapist should use objective language and should distinguish clinical data from opinions or hypotheses.

Regardless of a child's family circumstances, the therapist must determine which parent or guardian has legal authority to have access to and authorize release of a child's therapy records. The therapist must take care to record information in a manner that is objective and clinically useful without being inflammatory or prejudicial. The therapist must also be sensitive regarding the inclusion of sensitive material regarding a child's parents or family in the child's records. A therapist has a duty to protect the confidentiality of records pertaining to parents and family members as well as those pertaining to the child (American Academy of Child Psychiatry, 1982).

CONFIDENTIALITY

The therapist's obligation to keep conversations between therapist and patient confidential is based on both state law and professional ethical principles. Confidential therapeutic communication includes all material revealed during the course of a child's diagnosis and treatment. This material can be written or oral, and, in the case of children, can include actions and occurrences such as observations of the child's play and drawings. Communications by a parent about a child which are part of diagnosis and treatment are also confidential. Therapists have a duty to keep therapeutic communication secret and can be sued for revealing this information without appropriate authorization (parental consent or court order).

With regard to treatment of children and adolescents, the issue of confidentiality poses more complexity and challenge than is the case in the treatment of adults (Simon, 1992a). A child therapist often feels torn between the young patient who does not want information shared with either parent, and a custodial parent who has a legal right to access to therapeutic information. While child therapists must respect a parent's legal right to have access to a child's records, therapists usually try to offer a child some limited guarantee of confidentiality in order to facilitate therapeutic communication. Thus, a child therapist must balance the therapeutic and ethical duty to respect and maintain a child's confidential communication, including keeping therapeutic communication confidential from parents, with the therapeutic and legal duty to keep parents informed about the course of the child's treatment.

Therapists should attempt to negotiate these "confidentiality boundaries" between parent and child at the beginning of treatment as part of the treatment contract. Arrangements will vary with the age of the child, with adolescents usually requesting and requiring more explicit contracts around confidentiality. The therapist must address the question of access to records at the commencement of treatment. There must be explicit agreement concerning disclosure of information about the child or adolescent, whether orally or by access to records, to either parent. The therapist must seek to assure the child or adolescent patient that confidentiality is respected while at the same time respecting the custodial parent's right to have access to information about the child. In addition, there must be explicit agreement concerning whether a noncustodial parent, who may have no legal right to access of records, may nonetheless be granted some access to information about the child's therapy. Therapists should also note the exceptions to confidentiality between parent and child in these therapeutic contracts. Exceptions include situations in which the child or teenager is at risk to harm him or herself or others.

Child therapy typically involves collaboration with school systems, health and mental health professionals, and professionals in other institutions and agencies. Exchange of therapeutic information is often vital to these collaborations. A child therapist must determine which parent or guardian has legal authority to consent to release of confidential therapeutic records to third parties. When parents or others request release of confidential information, the therapist should obtain a specific written consent from the parent and child, when appropriate, before information is shared. Every effort should be made to limit the information released to that which is specific to the request, and to guard against the release of nonessential confidential information. In this era of managed care, insurance companies and health maintenance organizations make frequent requests for therapeutic information. Here too it is very important to obtain appropriate consent for release of information to insurance companies and to limit the information shared to that which is absolutely necessary.

EXCEPTIONS TO CONFIDENTIALITY

A therapist's duty to protect a child patient from harm and duty to warn and protect third parties from identifiable danger posed by a patient may create a clinical situation in which confidentiality is not maintained. Each clinical situation involves careful consideration of relevant therapeutic, legal, and ethical issues (Barnum, 1990).

Child protection statutes represent a major exception to principles of confidentiality. When a child or adolescent patient informs a therapist about physical or sexual abuse by an adult, statutory requirements for reporting govern over principles of confidentiality. Therapists are mandatory reporters under child protective statutes in every state (Brant, 1991; Barnum, 1990). Barnum reviews child abuse reporting laws in different states. States vary in defining reportable conditions, with some offering no definition of abuse and others specifying long lists of findings that indicate abuse or neglect. States also differ as to whether reportable conditions include those in which there is substantial *risk* of harm to a child, as well as situations in which harm has already occurred. All child therapists should be familiar with statutes on child abuse reporting in their state and should obtain clinical and legal consultation when necessary. If a therapist believes that a child's assertions of abuse are credible, the therapist must report the suspected abuse to the required state authorities. State authorities will investigate the reported abuse and may bring legal action to protect the child. Therapists who file reports of suspected abuse in good faith are protected from lawsuits brought by the suspected perpetrator of the abuse even if, after investigation, no abuse is shown. On the other hand, therapists can face civil or criminal penalties for failure to report child abuse (Barnum 1990; Newberger, 1992).

A therapist cannot offer a child or adolescent patient any promise of confidentiality if the patient reveals an apparent abuse situation. The therapist can determine when and how concern about abuse is shared with parents and legal or protective authorities and can strive to do so in a manner that minimizes risk to the child. A therapist can also keep a child informed about mandated protective actions which the therapist has taken and likely consequences.

When a child threatens harm to another person, a therapist must assess whether the duty to warn or protect a third party from danger requires a breach of therapeutic confidentiality (Barnum, 1990). The therapist must assess the extent to which the child or adolescent's clinical condition poses a likelihood of harm and whether there is an actual plan, whether the patient has a means to carry out the plan, whether the intended victim is identified, and whether the patient has access to the intended victim. If the therapist believes that an imminent threat to an identified person exists, the therapist must take action to prevent the threat from being carried out. Some state statutes or case law requires actual notification of the threatened person. Others require the therapist to protect such persons by involuntarily committing the patient (Simon, 1992a). Therapists must be aware of the law of the jurisdiction where they practice; when clinical risk is high and a potential victim is identified, a therapist must follow applicable state law on duty to warn or duty to protect. Clinical and legal consultation are often necessary in these high-risk situations.

Similarly, a therapist may take action when a child or teenager indicates a present intent to commit suicide. The therapist must assess the severity of the patient's condition and the likelihood that the patient will act in a hurtful manner. The therapist may notify parents if necessary to protect the patient from harm and may authorize having the patient involuntarily hospitalized.

TESTIMONIAL PRIVILEGE

Privilege statutes are a subset of laws which address confidentiality between patient and therapist. Testimonial privilege statutes limit *testimony* by therapists concerning therapeutic communication and require the consent of the patient or the patient's legal representative before a therapist can testify (Simon, 1992a). These statutes specifically apply to therapist testimony in judicial, legislative, and administrative proceedings. While laws vary from state to state, communications between patients and most licensed therapists are covered by privilege statutes.

Privilege statutes are exceptions to the general principle of law that all persons must testify to what they know about an event (Brant, 1991). In general, for the sake of justice, any witness with relevant testimony must provide that testimony in legal proceedings. However, some communications are considered so protected that a greater social value is served by keeping the communication private than by using it as evidence in a legal proceeding. These protected communications include those between spouses, penitent and priest, and patient and therapist. The patient has the *privilege* to refuse to disclose therapeutic information in legal, administrative, or legislative proceedings and has the *privilege* to prevent his therapist from testifying. Only the patient or his legal representative has the authority to waive testimonial privilege. However, a therapist has the standing to raise the issue (assert the privilege) as a defense against disclosing confidential therapeutic information which is subject to privilege. For example, if a child therapist receives a subpoena to testify about treatment of a child at a deposition, the therapist can assert that this is privileged information and await appropriate consent from the patient's legal representative or a court order before agreeing to testify. In the service of protecting the confidentiality of treatment records and in keeping with sound risk management, the therapist should assert any applicable privilege (Brant, 1991).

While a parent has legal authority to consent to the release of confidential therapeutic records for a child, a parent does *not* have legal authority to waive a child's therapeutic privilege. This represents an exception to the parent's usual legal right to consent to release of therapeutic records for a child (Herman, 1996). Thus, a therapist cannot testify in court about a child's treatment based on a parent's consent. This makes sense because child and parental interests are in conflict in many court cases. Termination of parental rights and custody proceedings are two examples. In some situations, a judge will appoint a guardian ad litem for the specific purpose of determining whether to waive or uphold a child's therapeutic privilege. The guardian ad litem will make a decision based on consideration of the relevance of therapeutic communication to the legal matter at hand, availability of nonprivileged sources of information, the extent to which the therapeutic relationship will be jeopardized by release of therapeutic information, and the child's preference, as well as risks and benefits of waiver, and the preference of the child's parent or guardian if a parent's interests are not at odds with those of the child (Ouelette, 1996). If the patient is a minor, the therapist cannot and should not testify without a court order or a guardian ad litem having waived the child's therapeutic privilege.

A court order, a formal court paper signed by a judge, should be distinguished from a subpoena. A subpoena is a demand for records prepared by an attorney in a case. Although the document may appear to be very formal and may have a court reference on it, a subpoena is not a court document signed by a judge. A subpoena does not waive the child's therapeutic privilege and does not give the therapist permission to release or testify about privileged information. A therapist is liable for improper release of confidential therapeutic information if the therapist shares confidential information based on a subpoena alone.

A therapist who receives a subpoena for a child's therapy records should contact the attorney who sent the subpoena and indicate that the records are confidential and will not be released without a court order. If the child has an attorney in the matter at hand, that attorney may act to quash the subpoena on the basis of the applicable patient-therapist privilege. A therapist needs the protection of appropriate consent or a court order to justify release of confidential information for a legal proceeding or testimony about treatment of a child. Because records of therapy involving child or adolescent patients may be used in highly contentious legal proceedings, such as divorce actions, a therapist must be very cautious before releasing information to a court.

EXCEPTIONS TO PRIVILEGE

Despite the existence of privilege statutes, many conversations between therapist and child or adolescent patients will become the subject of court testimony. This is because most privilege statutes have exceptions for many of the family situations which place a child at risk for physical or emotional harm. These exceptions to privilege include child abuse proceedings and child custody disputes. Some states require preliminary judicial determinations that the best interests of the child or adolescent favor having the testimony heard in court rather than kept private. Other exceptions to privilege include the following: involuntary hospitalization proceedings; court-ordered evaluations, as long as the patient is informed at the outset of the evaluation that privilege will not apply; cases in which the patient raises mental or emotional condition as part of the case (that is, the patient is seeking damages for emotional injury caused by trauma); and when the patient brings a claim against a therapist and disclosure is necessary for the therapist's defense (Simon, 1992a).

Malpractice Minefields

BASIC CONSIDERATIONS

Certain areas of practice require special care and vigilance to assure sound clinical and risk management practice. These areas of practice include high-conflict divorce, trauma and child abuse, and juvenile delinquency. They are most challenging because of the nature of the clinical work, the frequency with which these cases involve protective and legal issues, concerns about physical and emotional risk to children and others, and family and systems dynamics which are often adversarial and involve competing interests of parents and children. A therapist working with a child in these situations can be in a difficult position. By acting on behalf of the psychological and protective interests of a child, a therapist may be opposing the interests of one or both parents, as may occur in a child abuse case or a custody dispute. These situations can disrupt a therapist's alliance with a parent and threaten the ongoing work with a child. In more extreme situations, a parent can be angered by a child therapist's actions or opinions and may make a complaint or take legal action against the therapist.

There is a high demand for competent clinical care in these contentious areas. Clinicians who practice in these high-risk areas are often drawn to the complex, challenging, interdisciplinary nature of the work. In addition to attending to the basic issues of risk management outlined above, therapists involved in these clinical areas need to be aware of clinical and legal issues which are unique to each specialized area of practice. This awareness should lead to practice procedures and strategies which diminish a clinician's anxiety about liability issues and free the clinician to perform the challenging clinical work.

In some cases, clinicians will knowingly become involved in these complex clinical areas. In other instances, these clinical issues will unexpectedly arise in cases where they were not part of the initial presentation. Some of these areas of practice involve special skills and expertise. It is always important that clinicians practice within their areas of competence and seek additional education, consultation, or supervision before entering less familiar high-risk areas of practice. Very often, with appropriate clinical and legal consultation, a clinician will be able to proceed with a case. In some instances a clinical situation will take a therapist beyond the bounds of competence or into a realm where the clinician is overly anxious and apprehensive. Many of these cases are appropriately referred. The clinician must take care to follow sound methods and procedures in referring and transferring any case in general, and high-risk cases in particular.

It is always important for a child therapist to clarify role expectations in a particular case and to avoid conflict of interest. This is especially important in high-risk cases, which frequently involve clinical, protective, and legal issues. The child therapist, the parents, and the child must all be clear about the therapist's role. When a child therapist's role is clinical, the therapist's primary duty is to the patient. The therapist may be asked to speak to the child's teacher or may be summonsed to testify in a divorce proceeding. The clinician's response to these requests must always be grounded in clinical, ethical, and legal responsibilities to the patient. The clinician must carefully weigh and consider issues of consent, confidentiality, and privilege noted previously and be guided by a primary duty to the patient.

In contrast, a child therapist may also function in a forensic role. Forensic evaluations need to be distinguished from clinical evaluations. Forensic evaluations are conducted for an attorney or the court and are directed toward providing psychological data and opinions for legal proceedings rather than providing treatment for a patient. The child therapist is acting as a consultant to an attorney or the court and is not engaged in a clinician-patient relationship with the child or family. As a basic rule, a child therapist should not combine a primary clinical role with a forensic role in the same case.

Acting as a clinician, a child therapist can be a mandated reporter and can testify in and participate in legal proceedings as long as this is done within the clinical, legal, and ethical parameters of a primary clinical role. It is quite another matter for a child therapist to conduct a forensic evaluation by court order or at the request of an attorney. In this situation, the therapist is being employed by the attorney or the court and is not the child's therapist. Whether the therapist is functioning as a clinician or in a forensic role, informed consent requires that the child and family have a clear understanding of the role of the therapist and the limits of the role, and that the parents and child fully understand the distinction between clinical and forensic roles.

The therapist must set out these parameters at the beginning of an evaluation or treatment as part of the treatment or evaluation contract. The therapist must also clarify issues of confidentiality (or exceptions to confidentiality) at this time. For example, if the therapist is conducting a court-ordered evaluation of a child and family in a custody dispute, it must be made clear that the therapist is functioning in a forensic rather than clinical role and that the therapist's communications with the child and parents will be the subject of a report to the court and may be the subject of testimony in a legal proceeding.

Finally, sometimes child therapists are employed as consultants to schools, detention centers, or other agencies. The therapist may be requested to offer consultation regarding a particular child in a high-risk situation. During the consultation the clinician may meet with the child or parents. In such a situation it is again important to clarify the child therapist's role. In this case the therapist is being employed by the school or agency and is seeing the child as part of a consultation to the agency. The clinician is not functioning as the child's therapist but can facilitate referral of the child and family should they need clinical services.

HIGH-CONFLICT DIVORCE

High-conflict divorces create the likelihood of significant psychological risk for children (Johnston and Campbell, 1988; Nurcombe and Partlett, 1994). Children can also be exposed to physical or sexual abuse and interspousal abuse or violence in this context. Child therapists have a very important role to play in treating and evaluating children and parents in these stressful family circumstances. However, the child therapist must take care to avoid getting caught in the crossfire of parental conflict. For example, in a custody dispute, a child therapist may be pressured to side with one parent against another or may be asked to offer opinions about custody or visitation. A therapist often walks a tightrope between pleasing or angering one parent or the other. The following considerations should facilitate the goal of enabling a therapist to focus on the psychological needs of the child while maintaining neutrality in relationship to parental conflict.

To the extent possible, in the service of clinical flexibility and effectiveness, a clinician engaged to do child therapy should attempt to focus concern on the child's well-being, enlist the consent and cooperation of both parents, and remain neutral regarding the parents' conflict. A clinician can strive for this goal, but cannot always achieve it. Careful negotiation of a therapeutic contract at the beginning of treatment can help. It is important for the therapist to clarify physical and legal custodial arrangements and financial responsibility for treatment. The clinician should define the parameters and goals of treatment and the manner in which the child and each parent will be involved. Although consent is required from the parent or parents with legal responsibility, usually the custodial parent, ideally the therapist should obtain consent from both parents, unless this is clinically or legally contraindicated. It is especially important to clarify issues of access to records and confidentiality regarding the communications of the child and each parent in these high-conflict clinical situations. Finally, it is very important to clarify boundaries between a therapist's clinical role and a possible forensic role. It is not unusual for a parent to attempt to enlist the clinical services of a child therapist with the overt or hidden agenda of using the therapist to testify on the parent's behalf in a custody proceeding. Structuring a case in the manner suggested above, inquiring about the legal status of the case, and distinguishing clinical and forensic roles will help the clinician avoid pressure to serve as one parent's advocate rather than as the child's therapist.

When a therapist is engaged to perform a forensic evaluation in a child custody dispute, ideally the therapist should be appointed by the court or hired by a guardian ad litem as a neutral evaluator representing the best interests of the child. The evaluation should include the entire family, and the therapist should not enter as an advocate for one or another parent. The therapist should not combine forensic and therapeutic roles. A detailed contract must be negotiated before the evaluation proceeds. The contract should address informed consent regarding the method of evaluation, payment, waiver of confidentiality in the context of the evaluation and related court proceedings, and clarification about the report and the party to whom the report is released, usually the court (Herman, 1992; Nurcombe and Partlett, 1994).

TRAUMA AND SEXUAL ABUSE

Clinical practice in the area of child trauma and child sexual abuse requires specialized skills and training. Sometimes concern about trauma or sexual abuse will be present at the outset of treatment. A clinician can decide whether he or she has the required skills for evaluation and treatment or whether supervision, consultation, or referral for specialized sexual abuse evaluation and treatment is necessary. At other times concerns about possible trauma or sexual abuse emerge during the course of treatment. The clinician will need to determine whether the index of suspicion is sufficient to require a shift in therapeutic approach to a more focused clinical evaluation for suspected abuse or trauma (Sauzier, 1996). Clinicians may have the requisite skills for this shift to a trauma-evaluation mode, may require specialized supervision or consultation, or may decide to refer the case for evaluation.

The therapist involved in the evaluation and treatment of traumatized children in general, and sexually abused children in particular, faces significant clinical challenges. During the past fifteen years there has been a proliferation of clinical and research literature on child trauma and sexual abuse (Briere, 1992; Friedrich, 1990; Terr, 1990). National professional organizations have developed guidelines for clinical evaluation of sexually abused children (American Academy of Child and Adolescent Psychiatry, 1990; American Professional Society on the Abuse of Children, 1990). Specialized interdisciplinary programs for diagnosis and treatment of child sexual abuse have been developed in many communities. Expert consultation is also available. At the same time, the credibility of children's traumatic memories and disclosures of abuse is frequently challenged by defendants and their attorneys in legal proceedings. Therapists, too, are being challenged regarding their methodology and alleged bias in obtaining disclosures (Myers, 1994). In some cases therapists are being sued for implanting "false memories" of abuse in their patients.

In the age of the "backlash" it is important for therapists who evaluate or treat children making abuse allegations to protect themselves through sound clinical practice and risk management (Deutsch, 1996; Myers, 1994). Clinicians must have adequate training, consultation, supervision, and continuing education in the area of trauma and child abuse. They must be familiar with the evolving clinical and research literature and relevant professional guidelines for evaluations and use of diagnostic instruments such as anatomical dolls (American Professional Society on the Abuse of Children, 1995).

Clinicians must be aware of their assumptions and biases. They should strive for a methodology for interviewing children which promotes children's comfort and truthfulness in speaking about possible abuse while guarding against pressure, coercion, and influence on the child (American Professional Society on the Abuse of Children, 1990; Goodman and Saywitz, 1994). Clinicians must enter a case with an open mind, objectively gather and document clinical data, and consider alternative hypotheses to explain a child's symptoms, statements, and behavior.

Clinicians must practice within their area of competence and know their limits. Diagnoses and formulations should be supported by clinical data. When it is clinically appropriate, family members and other collaterals should be included in the evaluation in a balanced and neutral manner.

THE CHILD DELINQUENT AND OFFENDER

Child therapists face many clinical and legal complexities upon discovering that a child or teenage patient has broken the law, has threatened to harm himself or another, or is involved with drugs or alcohol. Clinicians must assess the risk that the child poses to himself or others. They must consider the family context and determine when parents need to be informed. They must determine the extent to which they can respond to a child's disclosure of endangering or criminal behaviors while maintaining confidentiality and when their duty to protect the patient or endangered third parties requires breach of confidentiality and notification of appropriate authorities (Barnum, 1990; Porter, 1996). (A therapist's duty to warn and duty to protect are discussed more fully in the section on exceptions to confidentiality.) Careful documentation and timely clinical and legal consultation are essential to sound clinical practice and risk management in these high-risk situations.

THE QUESTION OF BOUNDARY VIOLATIONS

In recent years much has been written about the maintenance and the violation of boundaries in the practice of psychotherapy with adult patients (Simon, 1992a, 1992b). Little has been written about appropriate boundaries in clinical work with children and adolescents (Koocher and Keith-Spiegel, 1990).

The circumstances and context of therapy and the age of the patient require reassessment of physical boundary issues with young patients. For example, it would rarely be appropriate for a therapist to take an adult patient out for coffee, while it may be entirely appropriate for a therapist to go to a snack bar with a resistant teenager or play with a young child at a playground. Physical contact with an adult patient should generally be limited to that which is medically necessary or very limited non-intimate contact such as a handshake or pat on the hand or shoulder. In contrast, a toddler may sit close to a therapist for physical comfort, spontaneously hug a therapist, or need assistance in washing hands or toileting.

Boundary issues related to a therapist's countertransference can occur in therapeutic work with adults or children. In therapeutic work with adults, frequent reference is made to feelings of sexual attraction which must be managed to avoid boundary violations (Simon, 1992a). Sexual feelings can also arise in therapeutic work with children and teenagers and must be managed so that they are not acted out. In addition, child therapists must contend with wishes or fantasies of becoming the protector, rescuer, or idealized parent of a child (Koocher and Keith-Spiegel, 1990). These countertransference issues must be addressed so that they do not lead to inappropriate interactions between a therapist and a child or adolescent. For example, a teenage patient has an argument with her parents, who, the therapist believes, are not able to understand the child as well as she can. The teenager shows up at the therapist's office after an argument at the end of the therapist's workday. The therapist considers bringing the girl home with her for the evening but has second thoughts. Here the therapist's countertransference toward the teenager and her parents could lead the therapist to inappropriately act out a rescuer role.

If a clinician has a question, concern, or anxiety about boundary or countertransference issues with a child or teenager it is always advisable to seek consultation and supervision. This is an area where therapists would be well served by more open discussion and development of guidelines within professional organizations.

/ / /

Clinical work with growing, developing children and teenagers can be stimulating, rewarding, and even fun. Child therapists can legitimately play in therapy with children. Yet this clinical work can lead to risky situations in which children or others are physically or mentally endangered and the therapist must negotiate complicated clinical, legal, ethical, and protective issues. Sound clinical practice, appropriate clinical and legal consultation, and implementation of risk management policies and procedures can strengthen our clinical effectiveness, protect ourselves and our patients, diminish our anxiety, and enhance our enjoyment of professional practice.

References

American Academy of Child and Adolescent Psychiatry (1990). *Guidelines for the Clinical Evaluation of Child and Adolescent Sexual Abuse.* Washington.

American Academy of Child Psychiatry (1982). *Principles of Practice of Child and Adolescent Psychiatry.* Washington.

American Professional Society on the Abuse of Children (1990). *Guidelines for Psychosocial Evaluation of Suspected Sexual Abuse in Young Children.* Chicago.

American Professional Society on the Abuse of Children (1995). *Use of Anatomical Dolls in Child Sexual Abuse Assessments.* Chicago.

American Psychiatric Association (1994). *The Principles of Medical Ethics with Annotations Especially Applicable to Psychiatry.* Washington.

American Psychological Association (1981). "Ethical Principles of Psychologists." *American Psychologist* 36: 633–638.

Barnum, R. (1990). "Managing Risk and Confidentiality in Clinical Encounters with Children and Families." In J. C. Beck, ed., *Confidentiality versus the Duty to Protect: Foreseeable Harm in the Practice of Psychiatry.* Washington: American Psychiatric Press.

Benedek, E. P. (1992). "Ethical Issues in Practice." In D. H. Schetky and E. P. Benedek, eds., *The Clinical Handbook of Child Psychiatry and the Law.* Baltimore: Williams and Wilkins.

Brant, J. (1991 and 1994 Supplement). *Law and Mental Health Professionals: Massachusetts.* Washington: American Psychological Association.

Briere, J. N. (1992). *Child Abuse Trauma: Theory and Treatment of Lasting Effects.* Newbury Park, Calif.: Sage.

Deutsch, R. M. (1996). "Your Practice Might Be in Jeopardy." Presentation at The Child/the Clinician/the Law, a continuing education course sponsored by Harvard Medical School, Boston, Feb. 10.

Friedrich, W. F. (1990). *Psychotherapy of Sexually Abused Children and Their Families.* New York: Norton.

Goodman, G. S., and R. J. Saywitz (1994). "Memories of Abuse: Interviewing Children When Sexual Abuse Is Suspected." In S. J. Kaplan and D. Pelcovitz, eds., *Child and Adolescent Psychiatric Clinics of North America: Child Abuse* 3, no. 4: 645–661.

Herman, R. (1996). "The Sheriff Brings the Summons." Presentation at The Child/the Clinician/the Law.

Herman, S. P. (1992). "Child Custody Evaluation." In Schetky and Benedek, eds., *The Clinical Handbook of Child Psychiatry and the Law.*

Johnston, J. R., and L. E. G. Campbell (1988). *Impasses of Divorce: The Dynamics and Resolution of Family Conflict*. New York: Free Press.

Koocher, G. P., and P. C. Keith-Spiegel (1990). *Children, Ethics, and the Law*. Lincoln: University of Nebraska Press.

Myers, J. E. D., ed. (1994). *The Backlash: Child Protection under Fire*. Thousand Oaks, Calif.: Sage.

Newberger, E. H. (1992). "Intervention in Child Abuse." In Schetky and Benedek, eds., *The Clinical Handbook of Child Psychiatry and the Law*.

Nurcombe, B., and D. F. Partlett (1994). *Child Mental Health and the Law*. New York: Free Press.

Ouelette, L. A. (1996). "You're Called: The Psychotherapist/Patient Privilege." Presentation at The Child/the Clinician/the Law.

Porter, S. G. (1996). "Your Patient Is a Child Offender." Presentation at The Child/the Clinician/the Law.

Sanzier, M. (1996). "The Child Begins to Speak of Trauma." Presentation at The Child/the Clinician/the Law.

Simon, R. I. (1992a). *Clinical Psychiatry and the Law*. Washington: American Psychiatric Press.

Simon, R. I. (1992b). "Treatment and Boundary Violations: Clinical, Ethical, and Legal Considerations." *Bulletin of the American Academy of Psychiatry and the Law* 20, no. 3: 269–288.

Terr, L. (1990). *Too Scared to Cry*. New York: Basic Books.

6

The Perspective of the Insurer

Peggy Berry Martin, M.Ed., A.R.M.

As a matter of survival, today's malpractice insurers have become service organizations, striving to be responsive to the cyclical nature of the liability insurance market, while providing unique services to the insured health care organizations and caregivers. This aspect of the business of professional liability insurance has created challenges for traditional commercial insurance companies and has led to the creation of a variety of new entities over the last fifteen to twenty years.

If the major challenge for many insurance companies is maintaining the balance between fiscal responsibility and a customer service philosophy, meeting that challenge may involve some new ways of relating to insureds. Some suggestions from a successful insurance program include the following:

Providing responsible leadership to caregivers as current risks change, new areas of liability emerge, and new delivery systems complicate the practice of medicine.

Maintaining focus on the quality of patient care rather than on defensive behavior that can further erode the patient/physician relationship.

Providing as much claims information as possible to insureds for educational purposes without compromising the privacy of the insureds or jeopardizing the attorney-client privilege.

Joining with the insureds in the effort to prevent losses and to successfully defend non-meritorious claims by providing support for using claims files for the development of guidelines.

One of the results of the so-called first malpractice crisis[1] of 1973–1975 was the creation of alternative forms of liability insurance for hospitals and health care providers. Later in 1973 commercial insurance carriers began to realize that the malpractice claims they were seeing and settling were only a fraction of the total number of potential claims. Published information such as the *Report on the Medical Insurance Feasibility Study* indicated that current claims figures represented "but a small portion of the iatrogenic injuries or potentially compensable events that occurred each year."[2] Insurers accurately concluded that the potential increase in claims was not as predictable as they needed it to be, and their profits depend on the accuracy of predicted losses.

At the same time that this information about potential claims rates was becoming public, an economic recession was beginning that endangered the investments of the insurers. Insurance carriers reacted to these related circumstances that threatened their profitability by either withdrawing from the professional liability market altogether or charging unreasonably high premiums for the coverage they continued to write.

Hospitals and physicians faced with two equally untenable situations— no coverage or outrageous premiums for the coverage they could get— sought alternatives to the commercial insurance market. Hospitals and physician groups entered the insurance business. By the end of 1979, 21 percent of the nation's nonfederal, acute-care beds were insured by "captives" (a form of self-insurance), a 75 percent increase from 12 percent in 1977.[3]

Broadly speaking, the fundamental difference between commercial insurance and the so-called self-insurance programs is that in self-insurance the owners of the insurance programs are also the insured. Hence, insureds are paying premiums into a pool, out of which losses (settlements, judgments against insured defendants, and expenses) are paid. The insureds decide who will be in the pool and who will be responsible for managing it. Most important, though, is the fact that the insureds' money essentially remains theirs to use for paying losses, reducing premiums if losses are small. Whereas with commercial insurance insureds pay a premium set by the insurance carrier, and that premium is gone whether or not an individual caregiver or insured institution has losses within the period for which the premiums are paid. The insurer does not refund any unused portion of the premium; it uses those dollars to fund losses greater than the premium collected or for profit to distribute to stockholders.

When care providers and hospitals entered alternative insurance arrangements, such as captives, loss prevention efforts became more important.

A captive insurance company is most easily defined as a wholly owned subsidiary of a group of participating hospitals organized for the purpose of insuring their own risks.[4] When hospitals entered into such arrangements, they became much more aware of the need to reduce losses, because they were, to a greater extent, losing their own money when losses had to be paid. This arrangement as well as a concurrent realization on the part of commercial insurers who were still in the market taught that existing risk management programs in hospitals may not have been effective to prevent losses.

The end of the 1970s and the beginning of the 1980s saw more research being done in the area of loss prevention—one element of a risk management program. The American College of Surgeons and others began to look at the iatrogenic injuries (those caused by health care providers) as opposed to the more traditional sources of financial risk to institutions such as safety issues related to the physical plant, and to recommend internal systems to prevent and reduce the severity of such injuries.[5] In addition, those hospitals that became part of self-insured programs were forced to provide internal risk management services for three reasons: (1) to better safeguard their own money by trying to prevent losses before they occurred (loss prevention); (2) to reduce the cost of claims once they were filed (loss control); and (3) to replace those risk management services that may have been provided by their previous commercial insurance company.

Concurrently with those changes, legislatures and accrediting bodies began to impose risk management requirements for hospitals and physicians. In the middle of the 1980s the Joint Commission on Accreditation of Healthcare Organizations (JCAHO) developed and released its Risk Management Standards.[6] Some states quickly followed by passing legislation that essentially mirrored those standards.[7] The Patient Care Assessment Regulations of the Board of Registration in Medicine in Massachusetts are an example of a state's attempt to legislate the structure of risk management programs in hospitals and other health care organizations such as clinics, HMOs, and nursing homes.[8]

Institutions and caregivers must operate within existing rules and regulations, such as those listed above, that have been established as a framework for the risk management function, since deviation from those standards could increase liability. Consequently insurers must assist their clients by helping them to develop ways to comply with those rules within the context of their daily practices. They help monitor changes in regulation and legislation, and communicate those changes to insureds in a timely manner.

In addition to new regulations, new treatment modalities are being developed at an alarming rate, especially in tertiary care and teaching facilities that routinely include major research components. Both loss prevention and claims management services must respond to claims that involve new procedures and treatment decisions. Loss prevention must incorporate the issues involved in such claims into educational material to share with insureds in an attempt to prevent potential liability situations with similar circumstances. Effective claims management techniques include retaining the best experts who have knowledge of the effectiveness of similar procedures and can help build a defense based more on hard science than on customary (and perhaps outdated) practice.

New health care delivery systems that are rapidly becoming the norm create other opportunities for insurers to provide specialized service to clients. At present, managed care systems engender special types of concern for potential and actual liability for both institutions and caregivers. Loss prevention services can be prepared to educate caregivers about realistic liabilities, sorting out the sensationalized coverage in the press from the actual circumstances of care that could lead to potential liability.

Changes in delivery systems have also been blamed for deterioration of the patient-physician relationship. While issues of health insurance coverage inevitably intrude into the partnership between the cared-for and the caregiver today, the relationship has always been a potentially difficult one. This is especially so when an adverse event occurs, preventable or otherwise. Loss prevention efforts that provide practice in communicating with patients in difficult circumstances, such as after an adverse event or interpersonal friction, can prove useful to caregivers when they are confronted with such circumstances in their daily encounters with patients.[9] In addition, education about the need for boundary setting and boundary maintenance with patients can help providers understand how misperceptions on the part of the patient can turn therapeutic encounters into potential liability situations. Suggesting appointments outside the normal business hours of the practice or in settings usually associated with social interaction in order to accommodate schedules of busy patients may be misconstrued. Any exchange of gifts between provider and patient, or any other action that seems to take advantage of the more powerful position of the physician in the therapeutic relationship, may lead to misperceptions, anger, and potential liability for the physician.

The insurer can best help the provider preserve and enhance relationships with patients if the focus of the insurer's loss prevention efforts remains squarely on helping the caregiver to provide better patient care rather than to be able to defend him/herself in court. While "good patient care is good risk management" is a cliché, building trust between provider and patient can be an effective deterrent to malpractice claims. A provider who maintains a defensive stance and views every patient as a potential plaintiff cannot hope to build the mutually trusting relationships with patients that are the core of effective claims prevention. The insurer has to reassure providers that coverage exists for good patient care, and that the insurer will back them to the extent possible if a claim is brought in spite of good-quality care.

One of the most valuable services insurers can render to their clients is to share malpractice claims information with them in an organized and meaningful way. Several advantages of using malpractice claims information should be emphasized:

In-depth study of individual cases can point to clinical and systems errors that may be preventable.

Analysis of aggregate data can suggest areas for further inquiry; for example, departments, specialties, institutions, or those claims with like allegations (such as failure to diagnose) can be targeted for further study.

Indemnity losses and expenses (for meritorious claims) may provide a measure of the "cost of poor quality."

While such data may be perceived as negative, causing defensive stances from caregivers, they capture attention and can stimulate discussion and interest in further inquiry.

The data frequently suggest some solutions—both long-term and short-term.[10]

While the sharing of malpractice claims data is one of the most important services that an insurer can render to insureds, certain disadvantages must be kept in mind:

Malpractice claims are the tip of the iceberg of medical injury. According to the Harvard Medical Practice Study, negligent adverse events in hospital patients occurred at a rate of 7.6 times that of actual claims—conclusions similar to those of a similar study done a decade earlier.[11]

Claims are often filed in the absence of negligence. Close to one-half of claims filed in the CRICO system are closed without any indemnity payment.[12]

The number of claims filed is small compared to actual patient encounters, making aggregation and comparison difficult.

Statistical analyses of claims often lack meaningful denominators, information that would, for example, indicate the total number of patient encounters out of which these claims have occurred. Knowing the percentage of claims for a specific number of physician-patient encounters would give the claims figures some perspective.

Claims data, fostered by the legal system, exemplifies the "bad apple" approach. Singling out individual caregivers for blame is not particularly useful for improving the quality of patient care, or for maintaining the dialogue with caregivers that is essential if the quality of patient care can be improved.

Analyses of closed claims are always retrospective.

Confidentiality of information and sensitivity to caregivers involved dictate that closed claims be used in the individual case studies prepared from claims; therefore, the material may be at least three and as much as ten or more years old.[13]

Even with the disadvantages noted, claims data are valuable in liability prevention and quality improvement efforts. In 1991 a RAND study of one malpractice insurer's claims set out to identify potentially preventable sources of medical injury in four specialties: obstetrics-gynecology, general surgery, anesthesiology, and radiology. One of the conclusions in articles reporting on the study was that claims data are useful for determining types of mistakes made in patient care, and for suggesting changes to be made.[14]

Aggregate data can be used to identify areas of preventable medical injury that could be targeted for improvement, and to provide a rationale for setting priorities. Individual case studies taken from malpractice insurers' closed claims files, which include the wealth of information gathered to fill insurance and legal needs, can be effective educational and analytic tools for implementing individual behavioral and systems changes. Case-method teaching and learning is familiar and engaging for physicians and other clinical staff. The presentation of carefully chosen information on malpractice claims nearly always guarantees a lively discussion. More important, if a particular scenario rings true with a group, immediate change in behavior or practice may result.

While the advantages of using actual care scenarios to alert providers to potential liability situations and loss prevention techniques that could prevent future similar claims (or render them more easily defensible) have never been verified with scientific study, such a link makes intuitive sense. The information can be shared with providers in a variety of ways, tailored to their needs and circumstances, such as: (1) having insurance company personnel present a detailed case and the providers respond to the issues in the case; (2) presenting several short scenarios from claims that all illustrate one issue (such as resident supervision or documentation problems); and (3) presenting cases in written or audio format for their own self-study.

The most effective way to get the claims information to the providers is for providers themselves to use information from closed claims with their colleagues. Insurers can take the lead in helping physicians and other providers have access to the information to present to colleagues, whether in conjunction with insurance company personnel or not. For instance, insurance personnel can help providers choose cases to present using simple guidelines like these:

Clinical facts must survive simplification. To be useful for discussion, claims abstracts must be short; therefore, clinical facts must be kept to a minimum necessary for participants to understand the case. However, enough pertinent information should be included so that participants do not feel that relevant facts were left out to trick them.

Loss prevention issues must logically follow from the case facts. What went wrong and what could have been done differently to avoid a claim should be clear.

Facts described should reflect current medical practice, be clinically correct, and make sense in this shortened version of the case. Outdated medicine or an unclear or confusing chronology of facts will lessen the credibility of the case, even if the loss prevention lessons are good.

Claims information that may cause embarrassment to certain participants must be avoided. Even though closed claims are used, the facts of a particularly emotional or well-publicized case may be recognizable. A less politically sensitive case that illustrates similar loss prevention lessons must be selected. If no single case on a particularly relevant issue is suitable to use, a composite of several similar claims can be created to illustrate the lessons to be covered. A case from another state that illustrates similar issues can be substituted, with a reminder to the physician-participants that similar cases have happened locally.

Claims in which the defendant prevailed can be used as well as those in which the caregivers or the institution were found negligent. Claims with verdicts in favor of the defendants can illustrate both what was done correctly that may have contributed to the favorable result and any issues that could have been a problem but that did not result in liability.[15]

Insurers can provide significant service to insureds by using individual claims as case studies, and by allowing groups of physicians access to closed claims files to extract preventable issues in an effort to create guidelines and standards based on actual liability situations. An example of this type of collaboration occurred in the early 1980s, when a group of anesthesiologists organized an effort to study malpractice claims to ascertain which incidents that led to claims were preventable. This effort was based on pioneering efforts by Dr. Jeffrey Cooper and colleagues at the Massachusetts General Hospital, who began rudimentary measurements of the quality of anesthetic care that involved the study of critical incidents in four Boston hospitals with identification of causes and outcomes.[16]

Armed with the Cooper studies, the chiefs of anesthesia at the nine Harvard teaching hospitals appointed a faculty committee chaired by Dr. John Eichhorn. This Risk Management Committee was charged to examine all insurance claims and major incidents on file with its malpractice insurance carrier for the period 1976–1984. The committee reported that "the majority of those incidents associated with major morbidity and mortality were preventable and, further, that appropriate monitoring should have been an important component in the management." The data from the claims led the physicians involved to believe that appropriate patient monitoring would prevent similar incidents in the future. To this end, the Harvard chiefs agreed to write and distribute to their departments a set of minimum monitoring standards.[17] Since their implementation, the number of anesthesia-related incidents has dropped. Insurers responded to this decrease in losses by lowering malpractice premiums for anesthesiologists.[18]

Two examples with more direct relevance to mental health practitioners are important to describe. In 1991 Harvard Risk Management Foundation formed the Suicide Risk Advisory Group (SRAG), a committee composed of psychiatrist representatives from the Harvard teaching hospitals. The impetus for the formation of the group came from a study of CRICO claims that revealed that lawsuits arising from patient suicides account for the largest single category of suits and the largest dollar amounts in settlements against psychiatrists.[19]

In an effort to better understand the care issues involved in suicide-related claims, the SRAG undertook a chart review of eleven such claims filed since 1985. This study, more descriptive than quantitative because of the small sample size, was undertaken to identify similar themes and pertinent loss prevention issues. For example, the review showed that the majority of physicians named as defendants in the claims sample were not psychiatrists, suggesting that physicians who have less familiarity with the management of suicidal patients may be at more risk for an adverse outcome.[20] The SRAG went on to develop guidelines for the identification and assessment of the suicidal patient in an effort to aid psychiatrists and others in the difficult task of determining the suicidality of a patient under their care.[21]

The second example addresses the reality that psychiatric patients often receive health care services concurrently from more than one provider. When these services are not coordinated, effective treatment may be compromised and liability may result. Many psychiatrists have expressed concerns about the ethical and practical clinical issues that arise when psychiatrists collaborate with other caregivers, but the ways in which care might be coordinated have not been formally addressed.[22]

A task force of Harvard Risk Management Foundation has considered these issues and developed guidelines for prescribing psychiatrists working with other caregivers. These guidelines offer a structure for approaching consultative, collaborative, and supervisory relationships.[23]

These efforts represent examples of the insurers' role—and responsibility—to convene the clinical expertise available to them and to provide the structure, support, and encouragement for those experts to create and disseminate working documents that may address some of the most common potential liability situations in their specialty.

While anecdotal evidence and common sense support the need for educational approaches to loss prevention, scientific evidence of the effectiveness of risk management programs has been scant, whether such programs are initiated by institutionally based risk managers or insurers acting in a consulting role. One study, though limited in scope, does give evidence that some of the basic assumptions of risk management do in fact hold true.[24] Published in 1991, the study correlates risk management activity at forty Maryland hospitals with the hospitals' claims experience, involving incidents that occurred in 1980 and 1981 and were resolved by 1987. In this study hospitals appear to have had fewer and less severe claims if they (1) educated physicians and nurses about their role in risk management; (2) had a policy of informing the clinical chief of staff when an adverse event occurred in his or her department; and (3) maintained a hospital board commitment for overseeing risk management and provided the board with regular reports on risk management activities.

This study is the first significant attempt to demonstrate the efficacy of some risk management strategies. The data show that hospitals involving clinicians in risk management seemed to have fewer claims than those that did not. The study also shows that educational programs on risk management and quality assurance issues correlate positively with lower claims figures.

Even with its acknowledged limitations, the study should encourage insurers to offer their own data from claims files to provide educational services to clients, with some evidence that the effort may help reduce the frequency and severity of claims. Case studies from closed claim files, aggregated and specific claim information for the chiefs of clinical departments to use, and claims data to report to the hospital governing body can all be provided by the insurer. The study mentioned all these uses for data as important elements in loss prevention.

While many insurers, as a matter of good business practice if not actual survival, will continue to provide such services to insured health care providers, it is important that the providers themselves help define what services they would find useful. Physicians and other health care professionals need to be willing to join with insurers in research projects, such as those that result in guidelines or standards. They need to be willing to use closed-claim statistics and summaries to help teach their colleagues about loss prevention.

Health care providers must also be actively involved in claims management by making themselves available to serve as expert witnesses for colleagues, and to review files and give opinions on cases for claims adjusters. They must invite the insurer to be involved, financially or otherwise, in research projects that may prevent claims and improve the quality of patient care. Insurers need to provide services; and insured physicians and institutions can help them to provide the services that are most needed.

Notes

1. J. E. Orlikoff and A. M. Vanagunas, *Malpractice Prevention and Liability Control for Hospitals.* 2nd ed. (Chicago: American Hospital Association, 1988).
2. California Medical Association, *Report on the Medical Insurance Feasibility Study* (San Francisco: CMA, 1977).
3. Orlikoff and Vanagunas, *Malpractice Prevention,* p. 27.
4. W. R. Kucera and N. Ator, "Risk Management: Five Alternatives to Commercial Insurance," *Hospital Financial Management* 32 (1978): 10.
5. American College of Surgeons, *Who Is Responsible for Patient Safety in Your Hospital?* Report of a pilot project by the ACS in consultation with the Maryland Education Institute (Chicago: ACS, 1978). Idem, in consultation with the Maryland Education Institute, *Patient Safety Manual: a Guide for Establishing a Patient Safety System in Your Hospital* (Chicago: ACS, 1979).
6. Joint Commission on Accreditation of Healthcare Organizations, *Risk Management Strategies* (Chicago: JCAHO, 1991).
7. U.S. General Accounting Office, *Health Care: Initiatives in Hospital Risk Management,* GAO/HRD-89-79 (Washington, July 1989).
8. 243 Code of Massachusetts Regulations (CMR) sec. 3.00.
9. J. Lindheim, "Role Playing Difficult Patients and Situations: A Workshop for

Physicians," *RMF Forum* 15, no. 3 (1994): 10–11. The Risk Management Foundation of the Harvard Medical Institutions (RMF), which is now known as Harvard Risk Management Foundation (HRM), was incorporated in 1979 as a charitable, medical, and educational organization. The Harvard medical institutions that are shareholders in the Controlled Risk Insurance Company (CRICO) have designated RMF to be their agent for the purpose of handling all claims matters. RMF also provides technical assistance in risk management, educational programs and publications, quality assessment, underwriting, and related research to the Harvard medical system.

10. P. S. Dasse, "Identifying Opportunities for Improvement: The Role of Malpractice Claims Data," *RMF Forum* 13, no. 4 (1992): 1.

11. L. L. Leape, A. G. Lawthers, T. A. Brennan, and W. G. Johnson, "Preventing Medical Injuries," *Quality Review Bulletin* 8 (1993): 144–149.

12. CRICO, owned by the Harvard-affiliated hospitals, was founded as an offshore captive in the Cayman Islands in 1976 to provide professional liability insurance coverage for the hospitals, their employees, and eligible physicians. In 1995 CRICO of Vermont (a risk-retention group) was established to take over the provision of professional liability insurance to the Harvard institutions, employees, and physicians. The company currently insures about 7,400 physicians.

13. Dasse, "Identifying Opportunities for Improvement," p. 2.

14. R. Kravitz, "Malpractice Claims Data as a Tool for Risk Management and Quality Improvement," *RMF Forum* 13, no. 4 (1992): 6–7.

15. P. B. Martin and M. Waterman, "Advice for Using Closed Malpractice Claims as Teaching Tools," *RMF Forum* 15, no. 3 (1994): 1–3.

16. R. J. Kitz, "Standards for Monitoring and Machines: Advantages," in J. S. Gravenstein and J. F. Holzer, eds., *Safety and Cost Containment in Anesthesia* (Boston: Butterworths, 1988).

17. J. H. Eichhorn et al., "Standards for Patient Monitoring during Anesthesia at Harvard Medical School," *JAMA* 256 (1986): 1017–20.

18. Studies are now under way to compare pre-standard claims with post-standard experience. Analysis of that data will be used to formulate loss prevention strategies which will be shared with anesthesiologists throughout the system. The information will also be shared nationally through the Anesthesia Patient Safety Foundation. "Anesthesia-related Professional Liability Claims," prepared by S. Trombly, RMF 1996, manuscript.

19. J. T. Maltsberger, "Commentary: Expanding Liability for Suicide," *RMF Forum* 14, no. 6 (1993): 1–2.

20. J. M. Ellison, "Risk Management Issues and Recommendations in the Care of Suicidal Patients," *RMF Forum* 14, no. 6 (1993): 3–4.

21. "Draft Guidelines for the Identification and Assessment of Suicidality," *RMF Forum* 14, no. 6 (1993): 14–19.

22. J. M. Ellison and L. I. Sederer, "Coordinating Multiple Providers of Mental Health Treatment," *RMF Forum* 17, no. 4 (1996): 10.

23. "Guidelines for Prescribing Psychiatrists in Consultative, Collaborative, or Supervisory Relationships," prepared by RMF Task Force on Psychiatrists in Clinical Practice Relationships with Other Clinicians, and C. Keyes, manuscript, RMF, 1996.
24. L. L. Morlock and F. E. Malitz, "Do Hospital Risk Management Programs Make a Difference?: Relationships between Risk Management Activities and Hospital Malpractice Claims Experience," *Law and Contemporary Problems* 54, no. 2 (Spring 1991): 21.

7

What Your Licensing Board Expects of You

Richard Waring, J.D.

Despite the fact that the federal government regulates and finances medical practice in the United States in an extensive way, the licensing and disciplining of physicians is exclusively a function of state government. All fifty states have established boards which perform the licensing and disciplinary functions, and board members are usually physicians.

Selection processes for board members vary from state to state. The members may, for example, be appointed by the governor, either at the governor's discretion or from a list submitted by the state medical society. In recent years some states have set aside one or more seats on the board for members of the public who are not physicians. It is thought that these nonphysicians will be less inclined to be protective of physicians appearing before the board than fellow physician members would be.

As Paul Starr notes in *The Social Transformation of American Medicine,*[1] state regulation of physicians has had a somewhat uneven history. Medical practice acts (the generic name for legislation which creates and empowers medical boards) were passed and then repealed by several state agencies in the early nineteenth century. Later in that century, state medical licensing boards were permanently established. In Massachusetts the Board of Registration in Medicine was created by legislation enacted in 1894.

At about the same time, the United States Supreme Court affirmed the states' authority to license and regulate physicians practicing within their borders. In *Hawker v. New York*[2] (1898), the Supreme Court upheld a New York State law prohibiting anyone who had been convicted of a felony from continuing the practice of medicine. The court said, "Character is as important a qualification as knowledge, and if the legislature may properly require a definite course of instruction, or a certain examination as to learning, it may with equal propriety prescribe what evidence of good character shall be furnished" (p. 194). The *Hawker* case is significant today in two respects. First, it upholds the states' authority to require a certain base of knowledge and technical competence for physicians in order to obtain a medical license. Second, it permits states to consider evidence of a physician's good moral character (or lack of it) in making licensing or disciplinary decisions. State boards may vary tremendously in how aggressively they use their powers to regulate the profession, but there is no doubt about the extensiveness of their authority. The *Hawker* case is still good law.

Perhaps because the United States is a highly mobile nation, where people frequently move from state to state, state medical boards have found it helpful to work together. To enhance their ability to work cooperatively, state medical boards in 1912 formed a private organization called the Federation of State Medical Boards, which serves as a central clearinghouse of information. Now located in Euless, Texas, a Dallas–Fort Worth suburb, the federation maintains files on physicians who have been disciplined by any state's medical board and also publishes a regular journal and a newsletter. The federation holds periodic meetings with representatives of member boards and may also form working groups to deal with specific issues.

The Licensing Function

The primary task of each state's medical board is granting licenses to physicians. States now grant both full licenses and limited licenses which allow a physician to practice under supervision during an internship or residency program. For many years, most physicians have obtained their medical licenses by obtaining the M.D. degree and passing the National Board examination. The National Board examination consists of two written tests given during medical school, parts I and II, and part III, a test of clinical competency. The National Board certificate, enabling a physician to be licensed, is not awarded until after successful completion of one year of training in an internship or residency. Obtaining the National Board certificate is a vitally important step in a physician's career, because many state boards will honor a National Board certificate forever, thereby enabling the physician to obtain a medical license in a new state many years after finishing medical school, without taking another examination. Some states may require more than one year of post-graduate training before granting the physician a full license. In addition to the National Board examination, there has been a second licensing examination, the Federation Licensing Examination (FLEX), for medical graduates who completed medical school in a foreign country where the National Board examination is not given. Graduates of American schools who for some reason did not take or pass the National Boards have also taken this examination.

While the National Board examination and FLEX have coexisted for many years as parallel routes to licensure, in 1990 the Federation of State Medical Boards and the National Board of Medical Examiners (NBME) agreed to establish a single, uniform examination that would be taken by all graduates. The new examination replaces the National Board exam and FLEX and is called the United States Medical Licensing Examination (USMLE). It is similar in content to the National Board and the FLEX. Any person concerned about how to comply with the new licensing examination program would be well advised to contact the appropriate state medical board's licensing section.

In addition to licensing recent medical school graduates, state boards are called upon to license individuals who have been out of school for many years and are now moving into a new state. Although many states will honor a National Board certificate forever, some will not and administer what is called the Special Purpose Examination (SPEX), a one-day multiple choice examination devised by the Federation of State Medical Boards.

While medical boards universally require a physician to have passed some sort of examination to obtain a license, boards are also concerned about the quality and quantity of medical education the candidate has received. Although graduates of medical schools located in the United States or Canada are licensed with minimal scrutiny of their schools' curricula, graduates of schools elsewhere must often establish exactly what courses they took in medical school, how often the courses met, and the extent of any clinical clerkships. Merely acquiring enough knowledge to pass a licensing examination does not satisfy medical boards. In fact, the Massachusetts Board of Registration in Medicine revoked the license of a physician in 1988 after it learned that his medical school program did not meet the statutory minimum of four academic years of at least thirty-two weeks each. The physician had been licensed in several states and was practicing in Texas when the Massachusetts board learned of the flaw in his education and commenced disciplinary action against him. Some states have Fifth Pathway programs to enable international medical graduates who may be unable to qualify otherwise to obtain licensure. The Fifth Pathway is essentially a fifth year of medical school in an American school. Information about Fifth Pathway programs may be obtained from the appropriate state's medical board.

Occasionally a state medical board will discover an outright impostor, who has no medical degree but has come up with a forged diploma and has passed the licensing examination. In 1987 the Massachusetts board was advised by a medical school in the Dominican Republic that a Massachusetts physician was using a forged diploma and had not graduated from medical school at all. The physician, a woman with two young children, had a background as a medical technician and had become board-certified in pediatrics at the time the Massachusetts board learned about her. She had become licensed in Connecticut and Massachusetts by passing the FLEX examination. When confronted by the Massachusetts board, the woman expressed surprise that her credentials would be questioned, but ended up stipulating that she did not possess the qualifications required by statute to be licensed as a physician in Massachusetts. Soon after learning about this physician, the Massachusetts board's staff discovered that her former husband was also licensed as a physician in Massachusetts (under a different surname) and was also using a diploma from the Dominican Republic school. Upon contacting the school, the board's staff was told that the husband's diploma, too, was forged. The board commenced disciplinary action against the former husband also, but he never appeared for a hearing and offered no explanation of the situation at all to the board. The board revoked his license. While impostors are rare, medical boards are understandably vigilant when reviewing candidates' credentials.

Once issued, medical licenses are not permanent in any state. Physicians must renew their licenses periodically. Some states also require physicians to obtain a certain number of hours of continuing education as a prerequisite to renewing the license. States may also require physicians to complete a renewal questionnaire covering such topics as malpractice claims, loss or limitation of hospital privileges, health statutes, and involvement as a defendant in a criminal case. The Massachusetts board requires physicians to certify that they have complied with all state tax laws as a prerequisite to renewing the medical license. This requirement is based on a Massachusetts statute that requires all licensed professionals (except attorneys) to comply with state tax laws as a condition of renewing their license.

Occasionally physicians who move from one state to another allow the medical license in the state they leave to expire. A physician who desires to reactivate an expired license should check with the appropriate board office to find out exactly what the reactivation process entails. Some states require extremely thorough documentation of the professional history of a physician who is seeking to reactivate an expired license. Boards are often concerned that physicians who relocate frequently, or late in their career, are trying to get away from professional difficulty. This is so because in some states, allowing a license to expire terminates the authority of the state board to pursue disciplinary action against the physician.

Some states maintain separate licensing boards for osteopathic physicians, whose professional degree is the doctor of osteopathy (D.O.). In states that do not have separate boards, one board licenses both M.D.'s and D.O.'s. A few states have separate boards for homeopathic physicians, as well. Some states have separate licensing and disciplinary boards.

The Disciplinary Function

In addition to licensing physicians, state medical boards maintain standards of practice which they expect physicians to follow. If a physician is found to have committed a serious violation of practice standards, boards have the authority to impose discipline, which may range from a verbal sanction, such as a reprimand, to revocation of the license. Boards may also take informal action against the physician, such as issuing a letter of warning. State medical practice acts usually contain a list of prohibited behavior. In Massachusetts, General Laws, ch. 112, sec. 5 lists the following grounds for disciplinary action: substance abuse, criminal conduct, fraud, malpractice, gross misconduct in the practice of medicine, mental illness, and assisting the unlicensed practice of medicine. (Those descriptions are not direct quotations of the statute.) Boards may also promulgate regulations and practice standards. Physicians practicing in Massachusetts are required to carry malpractice insurance of at least $100,000, pursuant to 243 CMR 2.07 (16), unless they practice solely in a government facility. Massachusetts physicians may interpret mammograms only if they meet specific training, continuing education, and experience criteria set out in 243 CMR 2.07 (24). In addition to statutory and regulatory grounds for discipline, some states have adopted standards set by professional organizations, such as the American Psychiatric Association, or have issued specific practice guidelines of their own.

Two areas have emerged as particular concerns of state medical boards in recent years: sexual exploitation of patients, and substance abuse by physicians. Alleged sexual abuse by physicians has become so prominent a concern that the American Psychiatric Association has issued highly specific ethical standards of conduct. Sexual activity involving a psychiatrist and an active patient is ethically prohibited, and so is sexual activity involving a psychiatrist and a former patient, no matter how much time has passed since the termination of the professional relationship. While there is no way of knowing how prevalent sexual exploitation truly is, the issue has been prominent in recent years.

A sensational case arose in Massachusetts in 1992. It was alleged that a female psychiatrist, Margaret Bean-Bayog, M.D., had engaged in sexual relations with a young Harvard medical student, who later committed suicide ten months after leaving Dr. Bean-Bayog's care. Exactly what transpired between Dr. Bean-Bayog and the student, Paul Lozano, was never proven in any tribunal. Mr. Lozano's family settled a civil malpractice action against Dr. Bean-Bayog for one million dollars. The doctor resigned her Massachusetts medical license rather than go through a hearing on charges the Massachusetts Board of Registration in Medicine had brought against her. The Massachusetts board's charges against Dr. Bean-Bayog did not include the allegations of sexual exploitation, because the chief witness against her, Mr. Lozano, was deceased. The allegation against Dr. Bean-Bayog in the board's proceeding centered on the quality of care she provided, not on sexual exploitation.

The Bean-Bayog case did serve as a catalyst. It led the Massachusetts board to convene a working group which drafted a set of guidelines to assist psychiatrists in maintaining proper boundaries in their treatment of adult patients. The document, entitled *General Guidelines Related to the Maintenance of Proper Boundaries in the Practice of Psychotherapy by Physicians (Adult Patients),* was issued in 1994. Developed with the Massachusetts Psychiatric Society, the Boston Psychoanalytic Institute, and the Massachusetts Medical Society, the guidelines are intended to apply to all physicians who provide psychotherapy, not just psychiatrists.

The guidelines are quite specific and are worth discussing at some length. While they are not binding on any physician practicing outside Massachusetts (and are only guidelines, not hard-and-fast rules, within Massachusetts), consideration of the issues raised by the guidelines should prove useful to physicians practicing psychotherapy anywhere. Departure from the guidelines, in appropriate circumstances, is not necessarily deviant.

The guidelines begin by stating that appropriate professional boundaries should commence early in therapy. Setting boundaries is the responsibility of the physician, not the patient. Maintaining the boundaries requires ongoing attention. Crossing of the boundaries should cause the physician to think about whether corrective action is required.

The guidelines specify that a physician practicing psychotherapy should see patients at the scheduled time, in the allotted period of time, and in the setting appropriate to psychotherapy. In general, the guidelines say treatment should occur during the physician's normal working hours and in an office setting. Home offices are not disfavored, as long as the office area is separate from the general living quarters. The guidelines recognize that certain situations do not allow for office treatment. Such situations might include visits to homebound patients, visits to patients confined to a hospital, or emergencies.

Billing practices are covered by the guidelines. They specify that fees, along with arrangements for missed sessions, canceled sessions, and telephone calls, should be worked out early in treatment. The parties need to agree on how insurance coverage will be handled. In particular, bills for psychiatric services should be accurate and should not be altered in an attempt to obtain insurance coverage that might otherwise be unavailable. In cases where there is small annual psychiatric benefit provided in a medical insurance policy, physicians have submitted bills in the names of family members who never saw the physician in an attempt to apply the other family members' coverage to pay for the patient's care. The guidelines also note that there is a long tradition of reducing or forgiving outstanding bills to assist patients who would otherwise be unable to afford care. Barter arrangements are viewed as problematic.

In addition to the economic relationship involved in billing patients, the guidelines discuss other financial relationships between physician and patients. For example, the guidelines state that physicians should avoid selling objects or services other than professional services to the patient. In one case, a psychiatrist sold two boats to a patient. The guidelines state that physicians should also avoid either employing or being employed by the patient and entering joint business ventures with the patient. The guidelines do note that certain economic relationships may be impossible to avoid. For example, a patient may own the only automobile repair shop within a reasonable distance. In that situation the physician is not expected to forgo the repair service, but is warned to be sure that using the repair service is not exploitative, confusing, or harmful to the therapy. The guidelines do not say what should be done if using the repair service would be exploitative, confusing, or harmful to the therapy. Other relationships are viewed as too remote to be of general concern, such as when a patient owns stock in a department store where the physician shops.

The guidelines note that physical contact between physicians and patients should be carefully limited. While such contact is appropriate for the purposes of conducting a physical examination and providing medical treatment, contact outside those parameters should generally be limited to a handshake at the start or end of a session, when this appears appropriate, and a comforting pat of reassurance on the hand or shoulder when the patient appears distressed. Beyond such limited circumstances, physical contact may be perceived as flirtatious or sexual and should be avoided. Outright sexual behavior or flirting is, of course, not permitted. The guidelines do recognize that some behavioral therapies may appropriately involve other forms of non-intimate physical contact in a public setting.

Self-disclosure, that is, physicians' revealing personal details of their own lives to patients, should be minimized, the guidelines say. Some self-disclosure is not only appropriate, however, but also necessary. An example would be a physician disclosing details of his or her own training or qualifications when a patient is deciding whether to enter therapy with him or her. In addition, in substance abuse treatment, the guidelines state, psychotherapists commonly disclose something about their own histories of substance abuse, if any. Finally, there may be other situations where, after careful thought, a psychotherapist may appropriately decide that some self-disclosure is in the patient's interest. It needs to be clear that the self-disclosure in these situations serves the needs of the patient and not those of the therapist. In particular, the guidelines state, physicians practicing psychotherapy should never discuss their own emotional problems or details of their own sexual lives.

The giving and receiving of gifts is another area covered by the guidelines. In general, the guidelines say that it is not inappropriate for physicians to accept gifts of minimal value from psychotherapy patients. Physicians should not accept gifts of substantial value or of a sexual or intimate nature, however.

Despite the cautions the guidelines contain with respect to gifts, they do state that there are occasions when it may be appropriate for a physician to make a gift to a psychotherapy patient. Small gifts may be helpful in establishing a therapeutic relationship with adolescent patients or with severely regressed adults, according to the guidelines. Moreover, gifts of small value may be appropriate to mark major events in a patient's life, such as the birth of a child. Gifts should never be extremely valuable, nor should they be of a sexual or other intimate nature.

Sometimes, particularly in small communities, social relationships outside the therapy may be impossible to avoid. This may be so in a small town or where the psychotherapist and the patient have a child in the same school. Even in these situations the physician needs to be careful to respect the patient's privacy and dignity. Such settings should not be used to encourage a personal relationship with the psychotherapy patient. In such close situations, a physician practicing psychotherapy should avoid having meals, sharing transportation, or attending social events where the patient might be present when the therapy might be compromised or when the patient might conclude that the physician has formed a romantic or sexual interest.

Not surprisingly, the guidelines also recognize that the therapist must avoid personal relationships with family members of the patient during therapy. A patient would naturally wonder what portions of the therapy were discussed with the family member.

A second major area of concern for medical licensing boards is substance abuse by physicians. For the period 1990–1993, 31 percent of the formal disciplinary actions taken by the Massachusetts board were in cases involving substance abuse. The substance abuse is most often alcohol or prescription (not usually street) drugs. Obviously, physicians can obtain access to prescription medication much more easily than the layperson can. This may account for the high proportion of drug abuse in disciplinary cases. The problem is widespread enough that a number of treatment facilities specializing in physicians have been established around the United States. A physician needing information about these centers can obtain it through the local state medical society. The amount of substance abuse by physicians is not necessarily higher than it is among the population in general.

While different state boards may have different procedures in place for dealing with substance abuse by physicians, the goal of all such programs is clear: to assist physicians to recover from their dependence and return to work in a way that eliminates any risk to the public. This can be done with ongoing treatment and monitoring of the physician. The Massachusetts Medical Society has an extensive program run by its affiliate entity Physician Health Services (PHS). Working closely with the Massachusetts Medical Board, PHS provides support and monitoring, and, when a physician is found to have relapsed, PHS reports to the medical board for whatever action is necessary. The board does sometimes find it necessary to suspend the license of a relapsing physician until the physician's recovery is again progressing. Substance abuse and relapses do not necessarily mean the end of a physician's career. In one Massachusetts case, a young physician relapsed several times before making what appears to be a successful recovery and progressing toward a return to practice in another state. The medical board in this new physician's new home state is aware of her problem.

Medical boards learn of physicians with substance abuse problems through various means. A Massachusetts statute, G.L.c. 112, sec. 5F, requires physicians to report colleagues whom they suspect may be impaired. Thus, a hospital chief of service may report a staff member who appears at the hospital while intoxicated. PHS reports physicians it is monitoring if it finds a positive screen for alcohol or for drugs the physicians are not being prescribed. Sometimes board staff members read in the newspaper about physicians being arrested for alcohol or drug offenses, and obtain further information from law enforcement authorities. Physicians sometimes report themselves to the state medical board, perhaps anticipating that the board will find out about their situation anyway.

In addition to abusing controlled substances, physicians sometimes run afoul of state and federal drug distribution laws, or violate prohibitions against prescribing certain classes of drugs to family members. The United States Drug Enforcement Administration (DEA) has promulgated very detailed regulations specifying how physicians should handle and keep track of controlled substances they use in their practices. The DEA requires physicians who possess controlled substances in their offices to keep records of their ordering and dispensing and to take inventory every two years. DEA investigators can and do visit physicians' offices from time to time and ask to see the drug record, particularly the inventory. If a physician has failed to keep the records, the DEA may take disciplinary action and then report the physician to the local medical board for further proceedings. Physicians who practice in relatively informal settings, such as a home office, may inadvertently overlook these DEA requirements. The DEA does survey local pharmacies and wholesale drug suppliers to find out which physicians have been ordering significant amounts of drugs and then visit those physicians to find out if the proper records are being kept. In Massachusetts, and perhaps other states, the DEA regulations have been incorporated into the board's own regulations by statute, so a physician who violates DEA regulations also violates the board's regulations.

A number of states, including Massachusetts, restrict physicians' ability to prescribe certain classes of drugs to family members. In Massachusetts physicians may not prescribe schedule II drugs to their family members or schedule II, III, or IV drugs to themselves. Examples of drugs in these schedules are Percocet, a schedule II; Fiorinal, a schedule III; and Valium, a schedule IV. It is thought that physicians' objectivity may be in question when they are prescribing for themselves or for family members. Other states have similar restrictions. On occasion, a well-meaning physician will obtain prescription drugs for family members through a wholesaler, at a lower price than a retail pharmacy would charge. If those drugs are in schedule II in the case of a family member, or in schedule II, III, or IV in the case of the physician, the physician has violated the prescribing restriction. In addition, the physician is not supposed to dispense drugs to a patient in more than a minimal amount, enough to treat the patient until the patient can have a prescription filled at a pharmacy.

States may also have their own restrictions on prescribing certain types of drugs. Until recently, Massachusetts prohibited physicians from prescribing anorectic drugs for weight-loss purposes. The Massachusetts board has now modified this restriction. Such restrictions may vary substantially from state to state, and over time, so a physician in doubt about the propriety of prescribing a certain drug for a certain purpose should check with the local medical board.

There is another highly specific situation in which a physician may act improperly. Some medical insurance policies contain low limits on the amount of care the policy will cover for a subscriber in one year. The limit may be as low as $500. Psychiatrists trying to assist a family in such a situation may bill the insurer for the first $500 of the patient's treatment and then submit a bill in the name of other family members up to the $500 limit for each of them, even if the psychiatrist has never met or treated them. The psychiatrist may believe this procedure helps the family by allowing it to obtain psychiatric care which would otherwise be financially burdensome, but billing for services rendered to family members the psychiatrist has never treated is fraudulent. In addition to being fraud on the insurer, such billing may also create a false record of psychiatric care of the nonpatient family member in the insurer's database. These inaccurate records may create problems in later years for the nonpatient family member, who may be called upon to explain the record of psychiatric treatment.

In 1996 a Massachusetts psychiatrist was convicted of 136 counts of mail fraud, witness tampering, and obstruction of justice in connection with a fraudulent billing scheme in which he billed insurers for psychiatric sessions which never took place, including times when he was out of the country on vacation. His sentence included forty-six months in federal prison and an order to pay a fine and restitution of more than $1.3 million.

In addition to the specific grounds for discipline of physicians, states often have a more general ground related to the physician's conduct showing lack of good moral character. That ground was cited in the *Hawker* case described earlier. The Massachusetts Supreme Judicial Court in 1982 issued an opinion, *Raymond v. Board of Registration in Medicine,*[3] which upheld that board's authority to revoke the license of Sherwin H. Raymond, M.D., based on his criminal conviction for possessing unregistered submachine guns. Such conduct, the court reasoned, showed that Dr. Raymond lacked good moral character, and formed the basis for the board to revoke his medical license.

Not to be overlooked is the fact that medical boards have the authority to discipline physicians for substandard care. Protection of the public from substandard care is, of course, one of the major reasons to have state medical boards in the first place. The extent to which state boards use that power varies. Some state boards have small staffs and may find it difficult to investigate and prove a case of substandard care against a physician. In addition, state boards must resolve the question of whether one egregious malpractice case is a sufficient basis for disciplining a physician, or whether a pattern of negligent practice needs to be established by showing that a physician has provided substandard care in a series of cases over time. Once the board has decided that a physician's practice has been substandard, it must decide what disposition is appropriate. The board may be reluctant to revoke permanently the license of a physician whose care is poor but who might benefit from further training or supervision.

All state boards provide the physician accused of any violation of the local medical practice act or board regulations with a hearing, in which the physician has the opportunity to put on a defense to the charges the board has made. If the board proves its case, despite the physician's defense, the board then has the responsibility to determine what sanction to impose on the physician. The board may revoke a license, suspend it, impose some form of verbal sanction, such as a reprimand or censure, or impose other restrictions on the physician's right to practice, such as supervision. After an adverse medical board decision, physicians have the right to appeal to the court system. In Massachusetts such appeals are heard in the state's highest court, the Supreme Judicial Court.

All final actions taken by the state board in formal disciplinary proceedings are reported to two places: the Federation of State Medical Boards, which maintains a data bank accessible to member boards, and the National Practitioner Data Bank, an entity created by the Health Care Quality Improvement Act of 1986. While neither bank is open to the public at this time, they serve a very useful purpose in protecting the public. State boards are able to obtain information about physicians from these banks and can use the information obtained in a decision to grant or deny a license. The information can also be used in a board disciplinary proceeding if the physician has been formally disciplined by another state's medical board. The existence of these data banks prevents the situation occurring when a physician is disciplined in state A for serious misconduct and then moves to state B and obtains a medical license without telling state B's medical board about the action taken in state A. In that sense, even though medical licenses are only good in the state where issued, one medical board's action can have consequences for the affected physician all over the United States.

/ / /

Because each state's medical board has its own policies, the discussion of licensing and disciplinary matters in this chapter has been extremely general. Examples from Massachusetts have been cited for illustrative purposes only and should not be interpreted as national policy. Physicians who need information about practice standards in their own state should contact the state medical board. Physicians would all benefit from obtaining and reading a copy of their state's medical practice act and board regulations soon after being licensed to practice. They should repeat the exercise from time to time. In that way, physicians will know what their medical board expects of them, and will never have to face the day when they receive a visit from a board investigator or a letter stating that their board is commencing a formal disciplinary action against them.

Notes

Richard E. Waring, J.D., the author of this chapter, is a Complaint Counsel for the Massachusetts Board of Registration in Medicine. The views expressed in this chapter are his and not necessarily those of the members of the Massachusetts Board of Registration in Medicine.

1. P. Starr, *The Social Transformation of American Medicine* (New York: Basic Books, 1982).
2. *Hawker v. New York,* 170 U.S. 189 (1898).
3. *Raymond v. Board of Registration in Medicine,* 387 Mass. 707 (1982).

Malpractice
Minefields

/ / /

8

Litigation Hot Spots in Clinical Practice

Robert I. Simon, M.D.

Certain aspects of psychiatric practice are associated with a higher risk of legal liability. Current and future hot spots include managing suicidal patients, violating boundaries in treatment, prescribing medications, prematurely releasing patients from hospitals, promoting recovered memories of childhood abuse, and practicing in managed care settings.

The chance of being sued in the 1980s was one in twenty-five a year (Benefacts, 1996). Currently, however, the odds have increased to about one out of every twelve psychiatrists. In some states, psychiatrists are sued at the rate of one out of six every year. Psychiatrists in Massachusetts have moved from twentieth to twelfth among the most frequently sued specialists within a period of three years.

The American Psychiatric Association (APA)–sponsored Professional Liability Insurance Program identifies a number of factors to account for the increase in malpractice suits:

1. Psychiatrists are treating "sicker" patients in managed care settings.
2. Media scrutiny of so-called recovered memories and ritual satanic abuse cases.
3. Failed tort reform legislation.
4. Psychiatrists are specializing in new practice areas such as geriatric psychopharmacology, adolescent addiction medicine, multiple personality disorder, pain management, and adult children of alcoholics.
5. Psychiatrists are providing more primary care such as the management of patients with diabetes and hypertension as well as a wide variety of acute general medical illnesses.

The legal liabilities associated with treating suicidal patients have been appreciated by clinicians for some time. Currently, however, managed care limitations on the frequency of visits and the duration of hospitalization dramatically increase the liability risk of treating the suicidal patient. The subject of reducing legal liability in the treatment of the suicidal patient is discussed in Chapter 11.

Treatment-boundary violations that disrupt the therapy of patients has become an area of prominent legal liability. There is a "natural history" of therapist-patient sex involving progressive, serious boundary violations that are precursors to eventual sexual involvement between therapist and patient. Even if a sexual relationship does not occur, boundary violations may interfere with the therapist's ability to correctly diagnose and treat the patient, increasing the risk of a bad treatment outcome and malpractice liability. This topic is discussed further in Chapter 13.

Prescribing Medications

According to the APA-sponsored Professional Liability Insurance Program, 13.2 percent of all closed malpractice claims involved medication problems (Macbeth et al., 1994). However, the clinician should recognize that bad outcomes do not necessarily result in a malpractice claim. Mistakes that occur in the absence of negligence are not legally actionable.

The basic elements of a malpractice suit can be described by the 4 D's—duty, deviation, damage, and direct causation. A doctor-patient relationship creates the *duty* of care. For example, prescribing for friends or neighbors will probably establish a doctor-patient relationship with its attendant duty of care. *Deviation* in care is established largely through expert testimony, the psychiatric literature, and the drug manufacturer's recommendations. If the deviation in care is the *direct cause* of damage to the patient, the elements of a negligence claim are in place. Damages may include both physical and psychological harm.

The plaintiff (individual bringing suit) still must prove that negligence occurred by a preponderance of the evidence (more likely than not). For example, in *Edwards v. United States* (1990), a federal district court held that loxapine prescribed at high doses of 300–500 mg per day was not the cause of a chronic schizophrenic's fatal heart attack. The drug manufacturer recommended not exceeding a daily dose of 250 mg. The Veterans Administration (VA) doctors found that the patient's delusions responded only to the higher doses. The plaintiff's complaint that prescribing the higher-than-recommended doses of loxapine was excessive and negligent did not succeed when the dosages could not be established as the cause of the heart attack. In the majority of malpractice suits brought against psychiatrists, the psychiatrist prevails because the plaintiffs must bear the burden of proof in cases where the standard of care may be highly variable.

Keeping thorough records of medication prescriptions is good clinical practice as well as a fundamental risk management technique. The clinician's records should indicate the medications prescribed, including dosage, amount, directions for taking the medication, and other instructions to the patient. Medications prescribed by other physicians, over-the-counter drugs, and the use of "street" drugs should also be recorded. Adverse drug interactions can harm the patient and bring about a lawsuit.

EXCEEDING RECOMMENDED DOSAGES

Some severely mentally ill patients may require the administration of psychoactive medications that exceed dosage guidelines. The reasons for making such a decision must be clearly documented in the patient's record. The patient should be made aware that drug guidelines are being exceeded. Generally, if very high levels of medication are required, the patient may need to be briefly hospitalized until a safer maintenance level can be achieved. The Food and Drug Administration (FDA) and the American Medical Association (AMA) have taken the position that prescribing higher-than-recommended doses remains at the physician's discretion.

Because drug tolerance may vary considerably from patient to patient, appropriate drug dosages may be difficult to assess. For instance, a young, acutely psychotic male may require 40 mg of haloperidol per day for management. However, an agitated, demented elderly patient may need only 0.5 mg of haloperidol per day for management. Therefore, it is difficult to ascertain when the patient has received an inappropriate dose. For example, in *Moon v. United States* (1981) a patient taking 20 mg of fluphenazine per day for a number of days while hospitalized drowned during an outing. The testimony of a forensic pharmacologist indicated that doses in excess of 20 mg per day should be administered only with the precautionary measures recommended by manufacturers and the *Physicians' Desk Reference* (PDR). A private-practice psychiatrist testifying on behalf of the plaintiff stated that when more than 20 mg per day of fluphenazine is given, vital signs should be checked frequently and a daily examination should be conducted to assess side effects. Based upon a review of the professional literature, the hospital's physicians testified that the dosage of fluphenazine was not excessive. The court, while acknowledging that a serious dispute over the appropriate daily dosage of fluphenazine existed, held that the drug treatment provided the patient was within allowable standards and was, therefore, not negligent.

The decision to prescribe medication that exceeds usual therapeutic limits should be made with the utmost care and consideration for the patient's psychiatric needs as well as the potential risks of treatment. Psychiatrists encounter liability problems when prescribing excessive medication where no reasonable medical rationale exists for such a prescription and where there is little or no monitoring of the patient's condition. For example, in *Dooley v. Skodnek* (1988), $1 million was awarded to a woman who became blind after being prescribed excessive doses of thioridazine, despite repeated complaints of deteriorating vision. Similarly, in *Fitrak v. United States* (1985), a VA extended-care facility was found liable for the death of a woman who originally sought treatment for gastrointestinal trouble. While a patient at the VA, she became psychotic and was treated with lithium. Appropriate lab work was never ordered, nor was the woman's lithium level monitored until she reached a fatal level of lithium toxicity. Her estate was awarded a judgment in excess of $100,000.

Psychiatrists who prescribe a large number of pills, particularly tricyclic antidepressants, to a known suicidal patient increase the risk of harm to the patient. Suicidal patients should be seen frequently and less than the minimal lethal dose of medication should be prescribed between appointments. Suicide cases in which patients are given lethal amounts of medication are difficult to defend in court. This problem exists because the psychiatrist often must prescribe medications that are capable of being abused by patients whose conditions predispose them to misuse and abuse. For instance, in *Argus v. Scheppegrell* (1986), the Louisiana Supreme Court held that a physician writing prescriptions for controlled substances in excessive amounts to a teenager who was addicted to drugs could be held liable for the patient's suicide. The court noted that the use of medication to commit the suicide was a consequence that the defendant should have foreseen.

As Appelbaum and Gutheil (1991) point out, focusing on the prescriber, rather than the patient, inappropriately shifts responsibility to the psychiatrist, producing an illusion of control. They state that life bristles with opportunities for self-destruction, including obtaining medication from other sources. Thus liability should not automatically result when determined patients circumvent all precautions to kill themselves. This includes overdosing with prescribed psychoactive medication.

On the other hand, prescribing less than the minimum lethal dose of medication may reassure the suicidal patient of the psychiatrist's concern.

Prescribing small amounts of medication to the suicidal patient, while important, often is not sufficient by itself to ensure safety. The emphasis with the patient should be on strengthening the therapeutic alliance. This ultimately provides the greatest hope to the patient and increases safety. The mere prescribing of medication apart from a working doctor-patient relationship does not meet generally accepted standards of good clinical care. It is a prime example of fragmented care. Such a practice will diminish the efficacy of the drug treatment itself or may even lead to the patient's failure to take the prescribed medication. Fragmented care, in which the psychiatrist functions only as a prescriber of medication while remaining uninformed about the patient's overall clinical status, constitutes substandard care that may lead to a malpractice action. Psychiatrists who prescribe medications only in a split treatment arrangement should be able to hospitalize the patient, if that should become necessary. If the psychiatrist does not have admitting privileges, then prearrangements should exist with other psychiatrists who can hospitalize patients if emergencies arise. Split treatment is increasingly utilized by managed care companies and is a potential malpractice minefield.

Often, a real danger to patient care is created by the patient's failure to renew prescriptions. Thus prescriptions that require frequent renewal may lead to nonadherence. In addition, a schizophrenic patient on long-term maintenance therapy may require very high doses of neuroleptic drugs. Such a dosage might appear to be a lethal dose for other types of patients. The psychiatrist should note these differences in the patient's medical record, including the fact that tolerance to the toxic effects of neuroleptic drugs develops quickly.

Psychiatrists who cover the practices of other psychiatrists may receive requests from their patients for large amounts of drugs. Unless a large volume of medication is specifically recommended by the treating psychiatrist, the covering psychiatrist should prescribe only enough medication for the patient until the treating psychiatrist returns. If the treating psychiatrist will be away for a longer period of time, the covering psychiatrist should consider seeing the patient directly. This will allow for adjustments to be made in the amount of medication that is provided according to the patient's observed clinical needs.

FAILURE TO MONITOR

The standard of care for prescribing medication requires that psychiatrists have a duty to possess that degree of skill and learning ordinarily possessed and used by members of the psychiatric profession who are in good standing and who are engaged in prescribing, dispensing and administering medication in the same or similar circumstances (Bies, 1984). Warning the patient of potential side effects, monitoring the patient, and treating undesired side effects in a timely manner all fall within this duty. As part of the working alliance with their patients, psychiatrists should inform patients of the potential side effects of medication, encouraging them to notify the psychiatrist if side effects arise that are of concern. Open communication about potential problems with medications enhances the therapeutic process through the establishment of trust and thereby reduces the problem of patient nonadherence.

Psychiatrists may be found liable for failing to diagnose treatable side effects or complications of psychiatric treatment (Simon, 1992). When the patient is under reasonable supervision, side effects or complications that arise from medications may be effectively treated by diminishing the dose, discontinuing the drug, or adding another treatment. The acute anticholinergic, autonomic, and extrapyramidal side effects of neuroleptic and antidepressant medications can be quite disabling. If these side effects are left unattended, patients may develop serious injury (*Dovido v. Vasquez* 1986) or, at the least, become noncompliant with drug therapy, which itself may be harmful.

In *Christy v. Saliterman* (1970), the plaintiff was able to argue successfully that the psychiatrist should have evaluated the patient before prescribing paraldehyde and should have advised the patient that the paraldehyde could have undesirable side effects. The patient, who was not warned of the soporific qualities of paraldehyde, fell asleep in a chair while smoking and set himself on fire, suffering serious burns.

Patients taking monoamine oxidase inhibitors should be warned against ingesting food and drinks that contain tyramine or taking drugs that interact adversely with the monoamine oxidase inhibitors (Anonymous v. Anonymous Psychiatrist, 1988). It is remarkable to observe how often these rudimentary warnings are not given despite the clear legal consequences that may arise (Sarno, 1986). Patients must be warned about driving or working around dangerous machinery if the medications they are taking produce drowsiness or slow reflexes. Similarly, the patient must be warned of the dangers of drinking alcohol while taking psychoactive drugs.

Psychiatrists have varying duties to report impaired patients to the Department of Motor Vehicles (DMV). A minority of states have mandatory reporting requirements while the remaining states have permissive requirements or no requirements at all. Usually, immunity from suit is provided in a number of reporting statutes. The APA, in an official position statement, states that the presence of mental disorder does not, by itself, imply an impaired capacity to operate a motor vehicle. The APA Position Statement advises that "accurate assessment of the impact of symptoms on functional abilities usually is not possible in an office or hospital setting because such an assessment typically requires specialized equipment or observation of actual driving, which goes well beyond the scope of ordinary psychiatric care. Moreover, psychiatrists have no special expertise in assessing the ability of their patients to drive" (APA, 1995, p. 819).

Nevertheless, psychiatrists must assess with the patient any impairment in driving caused by symptoms or medication effects. The patient should be reassured that required reporting of mental disorders to the DMV does not automatically result in losing one's license. Where reporting is discretionary, the record should contain the reasoning in deciding to report or not report a mental disorder to the DMV. Specifically, documentation should support the reasoning behind the clinical decision concerning whether a foreseeable risk of an automobile accident resulting from the patient's psychiatric condition is sufficient to merit reporting. Where reporting statutes are absent, some therapists have required the patient to self-report as a condition of continued treatment.

The proper monitoring of psychotropic medications requires that patients not be allowed to stay on prolonged drug therapy without improvement. Reevaluation of the patient's diagnosis, the indications for any given drug regimen, and the dosage levels of the drug are necessary when patients remain refractory to treatment. Generally, psychotropic medications should be withdrawn gradually, particularly if the drugs have been taken for more than a few months. Sudden withdrawal syndromes can occur that have severe sequelae and possibly serious legal consequences.

In monitoring medication, it is not necessary that the psychiatrist obtain serum blood levels for antidepressants as a matter of course (American Psychiatric Association, 1985). Drug plasma monitoring, however, can provide objective evidence substantiating the need for high doses of antidepressants in certain patients while establishing that the drug plasma levels are not in the toxic range. If toxicity from a tricyclic antidepressant is suspected, a plasma level should be obtained. Furthermore, medication compliance can be monitored by obtaining blood levels. When carbamazepine is used in the treatment of psychiatric disorders, regular serum level and hematological monitoring is necessary.

At present, research does not support the clinical utility of plasma levels in monitoring neuroleptic drugs (Schatzberg and Nemeroff, 1995). The value of neuroleptic serum levels is limited to assessing compliance with medication and differentiating between toxicity and the worsening of the patient's psychotic disorder. Psychiatrists may wish to order these tests when clinical conditions warrant, but should not do so because of any sense of legal concern. Obviously, monitoring lithium levels when therapeutic and toxic levels are relatively close is extremely important, particularly if patients are on low-salt diets or are taking diuretics. Neurotoxicity secondary to lithium therapy does not necessarily parallel lithium levels. Utilizing good clinical judgment rather than relying solely on laboratory reports remains essential.

The question frequently arises: How often should the patient be seen for medication follow-up? The answer is that the patient should be seen at a frequency that accords with her or his clinical needs. Since medication follow-up usually involves some sort of psychotherapy, the patient's need for psychological support must also be considered in determining the length of time between visits. Generally, most psychiatrists see their patients every thirty days to every three months.

INAPPROPRIATE INDICATIONS

Prescribing neuroleptics for patients who are not psychotically depressed or who suffer from neurotic anxiety may be an example of medicating inappropriately. However, the clinical needs of the patient are determinative. Psychoactive medications that are usually indicated for one type of psychiatric disorder may be empirically useful for a non-indicated disorder in certain patients. For example, low-dose neuroleptics may be indicated for some patients with borderline personality disorder.

The prescribing of multiple medications, or polypharmacy, has been much disparaged as a "shotgun" approach to treatment that may significantly increase the possibility of serious side effects. Nevertheless, under certain circumstances, some patients may benefit from such a regimen. Polypharmacy has become synonymous with negligent or inappropriate treatment, but judicious rational use of medication combinations in selected patients can be clinically useful. In bipolar disorders, when proper precautions are observed, good clinical practice may include various combinations of antidepressants, benzodiazapines, lithium, anticonvulsants, antihypertensives, clozapine, thyroid and estrogen replacement, calcium channel blockers, and adjunctive sleep medications (Simon, 1997). A significant number of patients are treatment-resistant to a single drug therapy.

The issue is not polypharmacy per se, but whether the drug combinations are chosen rationally. The use of multiple medications becomes clinically inappropriate and potentially actionable where no reasonable medical explanation for the use of each medication exists and where complications due to possible adverse drug interactions have not been evaluated. However, the art and science of psychopharmacology and psychiatric diagnosis have not progressed to the point where dogmatic positions can be taken about the drug treatment of patients. Psychiatrists should document their reasons for deviating from recognized guidelines in prescribing medication through a risk-benefit assessment. The specific treatment needs of the patient should also be adequately documented.

An attempt to impose social control on mentally ill patients through a "chemical straitjacket" is an inappropriate indication for psychoactive medications. This is especially the case when the objectionable behavior is not directly the result of a psychiatric disorder. For example, strong-willed, difficult elderly residents of nursing homes who are not accustomed to the constraints of institutional living may annoy staff or interfere with staff functioning. For the severely agitated elderly patient with dementia and psychosis, a neuroleptic may be lifesaving. However, neuroleptic medications ordinarily should not be prescribed to squelch objectionable behavior that is a long-standing aspect of the patient's personality rather than the symptom of a treatable mental illness. In addition, psychoactive drugs should never be used as a form of punishment (*Knecht v. Gillman,* 1973). Although chemical restraints raise issues of deprivation of liberty that can result in a civil rights suit, malpractice actions are much more likely.

A much less appreciated form of inappropriate administration of medication occurs when homeopathic doses are prescribed in the spirit of defensive medicine. Such practices deny a patient safe and effective clinical care. At the same time, they may expose the patient to the risks but none of the benefits of treatment while prolonging the disability and suffering of the patient. Rather than avoiding suits, defensive homeopathic prescribing may actually invite legal action (*Carter v. Dunlop,* 1985).

Another major problem area is the failure to prescribe psychotropic drugs for patients when they are clearly indicated. Patients suffering from severe, incapacitating depressions or severe anxiety disorders should be informed that drugs are available that may produce significant relief in a relatively short time. Subjecting such patients to long-term psychotherapy without first providing this information is a disservice to the patient and is potentially legally actionable (Malcolm, 1986).

Psychiatrists practicing in a managed care setting must not use medications inappropriately as a means of manipulating managed care reviewers. For example, in the treatment of inpatients, psychiatrists must resist any temptation to give medication that would otherwise not be given in order to convince managed care reviewers of the need for patient care.

Managed care drug formularies have become an increasing concern for psychiatrists. For example, a number of managed care formularies offer tricyclic antidepressants as first-line drugs because of cost-effectiveness. Selective serotonin reuptake inhibitors are available only if patients do not respond to tricyclics. Psychiatrists have successfully challenged certain managed care drug formulary recommendations in Massachusetts and California (Psychiatrists Speak Out, 1996).

"OFF LABEL" PRESCRIBING

Prescribing an approved medication for an unapproved use does not violate federal law (Macbeth et al., 1994). "Off label" prescribing of medications is at the discretion of the physician once a drug has been approved. The psychiatrist is not restricted by indications and labeling approved by the FDA. Restrictions apply only to the manufacturer's representations in advertising. In 1961 the FDA established regulations to provide a package insert for all prescription drugs (Simon, 1992). All drugs must contain adequate information concerning use, dosages, method of administration, frequency, duration, relevant risks, contraindications, side effects, and precautions in prescribing the drug. The FDA evaluates only the use that the drug company wants to place in the insert, thus not precluding other specific uses not mentioned in the insert. Failure to describe a particular use may mean only that the FDA has not been requested to review those data. Usually this occurs because the pharmaceutical company does not believe a market exists for a specific use, thus not justifying a need to prove its effectiveness to the FDA. The FDA abides by the principle that good medical practice requires a physician to prescribe medication according to the best information available. However, the physician who deviates from the package insert may have to explain such a departure should a lawsuit arise.

Few psychiatrists appreciate the treatment latitude they possess in regard to the PDR and the drug insert; most perceive FDA guidelines as absolutely authoritative. Could this be a symptom of defensive psychiatry (Simon, 1985)? A psychiatrist may prescribe a drug for a use that is not yet approved by the FDA. For example, no drug is currently approved by the FDA for the treatment of aggression. Yet a number of drugs, including neuroleptics, antidepressants, benzodiazepines, beta blockers, anticonvulsants, and lithium are all used effectively to treat violent behaviors. Furthermore, the use of carbamazapine and calcium channel blockers have not been approved by the FDA for the treatment of mood disorders (Schatzberg and Nemeroff, 1995). Only lithium and divalproex sodium have received official FDA approval for use as mood stabilizers. However, the psychiatric literature and clinical experience validate the usefulness of these drugs in the clinical management of violent and mood-disordered patients, respectively.

Similarly, few psychotropic drugs have received FDA approval for use in children under twelve years of age. As of this writing, excluding psychostimulants, only haloperidol, thioridizine, chlorpromazine, pimozide, imipramine, and clomipramine have received official approval. Although a significant scientific knowledge base does not exist for the use of other psychotropic medications in children, empirical trials and clinical experience provide a wide latitude for prescribing psychotropic medications for unapproved uses in children. Many drugs are not FDA approved for a new indication if the patent expires and no financial incentive exists to obtain FDA approval.

The decision to prescribe for nonapproved uses should be based on sound knowledge of the drugs backed by firm scientific rationale and peer-reviewed psychiatric literature. The psychiatrist should be able to cite texts or journal articles to substantiate the fact that the decision to prescribe for a nonapproved use was based on good clinical practice. For example, divalproex sodium was approved in 1995 by the FDA for the treatment of bipolar disorder. Nevertheless, before 1995 psychiatrists used this drug safely and effectively in the treatment of bipolar disorder based on scientific studies in the psychiatric literature.

The standard for obtaining informed consent is correspondingly heightened when a medication is prescribed for an unapproved use. The patient or guardian must be informed that the patient will be taking a drug for use that has not been approved by the FDA and should be warned of all possible, reasonably foreseeable risks. Although a consent form may provide added protection, the nature of the disclosure should be recorded in the patient's chart. Whether the disclosure is given orally or provided in a consent form, the chart notes should also contain an assessment indicating that the information was understood by the patient, that consent was freely given, and the note should state the rationale for using a medication for unapproved purposes. This procedure also should be followed when prescribing at higher-than-recommended doses.

The FDA does not have the power to dictate the practice of psychiatry, particularly when it comes to prescribing drugs. The use of a drug, once marketed, is the responsibility of physicians, and the drug is prescribed at their sole discretion.

The FDA does not consider its regulations to be legal documents, admissible as establishing the breach of the standard of care (Simon, 1992). Physicians are free to prescribe according to their best knowledge and judgment. The legal significance of the package insert or PDR, however, can vary with each medication, the facts of a given case, and the jurisdiction in which a physician resides.

Courts typically have not gone beyond declaring that a departure from a manufacturer's use or dosage recommendations establishes a prima facie case of negligence rebuttable by the physician (Macbeth et al., 1994). A prima facie case exists when the evidence in the case is "such as will prevail until contradicted and overcome by other evidence" (Black, 1990, pp. 1189–90). Thus, in *Mulder v. Parke Davis and Co.* (1970), the Minnesota Supreme Court stated that a physician's deviation from the drug manufacturer's recommendations for use, precautions, and dangers represented prima facie evidence of negligence. In addition, the court stated that the physician must disclose his or her reasons for such a deviation, leaving the issue to be settled by the trier of fact.

Courts appear to be more inclined to follow the rationale enunciated in *Ramon v. Farr* (1989). A malpractice action alleged birth defects from the injection of bupivacaine one hour before a child's birth. The fact that the PDR and the manufacturer's package insert indicated that the use of bupivacaine as a paracervical block was not recommended without further research was used as evidence to support the plaintiff's claims. The court rejected the plaintiff's contention that this information constituted prima facie evidence of the defendant's negligence. Instead, the court ruled that this information did not establish the standard of care but was to be considered by the court as additional evidence, along with the expert testimony to be weighed in determining whether there had been a breach in the duty of care.

Although the PDR is frequently used by attorneys in court, it would be a professional error for treating psychiatrists to regard the PDR as establishing the standard of care and as a constraint upon their clinical judgment. Psychiatrists are solely responsible for making informed decisions, taking into account their own clinical training, experience, and judgment as well as the relevant professional literature. They also must be prepared to justify their decisions based on professional standards. Because the PDR is not a textbook of psychiatry, patient care may be compromised if clinicians use the PDR as their primary source of professional guidance. Furthermore, the FDA and the AMA have taken the position that prescription for nonapproved indications or at higher-than-recommended doses should be based upon a physician's discretion (Archer, 1984).

INFORMED CONSENT

When prescribing medications for patients, the doctrine of informed consent requires the psychiatrist to disclose certain information to the patient, who must give competent, informed, and voluntary consent.

The psychiatrist is not required to inform the patient of every conceivable risk. A material risk is one that "a reasonable person, in what the physician knows or should know to be the patient's position, would likely attach significance to the risk or cluster of risks in deciding whether or not to forgo the proposed therapy" (*Canterbury v. Spence,* 1972). This definition has also been referred to as the *reasonable man standard.* Whether a risk is material depends on the severity and probability of the risk, the likelihood of treatment success, and the availability of alternative, less dangerous treatments. If necessary treatment presents minimal risks, the duty to disclose is not as rigorous as when a treatment presents a high risk and is dangerous or intrusive. When less dangerous but equally effective alternative treatments are available, the duty to disclose is heightened. For instance, if neuroleptic medication is prescribed for a patient's anxiety disorder when a benzodiazepine would be equally effective, the increased risk of adverse side effects from the neuroleptic medication requires a full disclosure.

Malpractice defense attorneys have recommended the "1 percent rule" as a guideline for physicians (Gibbs, 1987). If a particular risk of injury has a chance of occurrence greater than 1 percent, the risk is considered material and needs to be disclosed. This "rule" applies only in jurisdictions that have indicated some percentage in specifying what constitutes a material risk. As in all aspects of the informed-consent doctrine, uncertainty reigns. Courts have been inconsistent in deciding what is a major or minor risk.

Generally, doctors should provide patients with individualized information about the diagnosis, the nature and purpose of the proposed treatment, the risks and consequences of the proposed treatment, the probability that the proposed treatment will be successful, feasible treatment alternatives (including risks and benefits), and the prognosis if the proposed treatment is declined (see Table 8.1). Most psychiatrists probably fulfill a *subjective lay standard* when informing their patients of the risks and benefits if they approach every patient in an individualized manner (Simon, 1989). Furthermore, patients usually are given ample opportunity to ask questions in the give-and-take format of therapy. The information provided to the patient by the clinician and the patient's mental capacity to give a competent, voluntary consent to the proposed treatment or procedure should be memorialized in the medical record.

Table 8.1. INFORMED CONSENT: REASONABLE INFORMATION
TO BE DISCLOSED

Although there is no consistently accepted set of information to be disclosed for any given medical or psychiatric situation, as a rule of thumb, five areas of information are generally provided:

1. Diagnosis: description of the condition or problem
2. Treatment: nature and purpose of the proposed treatment
3. Consequences: risks and benefits of the proposed treatment
4. Alternatives: viable alternatives to the proposed treatment, including risks and benefits
5. Prognosis: projected outcome with and without treatment

Source: R. I. Simon, *Clinical Psychiatry and the Law,* 2nd ed. (Washington: American Psychiatric Press, 1992), p. 128.

All states require informed consent by either case law or statute (Malcolm, 1992; Brakel et al., 1985). Many states have statutes requiring informed consent for treatment (Solnick, 1985). The statutes may spell out instances when no consent is required beyond explaining the risks of anesthesia and surgery. For additional procedures, the state may specify what risks must be told to the patient and in what form they must be stated (oral or written). Under these statutes, only the disclosure of risks specified in the statute is deemed material as a matter of law (Meisel and Kabnick, 1980). Some statutes make compliance to the guidelines voluntary. Most state statutes classify failure to obtain informed consent as negligence rather than battery (Slovenko, 1989).

Premature Release of Patients

Important ethical and legal issues arise as a result of managed care decisions (Siebert and Silver, 1990). Psychiatric hospitals may be unable to provide long-term treatment to the dangerous mentally ill patient because of cost considerations. Psychiatrists may find themselves caught between a hospital wanting to discharge the patient for financial reasons and their professional and legal responsibility to provide appropriate care. The pressure for discharge under managed care may lead to an increase in premature discharges of dangerous patients. Furthermore, as the length of hospital stays is reduced, psychiatrists must become knowledgeable about the availability of community resources and the provision of quality aftercare. Malpractice cases involving the injury or death of patients because of the negligent release of a violent patient far exceed in number and frequency those cases involving outpatient *Tarasoff*-type duty-to-warn-or-protect situations (Simon and Sadoff, 1992).

In *Wickline v. State of California* (1986), the treating physician, Dr. Polonsky, requested an extended stay of eight additional days for his patient following surgery for Leriche's syndrome (occlusion of the abdominal aorta). The Medi-Cal reviewer granted four days. Ms. Wickline suffered complications following the premature release, necessitating amputation of her leg. She sued Medi-Cal. The jury ruled in her favor, but a California appellate court decided that the treating physician, who was not a defendant in the case, could be held liable, but not Medi-Cal.

In his testimony, Dr. Polonsky stated that he believed "that Medi-Cal had the power to tell him, as a treating doctor, when a patient must be discharged from the hospital." The appellate court noted that third-party payers of health care services can be held liable when appeals that are made on behalf of the patients for medical care "are arbitrarily ignored or unreasonably disregarded or over-ridden. The physician who complies without protest with the limitations imposed by a third-party payer, even if his medical judgment dictates otherwise, cannot avoid his ultimate responsibility for his patient's care. He cannot point to the health care payer as the liability scapegoat when the consequences of his own determinative medical decision go sour" (*Wickline*, 1986). The lesson is absolutely clear. Physicians are responsible for the medical care provided to their patients. The duty of the physician to exercise his or her best medical judgment on behalf of the patient is not dependent upon payment. Nor can this duty be abrogated to others.

In a subsequent case, *Wilson v. Blue Cross of Southern California et al.* (1990), a California appeals court did not follow the specific language of *Wickline*. In *Wilson*, a patient was hospitalized at College Hospital in Los Angeles suffering from anorexia, drug dependency, and major depression. The treating physician determined that the patient required three to four weeks of hospitalization. After approximately one and one-half weeks, utilization review determined that further hospitalization was unnecessary. The patient's insurance company refused to pay for further inpatient treatment. The denial of coverage was not appealed by the psychiatrist. The patient was discharged and committed suicide a few weeks later.

The Appellate Division of the California Court of Appeals held that third-party payers are not immune from lawsuits in regard to utilization review activities. The court determined that the insurer may be subject to liability for harm caused to the patient by premature termination of a patient's hospitalization. While the fact pattern of this case differs from that of *Wickline,* the decision in *Wilson* signals that a third-party payer may be held legally liable for a negligent decision to discharge the patient either separately or along with the patient's physician, depending upon the facts of the case. Although both *Wickline* and *Wilson* are California cases, they offer insight and, perhaps, precedence concerning future reasoning by other courts increasingly confronted with complex liability issues concerning utilization review decisions. The clinician must always remember that she or he has the moral, ethical, professional, and legal duty to provide adequate care for the patient (Simon, in press a & b). This duty cannot be abrogated by the economic priorities of managed care.

Litigation brought against physicians and managed care providers for premature release will likely burgeon in the future. Until now, the risk of suits against managed care companies for the negligent performance of utilization review has been suppressed by the Employee Retirement Income Security Act of 1974 (ERISA). ERISA preempts state laws and prohibits negligence claims in cases involving employer-sponsored health plans. However, recent cases have emerged where courts have held that the intent of ERISA was not to abolish the right of individuals to sue for negligence.

Recovered Memories of Childhood Abuse

It is critically important for the clinician to maintain a position of neutrality concerning recovered memories of childhood sexual abuse (Simon and Gutheil, 1997). An expectant position of listening that avoids polarization by the current rancorous dispute over recovered memories is essential. The clinician should neither discredit nor suggest sexual abuse memories. Asking the patient about childhood abuse as a legitimate aspect of taking a psychiatric history is important and entirely appropriate.

The therapist's role is to strive to understand the patient's psychological reality, so-called narrative truth, while not neglecting to consider the "historical truth" when such information is available. The treater is neither jury nor judge, attempting to determine the factual truth of the patient's story. The treater is an ally of the patient, and empathic listening is a validating experience for the patient. It says, "You are a person, important in your own right. I want to hear your story." A therapist's treatment role is quite separate and distinct from that of a forensic expert witness and should not be mixed (Simon, 1996).

Therapists who allege childhood sexual abuse of their patients had best be careful, and not only because they will have difficulty proving their allegations in courtrooms. In the years ahead, it is likely that therapists who zealously pursue sexual trauma from a patient's childhood, and who suggest that such trauma is the sole cause of a patient's emotional problems, will be pelted by a hail of lawsuits. Many of those accused of abuse by patients who have recovered abuse memories in therapy will sue the therapists for allegedly inducing those very memories. Even conservative therapists who conduct credible psychotherapy, in the course of which memories of abuse are recovered, will find themselves at increased risk of being sued. Recanters may also sue their therapists, sometimes joined by their families. Allegations of abuse can and do cause people to lose their reputations, careers, marriages, and families, and to be stigmatized for life. So it is to be expected that those who are accused of abuse will actively fight those charges.

In just such an early landmark case, *Ramona v. Isabella* (1994), a jury in Orange County, California, awarded $500,000 to a father who charged that his daughter's psychotherapists were responsible for "planting" her false memories of sexual abuse through the use of sodium amobarbital. Gary Ramona, age fifty, brought an $8 million malpractice countersuit against the therapists, the first case in the United States to allow a nonpatient family member to seek damages, after the daughter sued her father. Ramona attributed the loss of his $400,000-a-year salary as a winery vice president as well as the ending of his twenty-five-year marriage and the estrangement from his three daughters to charges leveled by his daughter in 1991 that he had sexually molested her. After Gary Ramona prevailed, the original suit brought by Holly Ramona against her father for sexual abuse was subsequently dismissed based on her father's victory in the malpractice suit. The dismissal was reversed by an appeals court (*Ramona v. Ramona*, 1995).

A mounting number of similar cases are in litigation or waiting to go to trial. In a December 1994 case in Dallas, Texas, a jury found that a psychiatrist committed slander when he accused a Seattle couple of past sexual abuse against their grown daughter (Hausman, 1995). The couple was awarded $350,000.

Lawsuits involving recovered memories of childhood abuse are proliferating rapidly. Strident advocacy by both supporters and disbelievers in the credibility of such recovered memories will likely fan the flames of litigation into the next century. As an example, a jury awarded nearly $2.7 million to the plaintiffs in a case alleging that the therapist implanted memories of sexual abuse (Grinfeld, 1995). In a second case, the plaintiffs brought similar allegations against the same psychiatrist with a comparable result. Other cases are expected.

The clinician must avoid the double-agent role of becoming an expert for the patient in any litigation. A forensic psychiatrist should be retained separately to perform that role. The therapist in court has many conflicts of interest that are likely to severely undermine his or her credibility (Simon, 1995). Almost certainly, the patient's treatment will be severely hampered or destroyed by the dual role of therapist and expert witness (Strasburger, 1987).

Above all, the clinician must not suggest abuse. On the other hand, it is defensive psychiatry at its worst to initiate therapy with a discussion about the uncertainties surrounding the concept of repressed memories as some have suggested (Managing the Risks, 1994). To do so will undermine the openness necessary for both therapist and patient to maintain their mutual observation of all psychological material produced by the patient. Psychiatrists also need to be able to ask about abuse when obtaining a patient's history without fear of being sued.

Careful documentation of the process of memory recovery using the actual words of the patient along with those of the therapist is necessary. Such a record will help establish that the therapeutic neutrality of the clinician was not compromised. As part of maintaining neutrality, the therapist must be able to tolerate uncertainty and ambiguity as the patient's story unfolds. It may not be possible to determine whether abuse occurred or, if it did, what kind of abuse and by whom. To reconstruct hypothetical childhood abuse prematurely or to suggest that the patient's symptoms indicate abuse is inappropriate when it circumvents the patient's ultimate judgment about what happened. It is prudent to maintain clinical focus on the patient's presenting symptoms. If the patient reporting recovered memories does not improve sufficiently within a reasonable period of time, a differential diagnosis should be undertaken and a consultation considered.

Psychiatrists should avoid the use of unorthodox treatment methods in a dogged effort to discover memories of abuse. Patients can become very suggestible under the influence of hypnosis or sodium amytal interviews. It is a relatively easy matter to implant false memories during altered mental states. If the patient appears to present difficult, complex problems that may require creative treatment approaches, a consultation should be obtained first.

It frequently happens that during the process of memory recovery patients become very upset. Especially at these times, the therapist must be able to help manage a patient's proclivity to act out anger toward important relationships. Major life decisions by the patient may need to be deferred until the psychological turmoil settles down. Moreover, with new patients, the clinician should neither blindly accept the diagnosis nor continue the treatment provided by a former therapist. The practitioner must conduct his or her own evaluation.

When supervising other therapists, a careful check of their credentials, licensure, and clinical experience is essential. Compatible treatment approaches reflecting agreement between supervisor and supervisee should be utilized. The supervising clinician must be alerted to the emergence of abuse memories. At this juncture, the supervisor should ensure that memories are not being suggested or debunked by the supervisee. A balanced treatment approach toward the patient is necessary. The supervisor also must make sure that the supervisee has adequate professional liability coverage. A receipt of the certificate of insurance should be obtained. The supervisor should also check to see if her or his malpractice policy covers supervisory relationships.

In order not to create an unintended doctor-patient relationship with family members or other third parties who attend a patient's session, it should be made very clear from the outset that they are not being seen as patients. The attendance of family members as adjuncts to the patient's treatment should be voluntary. Documentation of these clarifications is important. If a family member needs treatment, a referral to another practitioner should be made. Unless these measures are followed, the door is left open for the possibility of a nonpatient third-party suit later (Appelbaum and Zoltek-Jick, 1996). The third party may claim a doctor-patient relationship existed that creates the standing to sue the doctor.

Patients in managed care settings who are beginning to experience recovered memories of childhood abuse will probably need to be seen beyond a few sessions. It should be carefully explained to these patients that they will not be able to receive the extended care they will require under their managed care contract. A referral will probably be necessary for treatment outside the managed care plan.

The psychiatrist should maintain a position of neutrality concerning litigation against alleged abusers. It is a treatment issue for the patient whether to bring suit. The law is a blunt instrument. Although some therapists may encourage litigation as a means of empowering the abused patient, the legal arena can become a venue for revictimization.

Psychiatrists have an ethical and professional duty to maintain professional competence and stay abreast of new developments when treating patients who have recovered memories of childhood sexual abuse. Therapists can stay current by following new developments in the emerging field of memory science and in the evolving standards in the treatment of patients claiming sexual abuse.

Psychiatrists and other mental health professionals who enter into the public debate over recovered memories have to exercise caution and discretion. Encouraging a patient to make public accusations of sexual abuse against alleged perpetrators will significantly increase the risk of a slander suit (and perhaps other claims). In a number of jurisdictions, charges of slander may be brought against a therapist by accused third parties where only patients themselves can sue for malpractice. Therapists should avoid making public pronouncements about the veracity of sexual abuse reported by patients or other individuals. This caveat includes family members of the patient.

Prevention

Clinical risk management combines the professional expertise and intimate clinical knowledge of the patient with a clinically useful understanding of the legal issues governing psychiatric practice. Its purpose is to provide optimal care for the patient and, only secondarily, to reduce the risk of legal liability.

A few basic principles of clinical risk management can help the practitioner avoid the current and future litigation "hot spots" in psychiatric practice. Maintaining a clinical focus in providing good patient care is basic. A clinically useful understanding of the legal requirements governing the practice of psychiatry is essential, helping to dispel unduly defensive practices that may limit the clinician from utilizing a wide spectrum of effective treatments that are now available. Knowledge of the legal regulation of psychiatric practice also will enable the therapist to spot troublesome areas. Often, legal requirements can be incorporated into clinical interventions that help maintain good-quality care. Careful record keeping, open communications with patients, and obtaining consultation on problem cases are examples of basic risk management techniques that also constitute good clinical practice.

As a lifelong dedication, the practice of psychiatry is a privilege that should be enjoyed. Practicing without undue fear of litigation is an achievable goal. The words of Hippocrates are particularly applicable today: "May it be granted to me to enjoy life and the practice of the art respected by all men."

References

American Psychiatric Association (1985). "Task Force on the Use of Laboratory Tests in Psychiatry: Tricyclic Antidepressants: Blood Level Measurements and Clinical Outcome." *American Journal of Psychiatry* 142: 155–162.

American Psychiatric Association (1995). "APA Official Actions: Position Statement on the Role of Psychiatrists in Assessing Driving Ability." *American Journal of Psychiatry* 152, no. 5 (May): 819.

"Anonymous v. Anonymous Psychiatrist" (1988). *Medical Malpractice: Verdicts, Settlements and Experts* 4 (Dec.): 60.

Appelbaum, P. S., and T. G. Gutheil (1991). *Clinical Handbook of Psychiatry and the Law.* 2nd ed. Baltimore: Williams and Wilkins.

Appelbaum, P. S., and R. Zoltek-Jick (1996). "Psychotherapists' Duties to Third Parties: Ramona and Beyond." *American Journal of Psychiatry* 153: 457–465.

Archer, J. D. (1984). "The FDA Does Not Approve Uses of Drugs" (editorial). *JAMA* 252: 1054–55.

Argus v. Scheppegrell, 472 So. 2d 573 (La. 1985), cert. denied, 494 So. 2d 331 (La. 1986).

Benefacts (1996). "A Message from the APA-Sponsored Professional Liability Insurance Program." *Psychiatric News* (April 19).

Bies, E. B. (1984). *Mental Health and the Law.* Rockville: Aspen.

Black, H. C. (1990). *Black's Law Dictionary.* 6th ed. St. Paul: West Publishing.

Brakel, S. J., J. Parry, and B. A. Weiner. (1985). *The Mentally Disabled and the Law.* Chicago: American Bar Foundation.

Canterbury v. Spence, 464 F.2d 787 (D.C. Cir. 1972), cert. denied, 409 U.S. 1064 (1972).

Carter v. Dunlop, 138 Ill. App. 3rd 58, 484 N.E.2d 1273 (1985).

Christy v. Saliterman, 288 Minn. 144, 179 N.W.2d 288 (1970).

Dooley v. Skodnek, 1138 A.D.2d 102, 529 N.Y.S.2d 569 (1988).

Dovido v. Vasquez, no. 84–674 CA (L)(H) 15th Jud. Dist. Cir. Ct., Palm Beach City (Fla. April 4, 1986).

Edwards v. United States, 749 F. Supp. 1070 (D. Kan. 1990).

Employee Retirement Income Security Act of 1974 (ERISA). 1991. 29 U.S.C.A. §§1001–1461 (1988 and Supp. 1991).

Fitrak v. United States, no. CU81-0950 U.S.D.C. (E.D. N.Y. 1985).

Gibbs, R. F. (1987). "Informed Consent: What It Is and How to Obtain It." *Legal Aspects of Medical Practice* 15 (Aug.): 1–4.

Grinfeld, M. J. (1995). "Psychiatrist Stung by Huge Damage Award in Repressed Memory Case." *Psychiatric Times* 12, no. 10 (Oct.).

Hausman, K. (1995). "Psychiatrist Commits Slander in 'Recovered' Memories Case." *Psychiatric News,* Jan. 20.

Knecht v. Gillman, 488 F.2d 1136 (8th Cir. 1973).

Macbeth, J. E., et al. (1994). *Legal and Risk Management Issues in the Practice of Psychiatry.* Washington: Psychiatrists' Purchasing Group.

Malcolm, J. G. (1986). "Treatment Choices and Informed Consent in Psychiatry: Implications of the Osheroff Case for the Profession." *Journal of Psychiatry and Law* 14: 9–107.

Malcolm, J. G. (1992). "Informed Consent in the Practice of Psychiatry." In

American Psychiatric Press Review of Clinical Psychiatry and the Law, vol. 3, ed. R. I. Simon. Washington: American Psychiatric Press.

"Managing the Risks Involved in Cases of Recovered Memories of Abuse: Prescription for Risk." (1994). *Psychiatrists' Purchasing Group, Inc., Newsletter* 5: 1, 4.

Meisel, A., and L. D. Kabnick (1980). "Informed Consent to Medical Treatment: An Analysis of Recent Legislation." *University of Pittsburgh Law Review* 41: 407.

Moon v. United States, 512 F. Supp. 140, 146 (D. Nev. 1981).

Mulder v. Parke Davis and Co., 288 Minn. 332, 181 N.W.2d 882 (1970).

Physicians' Desk Reference. (1997). 51st ed. Montvale, N.J.: Medical Economics Data Production Co.

"Psychiatrists Speak Out against Managed Care Formularies—And Win." (1996). *Psychiatric News,* Jan. 19.

Ramon v. Farr, 770 P.2d 131 (Utah 1989).

Ramona v. Isabella, Rose and Western Medical Center, case no. C61898 (Cal. Super. Ct., May 13, 1994).

Ramona v. Ramona, no. B091052 (Cal. App. Dept. Super. Ct., Oct. 9, 1995).

Sarno, G. G. (1986). "Liability of Physician, for Injury to or Death of Third Party, Due to Failure to Disclose Driving-Related Impediment." *American Law Review* 4: 153–171.

Schatzberg A. F., and C. B. Nemeroff (1995). *Textbook of Psychopharmacology.* Washington: American Psychiatric Press.

Siebert, S. W., and S. B. Silver (1990). "Psychiatrists' Relationships with the General Public." In *American Psychiatric Press Review of Clinical Psychiatry and the Law,* vol. 2, ed. R. I. Simon. Washington: American Psychiatric Press.

Simon, R. I. (1985). "Coping Strategies for the Unduly Defensive Psychiatrist." *International Journal of Medicine and Law* 4: 551–561.

Simon, R. I. (1989). "Beyond the Doctrine of Informed Consent: A Clinician's Perspective." *Journal for the Expert Witness, The Trial Attorney, The Trial Judge* 4 (Fall): 23–25.

Simon, R. I. (1992). *Clinical Psychiatry and the Law.* 2nd ed. Washington: American Psychiatric Press.

Simon, R. I. (1995). "Toward the Development of Guidelines in the Forensic Psychiatric Examination of Posttraumatic Stress Disorder Claimants." In *Posttraumatic Stress Disorder in Litigation,* ed. R. I. Simon. Washington: American Psychiatric Press.

Simon, R. I. (1996). *Bad Men Do What Good Men Dream: A Forensic Psychiatrist Illuminates the Darker Side of Human Behavior.* Washington: American Psychiatric Press.

Simon, R. I. (1997). "Clinical Risk Management of the Rapid Cycling Bipolar Patient." *Harvard Review of Psychiatry* 4: 245–254.

Simon, R. I. (in press a). "Discharging Potentially Violent Psychiatric Inpatients in the Managed Care Era: Clinical Responsibilities and Duties." *Psychiatric Services.*

Simon, R. I. (in press b). "Discharging Potentially Violent Psychiatric Inpatients in the Managed Care Era: Standard of Care and Risk Management." *Psychiatric Annals.*

Simon, R. I., and T. G. Gutheil (1997). "Clinical-Ethical and Risk Management Principles in Recovered Memories Cases: Maintaining Therapist Neutrality." In *Trauma and Memory: Clinical and Legal Controversies,* ed. P. S. Appelbaum, L. Uyehara, and M. Ellin. New York: Oxford University Press.

Simon, R. I., and R. L. Sadoff (1992). *Psychiatric Malpractice: Cases and Comments for Clinicians.* Washington: American Psychiatric Press.

Slovenko, R. (1989). "Misadventures of Psychiatry with the Law." *Journal of Psychiatry and Law* 17: 115–156.

Solnick, P. B. (1985). "Proxy Consent for Incompetent Nonterminally Ill Adult Patients." *Journal of Legal Medicine* 6: 1–49.

Strasburger, L. H. (1987). "'Crudely, without Any Finesse': The Defendant Hears His Psychiatric Evaluation." *Bulletin of the American Academy of Psychiatry and Law* 15: 229–233.

Wickline v. State of California, 183 Cal. App. 3d 1175, 228 Cal. Rptr. 661 (Cal. Ct. App. 1986).

Wilson v. Blue Cross of Southern California et al., 222 Cal. App. 3d 660, 271 Cal. Rptr. 876 (Cal. Ct. App. 1990).

9

Supervisor, Supervisee, and Medical Backup

Thomas G. Gutheil, M.D.

There are several reasons why the risk management principles that apply to supervisors are important to review and consider. First, in malpractice litigation plaintiffs' attorneys are guided by what is known as the "deep pockets principle": you sue where the money is.[1] The relevance of this principle to the supervisory arrangement is that it is to the plaintiffs' attorneys' benefit if they can combine the insurance coverage of the supervisee with that of the supervisor by tarring both with the brush of negligence. This means a deeper pocket of potential reimbursement for the litigation.

The second aspect rendering this area an important one is the fact that supervision in some form is an intrinsic part of all professional training in America and elsewhere. One's specialty training, be it a psychology internship, a surgical residency, psychiatry residency, or psychoanalytic instruction, involves extended supervision phases during which active treatment, of course, is going on. Furthermore, the hierarchic structure of many institutions such as hospitals has implicit supervisory elements in the chain of command.

In psychiatry in particular, an extremely common model of health care delivery involves a nonmedical therapist such as a psychologist or social worker administering the therapy to the client or patient and a psychiatrist prescribing medication, serving, as it is termed, as medical backup.[2] This model may or may not involve the psychiatrist serving as supervisor to the nonmedical therapist. In an even more unfortunate and potentially risky situation in a liability context, the psychiatrist may be unaware that he or she is functioning as a supervisor and will be so considered by the court. The psychiatrist may envision himself or herself as merely a colleague and collaborator in the treatment. Portraying the psychiatrist in the supervisory rather than collegial role permits the plaintiff's attorney to extend the track of liability to the psychiatrist's usually much more extensive coverage—a particular version of the deep pocket.

With this background, let us look at the various structures of supervision as they relate to risk of liability.

The Two Models

In common clinical practice, supervision commonly adheres to one of two basic models. These might be styled the oversight model and the consultation model. These differ in significant ways in terms of both clinical practice and liability. In a direct oversight or hierarchic model of supervision, supervision is required and implicit because of the structural context in which it occurs. The classic example of this is the attending being responsible for direct oversight of the resident in a teaching-hospital setting. Whether or not the attending—as the fully trained, credentialed staff member—actually interviews the patient, prescribes the medication, or writes the clinical orders, the attending is structurally responsible for the care delivered by the trainee. As might be understood from this conceptualization, this form of supervision involves someone who is directly in the chain of command as it would apply to a particular patient.

This form of supervision has other implications. The first is that the supervisor may be responsible for hiring and firing under suitable conditions. If a supervisee under certain problematic circumstances refuses to perform some particular required action, the supervisor in this model may place the supervisee's job at risk. This is, again, a reflection of the authority over the supervisee that is held by the supervisor in this model. It is clear from this that the direct-oversight supervisor can issue or write orders on the care of the patient, either in the absence of the trainee or, under extreme circumstances, in direct countervention to the trainee's orders—for example, to admit or discharge a patient against the trainee's wishes. The ability to countermand the trainee's order is an illustration of the direct authority of that supervisor.

In addition to all the foregoing functions, the supervisor in this model usually has a direct performance-evaluation role, particularly clear for trainees, but arguably present in all hierarchic structures as regards credentialing. That is, senior staff, in general, are expected to monitor junior staff, even in treatment-delivery settings that are not formally designated as teaching hospitals. This evaluation role is peculiar to this model of supervision.

In economic terms, it is fairly unusual for this kind of supervisor to be paid by the supervisee. Rather, the institution as a whole usually handles the salary for the supervisor and hires into that role in a selective manner, attempting to choose individuals who, in addition to performing whatever service functions may be involved, are also good at teaching and have garnered high marks in the training context. Finally, the status of the supervisor and supervisee is clearly unequal, since one may be a trainee and the other an established staff member; the relative roles within the hierarchy may be that of junior in relation to senior. This unequal status is the final hallmark of this model of supervision.

The consultative model represents an entirely different approach to the question of supervision, although the term "supervision" is confusingly used for both models. The consultative model involves voluntary rather than required supervision. Very commonly, consultation is specifically or formally requested by the consultee (supervisee), although other precipitants for the consultation may also apply. In general the consultant is *not* in the chain of command within the hierarchy of the system and is invited to consult, in part, because of an independence and autonomy from the treatment staff or team. In part because of this relationship, the consultative supervisor rarely has any hiring or firing power or authority over the supervisee. He or she is an outsider to the structure of the organization and thus has no such control over the supervisee's actions.

The essence of the consultative supervisory model is that the only commodity dispensed is advice, rather than, under any circumstances, orders. This advice is given on a "take it or leave it" basis and is proffered to promote the understanding, level of care, or personal growth of the individual supervisee rather than to realize the goals of the institution or organization. In the same manner, these consultants are usually, but not always, nonreporting in relation to the supervisee. That is, unlike the hierarchic arrangement, these supervisors usually lack the evaluative function.

These individuals are usually paid by the supervisee in some manner. Since this is an elective and personal arrangement, reimbursement in the form of salary is less typical. Finally, these individuals are on a broadly equal footing with the supervisee. Some sort of peer consultation, in fact, may be included in this model of supervision, and the implication is that the relationships between consultant and consultee are more collegial than hierarchic, even though the consultant is usually chosen for particular skills or knowledge more extensive than those of the consultee.

In medicolegal consultative practice, I have found areas of confusion for psychiatrists about which of these two models directly applies. Psychiatrists working in small community clinics, for example, may assume that they are working *with* the social workers and psychologists who share the same building or suite of offices, but may discover in the context of litigation, to their dismay, that through unknown contractual arrangements the social workers and psychologists are considered to be working *for* the psychiatrists as supervisees. This is one of the more disturbing discoveries that clinicians can make shortly before trial.

The Liability Context

Liability in relation to supervision also occurs in two broad categories: negligent supervision and supervisory vicarious liability. *Negligent supervision* refers to the claim by the plaintiff in the case that certain harm occurred within the treatment duty because the supervision of the trainee was below the standard of care of the average supervisor in that specialty and situation. Here, for example, the attending is faulted for failing to exercise sufficient control and direction over the supervisee resident so that certain harm allegedly resulted to the patient being cared for. In this model the supervisor's own behavior is held up to scrutiny: the supervisor's own behavior is at issue.

The notion of *vicarious liability*, on the other hand, holds the supervisor responsible for someone else's behavior; the liability is not for the supervisor's own conduct, but for the vicarious responsibility tracking up the chain of command from the supervisee. The legal principle here is captured by the Latin phrase *respondeat superior*, which translates as "let the master answer for the deeds of the servant." This ancient legal principle still governs in supervisory constructs and may fault, vicariously, the attending for the resident's behavior, the unit head for the unit employee's behavior, the department head for the staff member's behavior, the institutional head for staff behavior, and so on.

The Medical Backup Arrangement

For the young psychiatrist starting out, choosing to serve as the psychopharmacologic member of a treatment team is a fairly common and popular role; often the physician in this situation also serves as liaison for a patient to the general medical community and as an "early warning system" for medical symptoms. Though extremely common in clinical practice, this function is scanted in the professional literature, for unclear reasons. However, it represents a potential exposure to certain forms of liability on either the negligent supervision or the vicarious liability model, largely because of lack of clarity about the nature of the arrangement and the agreements under which the arrangement will be carried out. To aid in more precisely defining this relationship and to offer some risk management protections, I have suggested the so-called Eight C's of medical backup:[3]

1. CLARITY

The respective roles of the parties involved must be clear from the outset. For example, is the psychopharmacologist, in addition to prescribing medications for the patient being treated in this joint model, expected to supervise the care in a manner which might require formal meetings to review the case at reasonably regular intervals? Who is expected to cover during vacations of either party? If supervision is required or desired, will that be administered by the psychiatrist on the case or from within the nonmedical therapist's own discipline from an entirely separate quarter? What is the arrangement during emergencies? Who should be called first? These and other questions should be carefully hammered out and documented before the arrangement is actually put into place with a patient.

2. CONTRACT

It is helpful, once clarity has been achieved, to enshrine the arrangement in a contractual form. This need not be an elaborate document bristling with legal boilerplate; rather, it should be a simple articulation of the arrangements. The preparation and drafting of this contract may well be a significant adjunct to the clarification of roles.

3. CONSENT

Though this step may be implicit in the medical backup arrangement, as with all other interventions, the patient's consent is required to have the treatment divided in the manner under consideration. That is, the patient should agree to whatever arrangements are relevant, including the sharing of the treatment by two parties. The patient should also be aware of the telephone and emergency hierarchies that have been decided upon by the parties in question.

4. COMPREHENSIVE VIEW

Because the prescribing psychiatrist usually has significantly greater malpractice coverage than practitioners in other disciplines, he or she is a far more likely target of litigation than the nonmedical therapist. On this basis alone, it is a sound risk management principle for that treating psychiatrist to maintain a comprehensive view of the case even though his or her pragmatic role may be limited to medication assessment and review of medical problems as they emerge. This means that the psychiatrist should arrange to be updated on the general state of the case on a regular basis, particularly in periods of decompensation or crisis or of significant life events (divorces, deaths) as they might impinge on the care. If, for example, the patient experiences a sudden trauma between physician appointments, the agreement should include the psychiatrist's being updated as to such life events even before seeing the patient the next time.

5. COMMUNICATION

This principle has several elements. First, it is extremely important that the patient's consent be obtained for the essentially limitless sharing of information between psychiatrist and nonmedical therapist. Any more restrictive arrangement hampers the capacity of this treatment dyad to respond quickly and decisively to crises and emergencies. The smooth delivery of care is also significantly hampered when the practitioners must pick and choose what information may freely be shared and what is proscribed. If a patient refuses to agree to this free sharing of information, serious consideration should be given to refusing to undertake the case, since most of the real difficulties that occur both clinically and in terms of liability flow from communicative difficulties and roadblocks. Second, some comfortable arrangement should be made for regular mutual communication about the progress of the case, such that both parties remain on top of clinical developments.

6. CREDENTIALING

Clinicians may be unaware of their responsibility for performing at least minimal credentialing before they sign on for a collaborative agreement. This may include such simple factors as being sure that the potential collaborator has a valid license in his or her discipline as well as whatever certification is required to practice and a valid diploma of graduation from the specialty school. Although such investigation can usually be abbreviated if the nonmedical therapist is well known to the psychiatrist, it is generally a good risk management principle to check on these basic documents.

An additional point should be made to cover the new contingency of a psychiatrist being responsible for credentialing a nurse who has been granted limited prescribing privileges under the new model currently in use in some states. It seems the issues here are in some ways far more complex. I would recommend a more systematic approach to credentialing, following the model suggested by James Hilliard, an attorney knowledgeable in these matters (personal communication). The credentialing of a prescribing nurse-clinician for whom one is supervising should include the following:

1. Proof of the nurse's registered nurse credential and licensing requirements for the expanded role of nurse prescriber.
2. DEA and FDA certificates.
3. $1,000,000–$3,000,000 liability coverage.
4. Two references specific to the expanded role as nurse prescriber.
5. Board of Registration disclosure relating to actions or claims against the nurse.
6. Sworn statement regarding substance abuse difficulties by the nurse in question.

7. CONTACT

The arrangement between the parties and the patient's consent should also govern the psychiatrist's freedom to have contact with the patient via a direct one-to-one interview at any point deemed necessary. The purpose of this might be to intervene in a decompensation or other crisis to evaluate a potential ongoing medical condition or other reasonable function. Once again, the agreement that this is within the arrangement from its initiation will save many difficulties later on in the course of the treatment.

8. CONSULTATION

Consultation is fully as appropriate for the treatment dyad (nonmedical therapist and physician) as for any other treater. When differences of opinion or conflicts arise, both parties may seek consultation with an appropriate source. Such consultation may or may not include the patient under certain circumstances. Such an approach may be extremely valuable not only in breaking up difficulties and logjams in the delivery of care but also in protecting the clinicians against the claim of liability.

Psychiatrists in the medical backup situation may not only write prescriptions for their patients but also be involved in signing or "signing off on" various insurance forms or other mechanisms of reimbursement. One pitfall that my consultative experience reveals is that psychiatrists tend to minimize or underestimate their role in the treatment, based on their perceived narrowness of their functioning. "I'm not really this patient's doctor," some psychiatrists may plaintively argue; "I *only* write prescriptions or sign off on insurance forms." For the purpose of risk management, however, I suggest that these measures are fully adequate to decree a legal duty in the eyes of the litigative process. The mnemonic I offer on this point goes: "If you sign, the case is thine." Psychiatrists should understand that this "mere signature" represents the taking on of full professional responsibility for the patient.

All too many psychiatrists, in addition, are unfamiliar with the APA's guidelines on psychiatric signatures.[4] It is valuable to have clear in one's own mind the fundamental issue addressed by those guidelines, namely, that a signature alone may be insufficient information to clarify the nature of the relationship and the responsibilities of the physician. Hence, the signature should usually be accompanied by explicatory prose. For example, "Case reviewed by (signature)," "Under the supervision of (name)," and the like, or "Treatment plan reviewed (patient not seen), (signature)." These additional statements eliminate the perilous ambiguity of the signature alone—an ambiguity into which plaintiffs' claims of duties and responsibilities beyond the imagination of the treating therapist might well flow.

In the medical backup context, if differences are irreconcilable between the two clinicians, the psychiatrist may have to withdraw from the case. Remember that since this is a treatment relationship in the fullest sense of the word, the psychiatrist must make reasonable efforts to replace him- or herself or to allow the nonmedical therapist adequate time to do so, so as to avoid the risk of abandonment of the patient, a risk which would be fully as applicable here as if the psychiatrist were the only practitioner in the case.

In the modern era, a special form of consultation/supervision has become relevant in certain parts of clinical practice. The market has made available a number of computer programs that offer certain guidance on medical decisionmaking, such as risk-benefit analysis of a decision or the compatibility of different drugs when used for a given patient, as well as selected treatment modality and choice of neuroleptic. These special consultations—though not as powerful a risk management and clinical decisionmaking tool as a consultation with an expert (human) colleague—are still an improvement over no consultation at all. The use of such programs should be carefully documented and in case of a malpractice allegation may serve as support for the idea that the clinician's decisionmaking comported with the average reasonable practitioner's level of care.

Risk Management Caveats for Supervisors

When one is responsible for a number of supervisees (as might be the case for the attending on a hospital unit, who may be responsible for several residents), it is somewhat risky to assume that all residents have uniform capability; that is, that all trainees can do all things. It is important to assign cases with some selectivity designed to meet the capacities of the trainees. This may require close scrutiny of the supervisee's skills before assigning treatment responsibilities.

One should be careful not to spread the supervision or the supervisors themselves too thin. While economic stresses and staffing problems at many institutions place considerable strain on the institution's ability to provide adequate oversight, the excessive dilution of the supervisory pool may be a false economy with significant elements of risk.

Finally, in the supervisory process it is important to listen carefully for "silences" in the form of omissions of important clinical data or failure to perform actual duties. Many difficulties and problem areas may be communicated "under silence" rather than under direct reportage to a supervisor. The attending or supervisor should also maintain a low threshold for direct interview with the patient, since few alternative sources supply information as valuable as this direct exploration.

In the sometimes rocky journey from trainee to full-fledged practitioner, supervisors may encounter a supervisee who appears to be indulging in risky conduct; that is, taking chances, indulging in shortcuts that may or may not be problematic. In the service of the delicate balance between acknowledging one's responsibility for trainees and fostering their autonomy as clinicians, supervisors should avoid the temptation to respond too quickly and too definitively for the requirements of the clinical situation. The supervisor should maintain a hierarchic view of the level of intervention required: counsel, recommend, threaten to report, report.

Counseling should be the first step in any supervisory interaction, since it is arguably the core of the supervisory process. The supervisor's experience and training are brought to bear on the situation in the form of suggestions. Should these fail, the supervisory intervention may move on to a recommendation, where the suggestion of what to do is couched in more formally and forcefully prescriptive terms. Should this fail and the quality of patient care appear to be endangered, the supervisor may have to invoke the threat of reportage to the academic or clinical senior staff. If even this fails, actual reporting to senior staff may be called for. The speed with which the supervisor traverses this sequence is determined by the safety and well-being of the patient in tension with the freedom of the trainee to make some safe mistakes in the service of learning.

Boundary Issues

Although the American Psychiatric Association proscribed sexual contact with supervisors in its 1988 revision of the code of ethics, this is an area that has not been extensively addressed in the clinical literature as yet. But it is one that may be an important focus of future litigation.

Four principles underlie the issue of boundaries in the supervisor/supervisee relationship. First, as a rule, the supervisor should take responsibility for the setting of appropriate boundaries. This issue has proven no less challenging than the comparable issue in clinician/patient settings. Is it appropriate for a supervisor to give a cocktail party for all his or her supervisees? Probably so. Would the same apply to a one-on-one dinner? Is the equation altered in any way if supervisor and supervisee represent potential social objects for each other (opposite sexes and a heterosexual context; same sex and a homosexual context)? It probably depends. In general, however, supervision has the qualities—a fiduciary relationship and a power asymmetry—that require consideration of boundary issues between the parties.

The principle of abstinence, so important in clinical work, is also relevant in the supervisor/supervisee relationship. The supervisor should keep the focus on the learning experience of the supervisee. Thus the supervisor "abstains" from direct primary gratification other than the satisfaction of doing one's job well. This principle will probably guide most interactions in a positive direction.

The duty of neutrality similarly may be applicable here. That is, the supervisor should remain neutral in the interaction such that the focus remains on the trainee's learning experience and educational growth. Such a position will, in general, preclude overly judgmental, overly personal, or social or romantic relatedness. However, the forced intimacy of the residency-attending relationship may make the boundaries somewhat looser than might otherwise be the case. For example, most clinicians regard it as nonviolative of any significant boundaries if attending and trainee (of same genders) share one on-call room when both are on duty.

Finally, the supervisor is to foster the personal and professional autonomy of the trainees. This means the supervisor should avoid behavior which increases the trainee's dependence on the supervisor.

How pervasive is this problem? The literature records a range of sexual contact with supervisors from 1.2 percent of male Canadian psychiatric residents to 22 percent of female doctoral students.[5]

Supervisory boundary violations include problems of role, where the supervisor merges into other functions such as date, therapist, patient, and so on; difficulties in adhering to times (omission of too many sessions, excessive extension of sessions); alterations of place (private home, social settings); difficulties around money (alterations in the fee agreements, failure to pay excessive charges); social, romantic, or sexual behaviors of various kinds based on violation of the propriety of the arrangement and the capacity to consent of the supervisee, who is in a fiduciary relationship where the supervisor's evaluation might affect his or her final grade and future career; self-disclosure by the supervisor in ways that are not didactic in purpose but turn the supervisee into a social confidant; the notion that "while other supervisors and supervisees could not have this kind of sexual relationship, it's okay for us because our connection is unique and our chemistry is special"; and the use of the supervisee by the supervisor for various institutional political purposes, such as the forging of alliances and oppositions.

All these situations pose questions similar to the therapeutic question of boundary crossings versus boundary violations in therapy.[6] It is useful to think of boundary crossings as benign deviations from strict role function (such as giving a tearful supervisee a tissue although that is not a strictly supervisory function) that do not harm—but may even enhance—the supervisory alliance. A boundary violation, in contrast, exploits the power differential of the supervisory relationship to take advantage of the supervisee for erotic, narcissistic, dependency, or other inappropriate goals. Supervisory boundary violations, then, may give rise to problems such as loss or damage to the supervisor; loss or damage to the supervisee; loss or damage to the patient; and loss or damage to others, including the clinical program. When a very senior supervisor married a former supervisee some time after the latter's completion of the training program, other staff members felt that the program had been compromised because they no longer felt safe.

A very common consultation question involves a supervisor's duties and responsibilities when a supervisee reports a boundary violation. I say "reports" deliberately, since commonly supervisees minimize or fail to report boundary violations with their patients out of shame, conflict, or—rarely but ominously—the wish to hide conscious wrongdoing.

Broadly speaking, such matters should be handled comparably to other missteps in the learning process, with an additional caveat: the supervisor should remain unthreateningly alert to mild boundary crossings and to possible issues between the lines of the report. Warning signs should provoke, not punitive criticism of the supervisee's character flaws, but an opening of discussion of boundary issues, the supervisee's avowed intent, the importance of context, and so on. Directed readings may be useful.

For more serious situations, more active solutions such as removal from a case, intensified supervision, case monitoring via one-way mirror, or recommendation for therapy for the supervisee may be called for. Case law on these situations tends to focus on what the supervisor knew and whether reasonable responses and remedies were employed.

Risk Management Approaches

The solutions to the above problems, though perhaps predictable, are worth reviewing here. First, supervisors should stay in their role and stay focused on the task at hand. Temptations and distractions should be filtered out for the protection of the clinical and educative work. Second, self-monitoring of the relationship similar to "countertransference hygiene" in clinical work should be a regular part of supervision. This would also be helpful to protect against other forms of excessively personal or judgmental engagement with the educational process. Next, vigilance as to preservation of the process should be an ongoing accompaniment of work with the supervisee. Here, the principles of abstinence and neutrality might be most clearly focused.

Consultation for the supervisor should be freely sought. Supervisors should also be familiar with relevant guidelines.[7] On occasion, consultation to the educational dyad of supervisor and supervisee may be appropriate, but much can be accomplished by presenting the supervision situation or dilemma to an experienced and knowledgeable colleague. Finally, education in principles of supervision or the resolution of supervisory impasses may be sought in the admittedly limited literature on this subject. Such continuing educational processes are as valuable in supervisory work as in the clinical sphere.

/ / /

In clinical work, supervision is a central component of the educational and clinical processes. The use of effective supervision is itself a risk management protection for the supervisee. With this protection, however, goes an increase in potential exposure to liability for the supervisor. If the risk management principles articulated in this chapter are followed, this risk may be successfully minimized.

Notes

1. P. S. Appelbaum and T. G. Gutheil, *Clinical Handbook of Psychiatry and the Law* (Baltimore: Williams and Wilkins, 1991).
2. R. G. Vasile and T. G. Gutheil, "The Psychiatrist as 'Medical Back-up': Ambiguity in the Delegation of Clinical Responsibility," *American Journal of Psychiatry* 136 (1979): 1292–96.
3. T. G. Gutheil, "Risk Management at the Margins: Less Familiar Topics in Psychiatric Malpractice," *Harvard Review of Psychiatry* 2 (1994): 214–221.
4. American Psychiatric Association, "Guidelines Regarding Psychiatrists' Signatures," *American Journal of Psychiatry* 146 (1989): 1390.
5. K. S. Pope, H. Levenson, and L. Schover, "Sexual Intimacy in Psychology Training: Results and Implications of a National Survey," *American Psychologist* 34 (1979): 682–689. M. L. Carr et al., "A Survey of Canadian Psychiatric Residents regarding Resident-Educator Sexual Contact," *American Journal of Psychiatry* 148 (1991): 216–220. R. D. Glaser and J. S. Thorpe, "Unethical Intimacy: A Survey of Sexual Contact and Advances between Psychology Educators and Female Graduate Students," *American Psychologist* 41 (1986): 43–51.
6. T. G. Gutheil and G. O. Gabbard, "The Concept of Boundaries in Clinical Practice: Theoretical and Risk Management Dimensions," *American Journal of Psychiatry* 150 (1993): 188–196.
7. E.g., American Psychiatric Association, "Guidelines for Psychiatrists in Consultative, Supervisory or Collaborative Relationships with Non-medical Therapists," *American Journal of Psychiatry* 137 (1980): 1489–91; P. S. Appelbaum, "General Guidelines for Psychiatrists Who Prescribe Medication for Patients Treated by Non-medical Therapists," *Hospital and Community Psychiatry* 42 (1991): 281–282.

10

The Violent Patient

James Beck, M.D., Ph.D.

Prudence Baxter, M.D.

The way to minimize your risk in dealing with violent patients is to maintain a focus on the clinical issues involved. Thinking about legal implications is likely to impair your capacity to carefully assess your patient. For that reason, this chapter is almost entirely about clinical risk assessment and has little to say about the law.

In recent years, research on mental disorder and violence has provided some useful information. There is now good reason to believe that there is an association between mental disorder and violence. This association is mediated by the presence of acute psychosis.[1]

When a person is acutely psychotic, whether or not that person is a patient, the person is at increased risk of violence. We can be even more precise. When a person is experiencing delusions of influence or control, violence is especially likely.[2] Among people who are mentally ill, as among people generally, alcohol and other substances are strongly associated with violence.[3]

There is considerable research on risk markers for violence in the population generally. Variables associated with violence include youth, male gender, low I.Q., coming from a subculture of violence, and a childhood history of violence in the family. However, it is important not to assume that these markers hold true for patients. The fact of being a patient may make a difference. For example, among patients brought to a psychiatric emergency service in a general hospital, violence was equally likely among men and women.[4] A person may be a patient in part as a result of having been violent. Therefore, the base rates of violence in particular demographic groups may or may not be relevant.

The assessment of potential for violence involves having a conceptual framework that helps dictate what information is important—and into which you insert the data that you gather. It is important to be aware of what research has documented, but this knowledge is a background for the assessment of the individual patient, not a substitute for this assessment. Careful assessment requires having a knowledge of demographics and diagnosis, making careful observations, being thorough, gathering history, and having the kind of curiosity about an individual and his or her history that will motivate you to delve beneath the surface.

It also requires the assessment of any violence that may already have occurred. This may seem obvious, but obvious things are frequently the things to which we pay insufficient attention. This notion—*that the assessment of potential for violence involves the analysis of violence that may have already occurred*—is central to our discussion.

Following an orderly process of assessment will allow you in the end to make informed predictions of the likelihood of whether—and under what circumstances—a patient will get into trouble, and thus to do treatment planning that makes sense.

A Philosophy of Assessment

It is easy to run around reading records, interviewing patients and family members, perusing criminal records if you have access to them, and so on. You may even convince yourself that this is productive activity. However, you may well be engaging in an effort that will neither yield all the information you need nor help you to interpret it in a useful way, if you do not go about it systematically. A systematic approach depends on having a conceptual framework into which to put the data you gather.

The conceptual framework is simple. *Individuals do not exist in a vacuum and violence does not occur in one either.* Rather, violent behavior results from the interaction of the person and a situation. Thus, the assessment task involves identifying *situational, interpersonal, and biological/diagnostic/mental-status factors*—specific to the individual you're evaluating—that affect his or her potential for violence. Ultimately, you will be weaving together the information that is specific to the patient's situation with demographic and research data. This will help you make informed decisions about how to manage the patient and the situation that has led you to be concerned about possible violence.

Another part of this conceptual framework involves delineating *factors that tend to increase or decrease the likelihood of violence.* These factors can be either internal—that is, related to the person's thoughts, perceptions, feelings—or external—that is, related to environmental or other situations that exist outside of the individual. The following are offered as examples on which you could no doubt expand:

Internal factors which make violence more likely: impulsivity, anger, frustration, rage, hostility, humiliation, fear, helplessness, jealousy, hate, grandiosity, paranoid delusions, command hallucinations. Any organic disorder, either diagnosed or unrecognized, involving the brain or affecting brain function secondarily.

External factors which make violence more likely: behavior/availability of target, stress, weapons, drugs/alcohol, lack of nonviolent options, facilitating environment.

Internal factors that tend to inhibit violence: learned values, empathy, moral/religious beliefs, feeling respected, absence of instigating symptoms.

External factors that tend to inhibit violence: fear of harm/punishment, social supports, mental health treatment (medication and other), inadequate means of attack, nonviolent options, chance to communicate concerns, being treated respectfully.

What We Mean by Violence

It is important in making assessments of potential for violence to *be specific*. To describe two different individuals—one who routinely shoves family members when acutely psychotic, and another who stalks and then kills someone for whatever reason—as "violent people" does justice to neither the person nor the word "violent." This leads to a corollary principle: violence is not an attribute of a person, like height or hair color: "tall woman, blond man, violent person." If it is sufficient to describe a person as violent, then it does not really matter how he or she is violent, or when, or why. That is, it allows you to bypass making assessments of potential for violence because you already have your conclusion—the person is violent.

You need to be specific when you are making assessments. In what way has the person been violent? What has she or he done? What happened? It is one thing to be violent toward a television set. It is another to be violent toward a person. It is one thing to be violent using a butter knife as a weapon, another to be violent using a Uzi.

The word "violent" standing on its own is not a useful piece of professional shorthand. Be careful of using the phrase "this is a violent patient" unless you are also prepared to be specific about what you mean.

Professional Contexts

You work on inpatient units, in crisis teams, in an office—either as part of a clinic or on your own. It is often the case that once someone is hospitalized, something violent has already happened (particularly in these days of tighter requirements for hospitalization). In an emergency room or crisis team, something may have already happened or there may be immediate concern that something may happen. You may learn that a patient has a history of some kind of violence. Or you may have a concern—which is more or less urgent—that your client may engage in a violent act. Working in these different settings, you will be approaching the assessment task from slightly different angles; you may have access to different amounts and kinds of information on an immediate basis, and you may feel more or less constrained—based on either legitimate or less-informed concerns about issues such as confidentiality—in seeking additional information.

It goes beyond the scope of this chapter to address issues about when and under what specific circumstances you have a right to get additional information without your patient's permission—beyond saying that as a general rule: *when you have a legitimate and immediate concern that your client may harm another person you should go about getting the information you need to make a good assessment regardless of whether or not you have permission from the client to do so.* It is preferable to be sued for a breach of confidentiality than for a wrongful death.

While you may be approaching the assessment task from slightly different angles, and for different reasons, the task at its core remains the same: to gather as much information as you can about the what, when, and why of the behavior that concerns you.

Assessing the Potential for Violence

A thorough assessment of potential for violence includes (1) an analysis of the violent episode, or set of circumstances such as threats, that leads you to have concerns about your patient's potential for violence; (2) a review of any past history of violence; (3) an assessment of the patient's insight into his or her behavior; and (4) verification of the patient's overall medical status—either ascertaining that the patient has had a medical work-up which would rule in or out relevant disorders, for example seizures, thyroid disease; or arranging for the patient to have a medical evaluation.

Violence is only rarely a function of an undiagnosed organic problem.

For this reason, mental health professionals often forget to consider the possibility. If you do not think about it, you will never make the diagnosis when the disease is there.

The steps outlined below draw heavily on an instrument developed by the Forensic Division of the Massachusetts Department of Mental Health. This instrument, called the Violent Behavior Assessment Form, has been used in the assessment of readiness for privileges or discharge of hospitalized patients with histories of violence. The information it calls for is also relevant to assessment in other settings.

If there has been a recent violent incident that has led you to have concerns about what lies ahead, the first task is to do an *analysis of the incident*. This involves not only describing what happened in as detailed a fashion as you can, but also looking at the context—social, interpersonal, physical—in which it occurred. Sources you can draw on include the patient, the victim, other witnesses, and possibly police reports. Note any discrepancies among these accounts.

In describing what happened, it is not sufficient to say that the patient hit someone. You need to know a number of things—from exactly what "hit" means (shove, slap, closed fist into the face)—to whether the other person was hurt, and if so, how seriously. Did the victim require medical attention?

Once you know what happened—and we can not stress enough the importance of this—you should gather data that will help explain and/or put in context what happened. First, look at *situational variables:*

Patient's living situation.
Patient's employment status. (Note: instability of housing and employment is correlated with higher rates of violence.)
Setting/location of the incident.
Presence of others at the time.
Use or presence of weapon. Exactly what type of weapon?
Did incident occur in the context of other criminal activity?
Stresses such as loss of job, relationship, housing, money.

Next, assess *interpersonal factors* at the time of the incident:

Who is the victim, and what relationship, if any, does he or she have to the patient?
Age and gender of victim.
Did the victim engage in any behavior that the patient interpreted in either a reality-based or a delusional way as a provocation or threat?

Are there any family issues involved, such as denial of mental illness or enabling of alcohol or drug abuse; estrangement/rejection; control over finances or some other aspect of the patient's life?

Were any social supports, such as friends, family, therapist, available to the patient at the time of the incident? Were attempts made to use them?

Finally, look at *biological, psychological, and mental-status factors:*

Mental status at the time—for example, delusions (especially persecutory or of control), hallucinations (especially command), mood symptoms such as euphoria, irritability.

Medication at time of incident—what, how much, how long? Was medication stopped—when, why? Any recent change in medication—dose or type?

Substance abuse, both in general and at time of incident. Be specific: what, how much?

Personality issues. Is the patient impulsive, narcissistic? paranoid? predatory? Did any of these traits appear to be a contributing factor?

Overall health status.

With all of this, you should be able to paint a detailed picture of the episode. Instead of saying "the patient hit his mother," you know that, for example, in the context of increased substance abuse, the patient discontinued his medication, spent all of his money, and was tossed out of his rooming house, and in a visit to his family's home, excitedly and apparently accidentally bloodied his mother's lip as he grabbed for the disability check for which she is payee.

Once you have a good understanding of the violent episode, you can move on to a *review of the patient's history of violence.* If common characteristics exist across past incidents, you will be able to identify them, and from this you will be able to identify risk factors.

Essentially, you will be conducting the same analysis of past incidents as you did of the present one. The more remote these are, the more difficult the task can be. But it is important—now as before—to be as specific as possible. Again, sources of information can include family members, records, and other members of the patient's treatment team.

What *situational factors* emerge across past incidents of violence? Have past episodes happened in the context of homelessness or unemployment? Have they followed losses in the patient's life? Have weapons been involved? Have they generally happened in the same place (for example, the family home), or the same kind of place (for example, homeless shelters, bars, inpatient units, or city parks)?

What *interpersonal factors* emerge across past incidents? What relationship did the victim have to the patient? Are the victims generally family members? the same family member? women who are not known to the patient? children? robbery victims? Was there conduct on the part of the victim that the patient perceived—either rationally or delusionally—as a provocation? Were social supports present or absent at these times?

Finally, what *biological and/or mental-status factors* emerge across the history? Was the patient apparently delusional in a paranoid way, was he or she taking prescribed medication (and if not, how long had it been, and what do you know about any pattern of decompensation when medication is stopped), was the patient under the influence of alcohol or drugs, or impulsive or paranoid?

Assuming that patterns have emerged across episodes—and in our experience they often have—you are now in a position to know and describe those patterns. You will also know when the patient appears to be at relatively lower risk.

Finally, you need to *assess the patient's insight* into his or her violent behavior. Here, we are speaking of something concrete and practical. You need to assess whether your patient can be an active participant in a plan to avoid violent responses in the future. If the patient's internal controls are not adequate, will additional external structure be required—supervised housing, medication, living apart from potential victims? There should be an emergency contingency plan in place in case all else fails.

Does the patient acknowledge the violence or other behavior that leads you to be concerned about potential for future violence?

If so, is the patient concerned about it? Does he express either regret or remorse for what happened? Does she minimize what happened, or externalize blame? Does he say he does not want it to happen again, not necessarily for empathic reasons but for fear of the consequences to him? Does she have a fear of losing control or of getting into trouble that may form the basis for a treatment alliance?

Does the patient feel justified in having acted violently, either because he felt threatened or because she felt the victim deserved it?

Does the patient understand—on any level—any relationship between the violence and his mental illness and/or substance abuse; between violence and situational and/or interpersonal factors? Does she acknowledge the need for medication, and if so, do you believe her? Clearly, the patient's assurance that she will take medication because of her understanding that without it trouble ensues is not worth much if she has a history of saying that but not following through.

Does the patient appear genuinely interested in managing the mental illness that may have contributed to the violence or concern about violence? Does he recognize the external precipitants and his own symptoms that are flags for future violence?

What does she say about managing the factors—either internal or external—that led to previous violence in a different way in the future?

If the patient has little or no insight, has medication changed the mental status that contributed to violence? What structures are in place to ensure that he will continue to take it? Will a new housing situation increase the likelihood that his condition will remain stable? Will a new payee result in less conflict with family members?

In our experience schizophrenic patients rarely have insight into the fact that they are mentally ill. These patients have an active denial of their symptoms and the effect of their illness on their actions. Given the belief that they are not ill, they do not see the need for medication, or the connection between mental illness and violence.

In contrast to schizophrenics, patients with bipolar disorder often understand that they are ill and have the kind of insight that permits a genuine alliance with you. Again, this is not the kind of alliance we talk about in dynamic psychotherapy. The patient may not have any interest in using the alliance to investigate his own past and how it may contribute to his current difficulties. He may well be interested in making a reasonable plan to stay out of future trouble.

Finally, you are in a position to *assess the patient's potential for future violence,* which is, after all, the point of the exercise. This assessment generally comes, in the case of an individual who has already committed a violent act, after some kind of therapeutic intervention—be it medication change or hospitalization or reinvolvement in treatment. This assessment is part of figuring out how concerned you should be about the potential for violence.

If the patient has already committed a violent act, and has subsequently received treatment, you will use all the information you have gathered to look at *what has changed* since the behavior. Are the patient's present circumstances—either internal (for example, change in mental status, or new insight into precipitants to violence), or external (for example, medication, housing)—different from those in which he or she acted violently in the past?

When the patient has been hospitalized after a violent act, nonviolence in the hospital is not a sufficient basis to conclude that the risk is over. The question is, what else, if anything, is different about the patient. If nothing much is different about the patient, what else will be different about the situation? If the patient has been seriously violent, and your assessment is that the patient and the post-discharge situation will be the same, discharge is contraindicated.

You want to look at the situational factors—where is the patient living, and where will he probably be living on discharge from the hospital? Will she have work or other ways to structure her time? Will he have access to the kinds of weapons he used in the past? Will the kinds of life stresses that led to past incidents be predictably present or not?

Will he have access to the same victim or kinds of victims—family members or small children? What about social supports? Has she reconnected with her family, and will they continue to support her as long as she takes medication? Does he have a case manager or therapist he knows and trusts? Is there someone she can turn to when she is feeling frightened or threatened?

Is his attitude toward the violence different now from in the past? Can she identify symptoms or stressors associated with her vulnerability to violent responses?

Using the Information You Have Gathered

You have what may be a mass of data. And presumably, the more serious either the recent violent incident or the threat of violence, the more thoroughly you've done your data gathering, and the more information you have. You know as much as possible about the recent violent incident or specific circumstances that led you to be concerned, you know a lot about past episodes, and you have a good handle on their features in common. You know what the patient thinks about it all, you know how you've treated him or her, you know the patient's current mental status. What do you do with all this?

There is no magic formula into which you can plug all this data and get an answer that will assure you now and forever that the patient won't be violent in the future. Equally, there is no way to predict with certainty that the patient will be violent. However, there are a few risk markers that you should particularly keep in mind:

The patient is angry.
The patient has a motive, either delusional or realistic, for harming someone.
The patient drinks.
The patient is now or has been delusional, especially if the delusions involve influence or control.

Any of these should raise your suspicion that violence may occur. The more that are present, the more concerned you should be.

This is where we return to the philosophy of assessment with which we started. What are the internal and external factors specific to your patient that tend to inhibit or encourage violence? Weighing the different components is clearly an exercise that is in part subjective. But in a rough sense, if the internal and external factors that inhibit violence appear to outweigh those factors which encourage violence, you have a less potentially risky situation. Understanding your patient and his or her situation will help you decide whether you need to provide more external inhibitors to violence, or to continue to shore up internal curbs.

The assessment of potential for future violence is—or should be—a data-driven and orderly process, built on a conceptual foundation. However, it ultimately rests on the exercise of clinical judgment, and this is where experience comes in.

So far we have not talked about any legal issues which violence raises. That is intentional. The way to avoid legal difficulty is to do your clinical work thoroughly. Paradoxically, one way clinicians get in trouble is by thinking about what they need to do to avoid being sued. When this kind of thinking drives behavior, it tends to obscure the clinical issues. The clinician who does the kind of assessment we have outlined and who documents carefully that she has done it will be as safe as one can be against legal liability, regardless of the outcome of the case.

One last comment: when you are unsure about how much danger a patient poses, consider getting a consultation. Two heads are often better than one. In the event that serious violence does occur in the future, the fact that you have obtained a consultation, and documented it, will further immunize you against possible legal consequences.

Patients with histories of serious violence are scary patients, no question about it. You can minimize your own fear and the likelihood of future violence by taking the time to do the kind of assessment we have outlined in this chapter.

A Case Example

Mr. D. was a hard-working, married father of two. He was well until his wife took a new job. He developed delusional sexual jealousy—his wife was having affairs with many men, including a U.S. senator, a famous athlete, and a movie star.

He was laid off from his long-time job. He developed ideas of reference and believed that surveillance devices had been planted in his house. He tried to strangle his wife on one occasion.

He became increasingly paranoid, fearful, and bizarre. He began to experience auditory hallucinations saying "Your wife is a prostitute." His wife separated from him, taking custody of their two children. He was hospitalized, but escaped.

He became increasingly delusional and disorganized. He began to write threatening letters to the persons about whom he harbored delusional beliefs. He lost visitation privileges when he stopped his support payments. He wrote one letter threatening to maim and torture his ex-wife. She obtained a restraining order. He was not charged criminally, but he was involuntarily hospitalized at the state hospital. There was no history of drug use or alcohol abuse.

Psychological testing revealed a paranoid core; a personality that could be explosive if overwhelmed, preoccupied with sexual matters; with a breakdown in boundaries of fantasy and reality.

At the hospital he was guarded and withdrawn. He maintained, and his family of origin supported his belief, that his troubles were all his wife's fault. He denied that he was mentally ill, or that he was a danger to his wife or anyone else. He was treated with antipsychotic and antidepressant medication. His family of origin was offered treatment, but refused.

After three months in the hospital without incident, staff were considering discharging the patient. They gave Mr. D. a grounds pass. He left the grounds, retrieved his car, and drove past his ex-wife's new home. When staff confronted him with this, he gave three different self-justifying stories about the reason he had done so. He continued to deny that his wife had any reason to feel threatened by him.

Staff reconsidered their discharge plan, and gave him a new individual therapist. The therapist and the psychiatrist together confronted the patient with the expectation that he must come to terms with his past behavior if he wanted to leave the hospital.

Over the next year, the patient made slow, steady progress in psychotherapy. He first was able to acknowledge he had a mental illness. He then was able to acknowledge that he had threatened his wife, and that he had been mentally ill and confused when he had done so. Slowly he acknowledged the extent of his past violence and took responsibility for it. He acknowledged that he needed to take medication in order to avoid again becoming confused. He acknowledged that his ex-wife had been reasonably frightened of him and that she was entitled to live her own life free of harassment from him.

He initiated an orderly plan to obtain supervised visitation with his children. He used grounds privileges and then off-grounds privileges without incident. He was discharged to a quarter-way house on the grounds with plans for an eventual transition to a community residence.

COMMENT

In this case, the pattern of violence was clear. First he developed delusional jealousy when his wife was more independent and had opportunities to meet other men. Next there was a realistic loss when he was laid off. Later there was a second realistic loss and a narcissistic injury: his wife left him.

The patient's delusional disorder worsened markedly. The delusions clearly related to his wife's rejection of him. The violence was related concretely to the delusions. In his violent behavior, he was retaliating against his rejecting wife.

This case illustrates a common error. The error is assuming that it is safe to discharge a patient because the patient is behaviorally stable in the hospital. When staff first gave Mr. D. grounds privileges, only his situation had changed. When questioned, Mr. D. continued to blame his wife for his difficulties.

This case also illustrates that medication alone was ineffective without psychotherapy. Only a long hospitalization with careful psychotherapeutic work plus medication led to improvement.

Finally, the case illustrates the kind of change that permits successful discharge. When Mr. D. was ultimately given privileges successfully, much had changed. He acknowledged his past violence, linked it to his mental disorder, and spoke convincingly of his need to continue on his medication in order to maintain his improvement. Now Mr. D. was ready to leave the hospital, and, slowly, to explore reentry into the community.

Risk assessment for the future suggests the importance of case management and adequate psychiatric follow-up. In a state with no outpatient commitment, it will be important to maintain a good working alliance with the patient. Should he break treatment or stop his medication, the risk of future violence would increase.

One external factor that encourages violence was not adequately addressed in this case. Members of the family of origin were offered treatment, but refused. Their attitude toward the ex-wife, if persistent, would tend to encourage violence. This in itself would not be a reason to hold up a clinically appropriate discharge.

In the current medical-economic climate, when there is pressure to discharge every patient quickly, it may be difficult for staff in some settings to provide appropriate treatment for a patient like this one. However, staff should not simply acquiesce to administrative pressure to discharge patients with a history of serious violence. Administrative pressures do not change clinical reality. In cases like this, it is important for staff to document the necessity for continued inpatient care and to resist attempts to discharge patients prematurely.

Notes

1. J. C. Beck, "Epidemiology of Mental Disorder and Violence," *Harvard Review of Psychiatry* 2 (1994): 1–6.

2. B. G. Link and A. Steuve, "Psychotic Symptoms and the Violent/Illegal Behavior of Mental Patients Compared to Community Controls," in J. Monahan and H. J. Steadman, eds., *Violence and Mental Disorder* (Chicago: University of Chicago Press, 1994).

3. J. W. Swanson, "Alcohol Abuse, Mental Disorder, and Violent Behavior," *Alcohol Health and Research World* 2 (1993): 123–132; Monahan and Steadman, *Violence and Mental Disorder;* P. Taylor, ed., *Violence in Society* (London: Royal College of Physicians, 1993); M. E. Rice and G. T. Harris, "Psychopathy, Schizophrenia, Alcohol Abuse, and Violent Recidivism," *International Journal of Law and Psychiatry* 18, no. 3 (1995): 333–342.

4. J. C. Beck, K. A. White, and B. Gage, "Emergency Psychiatric Assessment of Violence," *American Journal of Psychiatry* 148 (1991): 1562–65.

11

The Suicidal Patient

Robert I. Simon, M.D.

The evaluation of suicidal risk is one of the most complex, difficult and challenging clinical tasks in psychiatry. Patient suicides are all too common in the practices of mental health clinicians. Thus it is extremely important for the practitioner to understand how to conduct a competent suicide-risk assessment. Moreover, the practitioner must understand the appropriate use of contracts against suicide to try to lower suicide risk, to decrease the clinician's anxiety, and to provide a legal defense against a potential malpractice claim (Simon, 1991).

There are only two types of clinicians—those who have had patient suicides and those who will. Although it may seem counterintuitive, acceptance of the reality that some suicidal patients will kill themselves despite our best efforts may help diminish the inevitable anxiety associated with treating suicidal patients. The only certain way to avoid the terrible anguish that a therapist feels when a patient commits suicide is never to treat patients.

Risk Assessment versus Prediction

Professional standards exist for the assessment of suicide risk. However, no professional standards exist for the prediction of suicide, since this is not possible. When the clinician's interventions are informed by a competent assessment of suicide risk, it is more likely that both the patient's immediate risk of committing suicide and the therapist's attendant anxiety will diminish.

Suicide is a rare event with low specificity (high false-positive rates).

Murphy (1972) points out that it is not possible to predict suicide in the general population. One can only predict that certain groups or classes of people are statistically at high risk for suicide (Cross and Hirschfeld, 1986). For example, community-based psychological autopsy studies in a number of countries have found that major mental illness is a primary factor in approximately 93 percent of adult suicides. Major depression (40 to 60 percent of cases), chronic alcoholism (20 percent), and schizophrenia (10 percent) were the most common diagnoses for patients who commit suicide (Fawcett et al., 1993).

The inability to predict suicide was demonstrated by Pokorny (1983), who in a prospective study of 4,800 consecutive patients attempted to identify which psychiatric patients would commit suicide. Twenty-one items were used to identify a subsample of 803 patients who were considered suicidal risks. Of the 67 patients who committed suicide during the five-year follow-up period, only 30 were in the 803-patient subsample; 37 suicides (over 50 percent) were not among those identified as at risk. Furthermore, 766 of the 803 at-risk patients did not commit suicide. This overprediction of suicide risk and the high number of "missed" or undetected suicides are consistent with other "future behavior prediction" research (Melton et al., 1997; Pokorny, 1993). Pokorny (1993) reanalyzed his data using logistical regression. The results were the same as in his previous study.

Reasonableness, Foreseeability, and Prediction

The legal standard of *reasonableness* in assessing and treating suicidal patients preempts the thorny dilemma of "violence prediction." It judges professionals not on the absolute accuracy of their determinations but on whether their assessment *process,* which led to their final determination, was clinically reasonable (Simon and Sadoff, 1992). Mental health clinicians experience inevitable tension between their concerns about overrestricting a patient's freedom of movement versus not providing enough safeguards for the patient's immediate safety. This dilemma can be relieved by implementing a suicide "risk-benefit" analysis each time a significant clinical decision is made such as initial determination of risk, consideration for day pass, consideration for more freedom of movement (Simon, 1998).

When a risk-benefit analysis is noticeably absent, a court will be less able to evaluate the appropriateness of the decisionmaking process in assessing the risk of suicide. Clinicians should record all suicide assessments in the patient's hospital chart *at the time of evaluation.* For the outpatient who continues to be suicidal, an assessment should be made at each patient visit.

Whether a clinician deviated from the standard of care will be determined in a court of law, generally after hearing the testimony of experts for both the plaintiff and defendant. Thus practitioners who carefully document their reasoning process during the care of the patient will be in a better position to neutralize "after-the-fact second-guessing" by the plaintiff's expert.

Courts will closely scrutinize a suicide case to determine if the suicide was foreseeable. Foreseeability is a deliberately vague legal concept that has no comparable clinical counterpart. However, recording reasonable suicide-risk assessments that direct treatment interventions should more than adequately meet a fair legal interpretation of foreseeability.

Foreseeability must be distinguished from preventability. A suicide may not be foreseeable but, in hindsight, may have been preventable. Experts who testify in suicide cases should not confuse these two important but fundamentally different concepts. It would also be a serious mistake to equate foreseeability with predictability.

Risk-Benefit Analysis

Risk-benefit analysis provides a systematic assessment of the balance of clinical factors favoring or opposing the treatment intervention under consideration. A risk-benefit evaluation also allows the clinician more therapeutic latitude with vulnerable patients where fears of malpractice suits may inhibit appropriate therapeutic interventions. It is not unusual for the clinician to be so fearful of a malpractice action when treating a suicidal patient that the patient is unduly restricted to his or her therapeutic detriment. To protect themselves, practitioners need not *defensively* lock up suicidal patients, thus promoting despair and hopelessness.

In this era of open-door policies in psychiatric hospitals, courts recognize that suicidal patients cannot be treated like maximum-security prisoners (*Johnson v. United States,* 1976). If, after reasonable evaluation, the clinician feels that the benefits for the patient's recovery outweigh the specific risks for any given therapeutic intervention, these judgments should be recorded in a risk-benefit note in the patient's chart. The record should reflect what sources of information were consulted, what factors went into the clinical decision, and how the factors were balanced through the risk-benefit assessment (*Abille v. United States,* 1980). For example, when considering discharging the patient, the risks and benefits of both discharge and continued hospitalization should be noted. Risk-benefit notes are decisional road marks. When in doubt about a particular intervention, a risk-benefit analysis should be conducted and recorded.

In instances where the clinician has used reasonable care in evaluating and managing the suicidal patient but the patient nevertheless commits suicide, actionable negligence is unlikely since the risks were reasonably considered (*Katz v. State*, 1965). It is important for the practitioner's professional equanimity to understand that mistakes in clinical judgment do not necessarily constitute negligence. This knowledge may help the practitioner treat suicidal patients without experiencing crippling fears of litigation that can interfere with the provision of good clinical care (70 C.J.S., 1987).

When a practitioner fails to describe his or her decisionmaking process, such as in a risk-benefit analysis note, the court may be unable to clearly evaluate the complex issues involved in the determination of the suicide risk. This omission by the clinician tends to encourage the courts to narrowly focus only on certain aspects of the case at the expense of the many clinical complexities that exist with every suicidal patient.

Discharging a patient from the hospital tends to represent a much more difficult decision than that of admission. For example, at the time of a pass or discharge, the patient's anxiety about separating from the security of the hospital and facing the burdens and responsibilities of outside life may precipitate a crisis. The psychiatrist should evaluate this issue carefully through risk-benefit analysis. Although keeping the patient hospitalized may lessen the chance of suicide and diminish the clinician's anxiety, resumptions of the patient's usual life-style as soon as it is clinically feasible can be very reassuring and therapeutic for the patient.

Suicide-Risk Indicators

A clinical aphorism states that there is no such thing as a suicidal patient, there is only the patient at suicide risk. No pathognomonic *predictors* of suicide exist. Some of the many clinical indicators of suicide risk reported in the psychiatric literature are included in Table 11.1. This list, by no means exhaustive, separates variables into short-term (statistically significant less than one year after assessment) and long-term categories. Fawcett and colleagues have identified several statistically significant, short-term suicide indicators such as panic attacks, psychic anxiety, loss of pleasure or interest, alcohol abuse, depressive turmoil, diminished concentration, and global insomnia (Fawcett et al., 1987, 1990; Fawcett, 1988). A recent

Table 11.1. SUICIDE RISK VARIABLES

  I. Relationship Potential
    1. Lack of therapeutic alliance with a therapist
    2. Absent or limited meaningful supportive relationships
    3. Not living with a child under 18 years of age
  II. Suicidal History
    1. Prior suicide attempts, particularly recent
      a. High lethality potential of attempt[s]
      b. Presence of specific plan
    2. Current suicidal ideation
      a. Presence of specific plan
      b. Accessibility of lethal means
      c. Suicidal impulses—syntonic or dystonic
      d. Behavior suggestive of decision to die (severing relationships, giving away valued possessions, inappropriate sense of peace, calm, or happiness)
      e. Patient wants to die or is considering suicide
      f. Family history of suicide
 III. Psychiatric/Medical Factors
    1. Chronic psychiatric disorder (severe depression [with feelings of despair]; anhedonia, mood cycling, psychosis [command hallucination], or thought insertion)
    2. Mentally incompetent (impacts judgment, impulse control, relationship development)
    3. Recent discharge from psychiatric hospital (within 3 months)
    4. Remission of psychiatric episode but continuance of secondary depression
    5. Impulsivity (violence toward others and self, reckless driving, spending money)
    6. Physically ill, particularly if chronic
    7. HIV diagnosis
    8. Alcohol abuse
    9. Drug abuse
 IV. Demographic—Actuarial
    1. Ages 15–24 or advancing age for men
    2. Marital status
    3. Sex
    4. Race
    5. Socioeconomic group
    6. Religion
    7. Ethnicity
    8. Suicide base rates
  V. Short-term Variables (within one year of assessment)
    1. Panic attacks
    2. Psychic anxiety
    3. Loss of pleasure and interest
    4. Alcohol abuse
    5. Depressive turmoil
    6. Diminished concentration
    7. Global insomnia
    8. Recent discharge from psychiatric hospital (within 3 months)

Source: R. I. Simon, *Clinical Psychiatry and the Law,* 2nd ed. (Washington: American Psychiatric Press, 1992).

discharge from a psychiatric hospital (within three months) has been found to be statistically significant by others (Roy, 1982, 1985; Frances et al., 1987).

Suicide is the result of a complex interplay of factors and thus is a multi-determined act. Practitioners rely upon many clinical variables in assessing the suicide potential of patients. Some of the variables are vague and difficult to interpret. Furthermore, it is extremely difficult for the clinician to determine the weight to be given to the various factors that might signal suicide risk. Risk variables identify too many false-positive patients to be useful in long-range suicide prediction. Nevertheless, they are useful for short-range assessment of suicide risk, especially if the patient is undergoing an acute suicidal crisis.

The Weather Forecast Model

The weather forecast model is a time-driven method of suicide-risk assessment (Simon, 1992). Since time weakens assessment reliability, the weather forecast analogy is applicable to the assessment of suicide risk. Like weather forecasts, short-term suicide-risk assessments are much more accurate than long-term assessments because, in the short term, the parameters (suicide-risk factors) that influence future occurrences can be specified with greater precision. Clinicians cannot *predict* when or if a patient will actually commit suicide. At best, they can only assess the degree of suicide risk after an adequate psychiatric evaluation of the patient. As time passes, the ability to specify both psychological and environmental determinants of behavior diminishes. As a result, assessment accuracy becomes less and less reliable beyond the immediate, short term (24–48 hours).

The assessment of suicide risk is a here-and-now determination in regard to a specific clinical decision or intervention being considered by the practitioner. Every suicide is a unique event that defies easy analysis, even in retrospect. Accordingly, patients undergoing a suicidal crisis should be seen frequently and the suicide risk assessed from session to session. Like a weather forecast, suicide-risk assessment needs to be updated often. The clinician must remember that the systematic assessment of suicide risk is good clinical practice and, only secondarily, a risk management technique.

Method of Assessment

Before an adequate suicide-risk assessment can be done, the clinician must obtain a complete psychiatric history and a thorough mental-status examination. Records of prior psychiatric treatment should be obtained whenever possible. Frequently, obtaining the actual records will require considerable time. The clinician should attempt to call previous treaters if the patient or guardian provides a competent authorization to release information. Even if the patient refuses to produce an authorization, former treaters may decide to provide clinical information for the sake of the patient's treatment. Liability for such disclosures is likely to be minimal. Also, the past psychiatric history may be released when an emergency exists on the basis of the emergency exception to patient consent and authorization. The psychiatrist should record attempts to obtain records if they cannot be obtained. With hospital patients, psychiatrists must carefully review all notes and protocols written by caregivers in the current hospital record.

Assessing suicide risk involves three separate steps:

1. Identifying patients with certain clinical and epidemiologic risk factors associated with suicide.
2. Assessing the overall risk of suicide based on the rating of specific risk factors.
3. Implementing therapeutic interventions that bear a logical nexus to the overall suicide-risk assessment.

After all relevant information is gathered, the clinician should make a probability determination of suicide risk as low, medium, or high (Table 11.2). Once that is made, clinical interventions appropriate to that determination must be initiated, such as hospitalization, more frequent patient visits, or medication adjustments (Table 11.3). No one suicide-risk variable can be counted upon exclusively in the assessment of suicide potential. Instead, the clinician should consider all of the relevant factors and weigh them accordingly. In Table 11.2, suicide-risk factors are not listed in order of clinical importance. Such a determination depends upon the patient's clinical presentation. In a crisis, when consultation is desired but unavailable, the suicide-risk and intervention tables can be completed in lieu of consultation.

The method of assessment of suicide risk in Table 11.2 is only one example of a systematic risk assessment. A number of other assessment methods exist (Motto, 1991; Maris et al., 1992; Chiles and Strosahl, 1995; Jacobs, 1992). Certain patients may present recurrent, unique clinical risk factors that need to be more closely evaluated. The assessment of the standard risk factors for suicide may be insufficient in these cases. For example, a patient with a profound stutter would begin to speak clearly as he became

Table 11.2. ASSESSMENT OF SUICIDE RISK

Risk Factors	Facilitating suicide	Inhibiting suicide
Short-term*		
Panic attacks		
Psychic anxiety		
Loss of pleasure and interest		
Alcohol abuse		
Depressive turmoil		
Diminished concentration		
Global insomnia		
Recent discharge from psychiatric hospital (within 3 months)		
Long-term		
Therapeutic alliance—ongoing patient		
Other relationships		
Hopelessness		
Psychiatric diagnoses (Axes I and II)		
Prior attempts		
Specific plan		
Living circumstances		
Employment status		
Epidemiologic data		
Availability of lethal means		
Suicidal ideation: syntonic or dystonic		
Family history		
Impulsivity (violence, driving, money)		
Drug abuse		
Physical illness		
Mental competency		
Specific situational factors		

Rating System: L = low factor; M = moderate factor; H = high factor; 0 = nonfactor.
   * Short-term indicators are risk factors found to be statistically significant within 1 year of assessment.
   Note: Clinically judge as high, moderate, or low the potential for suicide within 24–48 hours from assessment of suicide.
   Source: Simon, *Clinical Psychiatry and the Law,* 2nd ed.

acutely suicidal. Clear speech was a unique suicide-risk factor in this patient.

In Table 11.2 the risk factors to be assessed are arranged in one column at the left. (Short-term risk factors should be considered significant within one year of assessment.) At the right, the clinician assesses each factor as either facilitating or inhibiting suicide. Each risk variable is estimated as a

Table 11.3. ASSESSMENT OF SUICIDE RISK AND EXAMPLES
OF PSYCHIATRIC INTERVENTION OPTIONS

Suicide risk	*Psychiatric interventions*
High	Immediate hospitalization
Moderate	Consider hospitalization
	Frequent outpatient visits
	Reevaluate treatment plan frequently
	Remain available to patient
Low	Continue with current treatment plan

Note: Tables 11.2 and 11.3 represent only one method of suicide risk assessment and intervention. The purpose of these tables is heuristic, encouraging a systematic approach to risk assessment. The therapist's clinical judgment concerning the patient remains paramount. Given the fact that suicide risk variables will be assigned different weights according to the clinical presentation of the patient, the assessment method presented in these tables cannot be followed rigidly.

Source: Simon, *Clinical Psychiatry and the Law,* 2nd ed.

low, medium, high, or a non-factor prior to assessing the overall risk of suicide. Table 11.3 indicates a few examples of the appropriate clinical interventions corresponding to the assessment of overall suicide risk.

Practitioners use a variety of risk assessment methods based upon their training and clinical experience (Truant et al., 1991). No one method of suicide-risk assessment can be said to be inferior to another as long as it is conducted reasonably. When clinicians fall below the standard of care in suicide assessment, they usually do so not because the method of assessment was unacceptable but because no suicide-risk assessment was done at all. As an example, a significant degree of past suicidal behavior is not recorded by clinicians in inpatients with a diagnosis of major depressive episode (Malone et al., 1995).

The Contract against Suicide

The contract against suicide frequently is used in clinical practice as a suicide-management tool (Stanford et al., 1994). Through such an agreement, the practitioner attempts to therapeutically engage suicidal patients so as to prevent them from committing suicide. No harm contracts appear to be used more in outpatient settings since less control can be exerted upon the suicidal patient. Contracts against suicide also are used in psychiatric hospitals, particularly at the time of admission, passes, or discharge.

The contract against suicide may be either oral or written, but it is always an express rather than implied agreement. That is, the terms of the contract are specifically declared and agreed upon, usually at the time it is made, either orally or in writing. Since an implied contract is one that is not put into words, it is of no practical value to the clinician or the suicidal patient.

Frequently, the contract against suicide is generated as a risk management device to defend against a potential malpractice suit, in case the patient commits suicide. The appropriate and inappropriate uses of the contract against suicide both as a clinical tool and as a risk management strategy will be discussed later.

Suicide Risk and the Therapeutic Alliance

The therapeutic alliance is defined as the conscious task-oriented collaboration between therapist and patient to help the patient with his or her problems (Karasu, 1995). The therapeutic alliance also contains unconscious and affective elements. One type of therapeutic alliance occurs when the patient's consciousness splits into an observing and an experiencing part. The observing part is allied with the therapist when the patient asks such questions as "Can I understand why I feel suicidal?" or "Will you be available to me if I can't control myself?" The presence of a therapeutic alliance is a fundamental indicator of the patient's willingness to seek help and sustenance through personal relationships during serious emotional crises.

A therapeutic alliance with the suicidal patient is exemplified by the healthy part of the patient's personality that is willing to work with the therapist based upon a life-affirming statement such as "I believe you can help me learn to cope better and be happier." This is the antithesis of hopeless feelings that impair the therapeutic alliance where the patient says "There is no hope for the relief of my pain; I am going away."

The therapeutic alliance often is used by clinicians as a here-and-now indicator of the patient's suicidal state. However, there are patients who, because of their illness, may not be able to form or sustain such an alliance. Borderline patients can rapidly fluctuate in and out of a working alliance. Schizoid patients may have great difficulty in reaching out to anyone. Paranoid patients tend to treat any close relationship with extreme fear. Nonetheless, unless bent on committing suicide, even these patients usually maintain at least the modicum of a relationship with someone. The paranoid patient often tries to find one person to trust. In the hospital, the staff can be extremely important in providing supportive relationships at the time of a suicidal crisis.

On occasion, a patient who appeared to have a working therapeutic alliance with the therapist commits suicide. The therapist is dumbfounded. The therapeutic alliance which seemed solid during the therapy can break down between sessions because of sudden exacerbations in the patient's psychiatric condition. More frequent visits and telephone contacts between sessions may be necessary with the suicidal patient whose clinical condition is unstable and with whom the therapeutic alliance is tenuous.

There are some notable exceptions to the general rule that the presence of a strong relationship with the therapist or another person inhibits suicide. Some patients may develop intense relationships based on anger. In the presence of a borderline personality disorder, splitting defenses may turn the rage meant for others toward oneself. The other person is valued but the self is suicidally devalued (Gutheil, 1985). Psychotic fusing and merging with a virulently hated person may lead to suicide. Patients with intense relationships may make a suicide pact with their partner or induce the partner to join in a double suicide. Social isolation, dominance, and aggression seem to characterize persons who form suicide pacts (Simon, 1992).

The Contract against Suicide and the Therapeutic Alliance

Some therapists attempt to formalize the therapeutic alliance by an oral or even a written contract with the patient agreeing to call upon the therapist if doubts about control of suicidal impulses arise. The contract may promise too much if it states that the clinician will be available at all times—an obvious impossibility.

A simple agreement intended to address the patient's clinical needs and circumstances may read as follows:

> We (doctor and patient) agree that you (patient) will call me if you find that you are worrying about harming yourself. I will get back to you as soon as I am able. If you feel you need immediate help and cannot reach me at that moment, you will go directly to the emergency room (specifically designated). I will then be in touch with the emergency room. If you need to be seen between appointments, I will be available to see you.

Some therapists require the patient to sign such a statement, but the patient's signature is not critical. The therapist also may obtain an oral agreement against suicide. The existence and terms of an oral agreement should be recorded in the patient's chart.

Although some patients will accept a suicide contract, some will state openly that they cannot be sure that, if self-destructive impulses threaten, they can or will want to call. The problem with the patient contract against suicide is that it may falsely ease the therapist's concern and lower the clinician's vigilance without having any appreciable effect on the patient's suicidal intent. Forensic psychiatrists who have reviewed numerous suicide cases can attest that the road to suicide is strewn with broken contracts and unkept promises against suicide by patients. Often such contracts reflect the therapist's attempt to control the inevitable anxiety associated with treating suicidal patients.

In a Massachusetts case, the psychiatrist thought he had a "solid pact" with a manic-depressive patient to contact him if the patient felt suicidal (*Stepakoff v. Kantar*, 1985). In fact, the patient did contact the psychiatrist or his designated replacement on several occasions. Given a favorable telephone assessment of the patient's mental stability and the patient's defense mechanisms, the psychiatrist felt the patient was unlikely to commit suicide. The patient committed suicide anyway. The Massachusetts Supreme Judicial Court found in favor of the psychiatrist in affirming that the psychiatrist's legal obligation to the patient was to treat him according to the standard of care and skill of the average psychiatrist. Presumably, having a "solid pact" with the patient against suicide fell within such a standard. However, there was no expressed commentary by the court addressing suicide-prevention pacts.

Courts appear unlikely to place much credence on contracts against suicide if significant deviations in the standard of care were present and the patient attempted or committed suicide. The psychiatrist in the Massachusetts case was able to demonstrate that he provided clinically appropriate care and procedures through frequent contact and assessment of the patient, documented consideration of involuntary hospitalization, and used an "active" substitute therapist while he was on vacation.

Some therapists gauge the patient's suicidal intent by the patient's willingness or unwillingness to formalize the alliance into a written contract. Contracts against suicide may be useful in certain instances in reaffirming the therapeutic alliance, but their limitations should be clearly understood. Suicidal patients who refuse outright to accept suicide contracts at least disabuse the clinician of a false sense of security associated with such contracts. Although the refusal to sign may not mean that the patient is suicidal, certainly the state of the therapeutic alliance should be reassessed.

Is It a Legal Contract?

A common question raised by therapists who use suicide-prevention contracts is what legal authority these agreements have, if any. Put another way, will a written or oral agreement with a patient not to kill nor harm himself immunize a therapist from a lawsuit if the patient subsequently attempts suicide? The answer is that a therapist's presumed defense of "breach of contract" is not likely to be sustained for several reasons. Each reason, on its own, serves as a basis for rejecting the clinician's pseudo-contract as legally enforceable.

A contract can be defined as "an agreement between two or more persons which creates an obligation to do or not do a particular thing" (Black, 1981). Some of the general requirements that are essential to making a contract or agreement legally enforceable include the following:

1. The parties to the contract must be legally competent parties. A person must have sufficient cognitive capacity—or ability to understand the nature and consequences of a proposed transaction—to be considered competent to contract (*Cundick v. Broadbent*, 1968). A contract is voidable if the party "by reason of mental illness or defect . . . is unable to act in a reasonable manner in relation to the transaction and the other party has reason to know of this condition" (Restatement Second, Contracts, 1969).

There is a legal presumption that all adults are competent. However, in the case of psychiatric patients, especially those who are suicidal, serious questions certainly would arise regarding the legal competency of these patients to enter into an agreement, such as a suicide-prevention contract, with their therapists. Other factors such as medication effects and transference phenomena in an already mentally compromised individual would probably undermine any conclusion that a patient was sufficiently competent to contract (Sharpe, 1957; *Williamson v. Matthews*, 1980; *McPheters v. Hapke*, 1972). A severely depressed or agitated patient may be functionally incompetent (affectively incompetent) and lack the mental capacity to enter into any type of contract (Bursztajn et al., 1991).

2. The agreement or contract must include a valuable consideration—an inducement for each party to carry out his or her part of the bargain. Consideration is something of value (money) requested by the psychiatrist in exchange for the psychiatrist's promise to provide professional services to the patient. In the case of any agreement between a therapist and a patient specifically "not to commit suicide," no additional consideration is given by either the psychiatrist or the patient.

3. A mutual obligation must be imposed on each party. As noted earlier, in a suicide prevention pact, the only party actually agreeing to forbear or not do something that he or she is under no legal obligation to give up is the patient. The patient agrees not to attempt suicide or agrees to call the therapist if he or she feels suicidal. But the patient has no contractual obligation beyond payment for professional services received. The therapist's promise to be available for the patient is nothing more than an extension of the duty of care that is already owed the patient. Therefore, the therapist's obligation stated in a suicide-prevention agreement is superfluous. Moreover, the fiduciary nature of the therapist-patient relationship where the therapist holds a significant power advantage over the patient would probably nullify the legal validity of a no harm contract between the parties.

4. The contract must not contravene public policy (Roy v. Hartogs, 1975). A suicide-prevention "contract" is a classic illustration of an "exculpatory clause." (*Porubiansky v. Emory University*, 1981; *Meiman v. Rehabilitation Center*, 1969; *Olson v. Molzen*, 1977). There is general agreement that persons may not enforce contract terms that would relieve them from liability for any harm caused by their negligence. Therefore, a suicide-prevention agreement with a patient would not immunize a therapist from liability if the therapist's conduct was negligent and it was this negligence that proximately caused the patient's suicide death or injury. Doctors cannot contract to provide less care than what is normally owed, regardless of whether a patient implicitly or explicitly agrees to the arrangement. To do so is a violation of public policy. Negligence cannot be "contracted" away. Furthermore, although suicide is no longer a crime in any state, suicide itself is against public policy (*Bouvia v. County of Riverside*, 1983; *In Re Conroy*, 1985). Thus a contract written to prevent an act, which already has been declared to be against public policy, is a meaningless contract.

Clinical Risk Management

Therapists who look upon no harm contracts as valid legal instruments that bind the patient not to commit suicide make a twofold error. First, the idea that a legal document could prevent a patient from committing suicide is naive and self-delusive. Clinicians who are under considerable pressure in managing difficult suicidal patients may regressively grope at any straw for reassurance. Second, in court, waving around a no harm contract signed by a deceased patient will not immunize the therapist against legal liability. On the contrary, unless the therapist has performed an adequate assessment of suicide risk and made adequate risk-benefit assessments prior to her clinical decisions, the contract against suicide could indict the therapist who relied solely on it to prevent a patient's suicide.

Simply asking patients if they are suicidal and obtaining a no harm contract is insufficient. Especially with new patients, there is no credible basis for relying upon such reassurances. A layperson could just as easily ask these same questions. The clinician's special expertise is taking an adequate psychiatric history and performing and recording competent suicide-risk assessments that inform appropriate clinical interventions.

No harm contracts are useful clinical risk management stratagems only when they facilitate good clinical care. Some patients are very reassured by the psychiatrist's interest and availability. The therapeutic alliance may be greatly strengthened thereby and the suicide threat may be averted. Good risk management is always a derivative of good clinical care.

Contracts against suicide also may be used to assess the competence of patients to collaborate with treatment and management decisions. The ability to reach out to another person in a time of crisis indicates the presence of a basic level of adaptive competence. Patients with Axis I disorders, particularly acute schizophrenic and affective disorders, may not possess the mental capacity to enter into a behavioral contract. Patients with Axis II personality disorders usually possess the mental capacity to collaborate with psychiatric treatment. However, due to maladaptive character structures and psychological defenses, the ability to cooperate with a behavioral contract may be impaired. Gutheil (1984) recommends that clinicians should specifically evaluate the patient's competence to participate in clinical decisions. Patients who are not competent to collaborate with the psychiatrist require even more conservative management.

Clinical Vignette

A thirty-six-year-old divorced man with the diagnosis of borderline personality disorder has been treated by once-a-week psychotherapy for one year. His main difficulties include chaotic relationships, poor work performance, lack of clarity in personal identity and life goals, recurrent depression, and frequent suicidal ideation.

Currently, the patient is experiencing increasingly frequent thoughts of suicide following the breakup of yet another relationship. No previous suicide attempts have been made. Vegetative signs of depression such as insomnia, loss of appetite, and psychomotor retardation are present. Nevertheless, the patient is able to work. Intense rage combined with a serious depression threatens to disrupt the therapeutic alliance.

After careful assessment of suicide risk and evaluation of both the risks and benefits of psychiatric hospitalization versus outpatient treatment, the psychiatrist concludes that continuing outpatient care is the best option. The psychiatrist asks the patient to enter into a no harm contract in lieu of hospitalization. Additionally, the psychiatrist hopes to enhance, as well as test, the faltering therapeutic alliance by directly engaging the patient through an expressly stated mutual agreement of cooperation. The psychiatrist records the diagnosis of borderline personality disorder and major depressive episode.

The patient signs a written document that clearly spells out the psychiatrist's availability to help him at any time. The contract also states the patient will call the psychiatrist at any time if suicide thoughts or impulses threaten him. Although the patient signs the agreement, he is not sure if he can comply because, "I may want to kill myself."

The thoughts of suicide have been comforting to the patient as a possible means of controlling or escaping extremely painful feelings. The therapeutic alliance appears strengthened during the patient's sessions, but his life outside of therapy is chaotic. One month after signing the contract, the patient takes an overdose of a tricyclic antidepressant prescribed by his psychiatrist. It is discovered later that he had been hoarding antidepressants for some time. The patient recovers from the overdose but is left with mild brain damage. A malpractice suit is brought against the psychiatrist.

At the time of trial, the no harm contract is used in the psychiatrist's defense. The psychiatrist's expert asserts that the contract against suicide was used as part of the assessment of suicide risk. The patient's willingness to enter into a no harm agreement was evidence that he had formed an essential therapeutic alliance with the psychiatrist. It was additional evidence that the psychiatrist had met the standard of care in appropriately assessing and treating this suicidal patient. The plaintiff's psychiatric expert stated that the no harm contract that was ambivalently agreed to by the patient was worthless and could not be relied upon in managing a seriously suicidal patient. Furthermore, the psychiatrist relied upon a behavioral contract instead of hospitalizing the patient. The expert was critical of the psychiatrist's reliance on a tenuous therapeutic alliance when the patient's life was falling apart between sessions. The expert concluded that the patient's diagnoses and clinical condition required psychiatric hospitalization.

The psychiatrist in the clinical vignette did not rely upon the no harm contract to replace adequate suicide-risk assessment. This is a very important point. The plaintiff's expert is in error in asserting that the no harm contract was worthless in this case. The most important clinical use of the suicide contract is to assess the state of the therapeutic alliance. Although patients who are intent on committing suicide may sign such a contract in order to deceive the clinician, basic elements of the therapeutic alliance usually will be absent. For example, therapy may be stalemated or a feeling of "unrelatedness" may be sensed by the therapist in working with the patient. In the clinical vignette, the psychiatrist used the contract to assess the therapeutic alliance. The patient openly stated that he did not know if he could comply with the contract, rather than attempting to deceive the psychiatrist. The patient's candor was viewed by the psychiatrist as a positive collaborative sign.

The psychiatrist did state clearly that he would be available to the patient at all times. Although the patient did not call prior to his suicide attempt, he could have called when the psychiatrist was unavailable. Some patients do find suicide contracts very helpful and reassuring during a time of emotional crisis. They will call as promised. In establishing the contract against suicide, the therapist must indicate that he or she may be unavailable for brief periods of time. Obviously, the therapist cannot be available all of the time. Promising to be available to the patient is unrealistic and potentially disastrous if a suicidal patient calls and cannot reach the therapist. If the patient needs immediate help, and the therapist cannot be reached, he should have emergency resources available such as a suicide hotline, the telephone number of an available friend, or instruction to go to a nearby emergency room. This option should be clearly stated in the contract. If the patient cannot tolerate brief absences of the therapist, then psychiatric hospitalization should be seriously considered.

The psychiatric defense expert asserted that the defendant psychiatrist's use of a no harm contract met the standard of care. The psychiatrist used the contract in the context of a full assessment of suicide risk and risk-benefit analysis. The contract also was a means of affirming the psychiatrist's availability to the patient. It was not used in the service of inappropriate defensive psychiatry, providing false reassurance to the psychiatrist and inadequate care to the patient. Nor did the contract take the place of hospitalization. The decision not to hospitalize the patient was based upon sound clinical risk-benefit analysis.

The plaintiff's expert psychiatrist focused on the no harm contract itself, testifying that any reliance upon it was poor clinical practice and below the standard of care. The expert argued that the behavioral contract promising the psychiatrist's availability was a sham transaction since the psychiatrist could not possibly be available to the patient at all times. Also, the patient openly expressed his reservations about complying with the contract. The plaintiff's expert further asserted that had such a contract not been relied upon, the patient likely would have been hospitalized immediately, given the seriousness of his diagnoses.

The court found in favor of the defendant psychiatrist. The court reasoned that the presence or absence of the no harm contract was not, by itself, material to the determination of the standard of care provided by the psychiatrist. Finding that the psychiatrist's assessment of suicide risk and subsequent risk-benefit analysis met the standard of care, the court found the decision that the patient could be treated as an outpatient to be a valid exercise of professional judgment.

Summary

Psychiatrists who make clinical decisions and interventions based upon the treatment needs of the patient do not need to be overly concerned about defensive practices. A no harm contract established with a patient struggling against suicidal impulses can be an important part of the clinical care provided. However, if a behavioral contract is used in the place of adequate clinical assessment of suicide risk, the patient may be harmed. The no harm contract can be an important aspect of good clinical care but never a substitute for it. The clinical care provided after a no harm contract is created is much more important than the mere presence of a contract in hand. An additional danger posed by no harm contracts is their delusively defensive use by therapists to allay realistic anxieties in treating difficult suicidal patients. Therapists must be able to adequately manage their own fears with suicidal patients or they should not treat them. In order for the clinician to sleep well at night, she or he must know how to adequately assess and manage suicidal patients, not merely clutch at a piece of paper signed by the patient. Furthermore, it is a serious error to view such contracts as an absolute legal defense to a subsequent malpractice suit if the suicidal patient failed to comply with the terms of the contract.

Can the no harm contract save the psychiatrist in court? When used by itself, the answer is no. When a behavioral contract is used as part of the provision of good clinical care to the patient, the good clinical care will be the best defense against an allegation of malpractice.

References

Abille v. United States, 482 F. Supp. 703 (N.D. Cal. 1980).

Black's Law Dictionary, 5th ed. (1981). St. Paul: West Publishing.

Bouvia v. County of Riverside, no. 159780, 8 MPDLR 377 (Cal. App. Dept. Super. Ct., Dec. 16, 1983).

Bursztajn, H. I., et al. (1991). "Beyond Cognition: The Role of Disordered Affective States in Impairing Competence to Consent to Treatment." *Bulletin of the American Academy of Psychiatry and Law* 19: 383–388.

Chiles, J. A., and K. D. Strosahl, eds. (1995). *The Suicidal Patient: Principles of Assessment, Treatment, and Case Management.* Washington: American Psychiatric Press.

Cross, C. K., and R. M. Hirschfeld (1986). "Epidemiology of Disorders in Adulthood: Suicide." In J. O. Cavendar, ed., *Social, Epidemiologic and Legal Psychiatry.* New York: Basic Books.

Cundick v. Broadbent, 383 F.2d 157 (10 Cir. 1967) cert. denied 390 U.S. 948 (1968).

Fawcett, J., et al. (1987). "Clinical Predictors of Suicide in Patients with Major Affective Disorders: A Controlled Prospective Study." *American Journal of Psychiatry* 144: 35–40.

Fawcett, J. (1988). "Predictors of Early Suicide: Identification and Appropriate Intervention." *Journal of Clinical Psychiatry* 49, no. 10, suppl.: 7–8.

Fawcett, J., et al. (1990). "Time-related Predictors of Suicide in Major Affective Disorder." *American Journal of Psychiatry* 147: 1189–94.

Fawcett, J., D. C. Clark, and K. A. Busch (1993). "Assessing and Treating the Patient at Risk for Suicide." *Psychiatric Annals* 23: 244–255.

Frances, R. J., J. Franklin, and D. Flavin (1987). "Suicide and Alcoholism." *American Journal of Drug and Alcohol Abuse* 1: 327–341.

Gutheil, T. G. (1984). "Malpractice Liability in Suicide." *Legal Aspects of Psychiatric Practice* 1: 1–4.

Gutheil, T. G. (1985). "Medicolegal Pitfalls in the Treatment of Borderline Patients." *American Journal of Psychiatry* 142: 9–14.

Halleck, S. L. (1980). *Law in the Practice of Psychiatry.* New York: Plenum.

In Re Conroy, 98 N.J. 321, 486 A.2d 1209, 1222–1223 (1985).

Jacobs, D., ed. (1992). *Suicide and Clinical Practice.* Washington: American Psychiatric Press.

Johnson v. United States, 409 F. Supp. 1283 (M.D. Fla. 1976), rev'd on other grounds 576 F.2d 606 (5th Cir. 1978) further appeal 631 F.2d 34 (5th Cir. 1981) cert. denied 451 U.S. 1018; *Lucy Webb Hayes National Training School v. Perotti,* 136 App. D.C. 122, 419 F.2d 704 (D.C. Cir. 1969).

Karasu, T. B. (1995). "Psychoanalysis and Psychoanalytic Psychotherapy." In

Comprehensive Textbook of Psychiatry, 6th ed., vol. 2, ed. H. I. Kaplan and B. J. Sadock. Baltimore: Williams and Wilkins.

Katz v. State, 46 Misc.2d 61, 258 N.Y.S. 2d 912 (1965).

Malone, K. M., et al. (1995). "Clinical Assessment versus Research Methods in the Assessment of Suicidal Behavior." *American Journal of Psychiatry* 152: 1601–07.

Maris, R. W., et al., eds. (1992). *Assessment and Prediction of Suicide*. New York: Guilford.

McPheters v. Hapke, 94 Idaho 744, 497 P.2d 1045 (1972).

Melton, G. B., et al. (1997). *Psychological Evaluations for the Courts*. 2nd ed. New York: Guilford.

Motto, J. A. (1991). "An Integrated Approach to Estimating Suicide Risk." *Suicide and Life-Threatening Behavior* 21: 74–89.

Murphy, G. (1972). "Clinical Identification of Suicide Risk." *Archives of General Psychiatry* 27: 356–359.

Olson v. Molzen, 558 SW3d 429 (Tenn. 1977).

Pokorny, A. (1983). "Prediction of Suicide in Psychiatric Patients." *Archives of General Psychiatry* 40: 249–257.

Pokorny, A. D. (1993). "Suicide Prediction Revisited." *Suicide and Life-Threatening Behavior* 23: 1–10.

Porubiansky v. Emory University, 156 Ga. App. 602, 275 S.E. 2d 163 (1981); *Meiman v. Rehabilitation Center*, 444 SE 2d 78 (Ky. App. 1969); *Olson v. Molzen*, 558 SW3d 429 (Tenn. 1977).

Restatement Second, Contracts §15; *Ortelere v. Teachers' Retirement Board of the City of New York*, 25 N.Y. 2d 196, 303 N.Y.2d 362, 250 N.E.2d 460 (1969).

Roy, A. (1982). "Risk Factors for Suicide in Psychiatric Patients." *Archives of General Psychiatry* 39: 1089–95.

Roy, A. (1985). "Suicide and Psychiatric Patients." In *Self-Destructive Behavior*, ed. A. Roy. *Psychiatric Clinics of North America* 8: 227–241.

Roy v. Hartogs, 366 N.Y.S. 2d 297, 301 (Civ. Ct. 1975).

70 C.J.S., *Physicians and Surgeons* §73, at 474 (1987).

Sharpe. (1957). "Medication as a Threat to Testamentary Capacity." *North Carolina Law Review* 35: 380.

Simon, R. I. (1991). "The Suicide Prevention Pact: Clinical and Legal Considerations." *American Psychiatric Press Review of Clinical Psychiatry and the Law*, vol. 2, ed. R. I. Simon. Washington: American Psychiatric Press.

Simon, R. I. (1992). *Clinical Psychiatry and the Law*. Washington: American Psychiatric Press.

Simon, R. I. (1998). *Concise Guide to Psychiatry and Law for Clinicians*. 3rd ed. Washington: American Psychiatric Press.

Simon, R. I., and R. L. Sadoff (1992). *Psychiatric Malpractice: Cases and Comments for Clinicians*. Washington: American Psychiatric Press.

Stanford, E. J., R. R. Goetz, and J. D. Bloom (1994). "The No Harm Contract in the Emergency Assessment of Suicidal Risk." *Journal of Clinical Psychiatry* 55: 344–348.

Stepakoff v. Kantar, 393 Mass. 836, 473 N.E. 2d 1131 (1985).

Truant, G. S., M. B. O'Reilly, and L. Donaldson (1991). "How Psychiatrists Weigh Risk Factors When Assessing Suicide Risk." *Suicide and Life-Threatening Behavior* 21: 106–114.

Williamson v. Matthews, 379 So.2d 1245 (Ala. 1980).

12

Pitfalls of Prescribing Medications

James Hilliard, J.D.

Physicians registered to practice medicine in the United States who write prescriptions for controlled substances are required to be registered with the Federal Drug Enforcement Agency (DEA) and, in most states, are also required to be registered with their state Department of Health. In many states the case law and regulations are much more stringent than the federal law and will not allow certain practices which may be authorized under federal law. This chapter will discuss the various aspects of the federal law. It will point out those areas where most physicians have tended to run afoul of the law, leading both state and federal enforcement agencies to levy sanctions or penalties, including the revocation of the violating physician's license to prescribe controlled substances.

Controlled Substances

All prescriptive drugs are considered controlled substances and are categorized in classes or schedules I through VI (see Table 12.1).[1] Schedule I drugs (for example, heroin, mescaline) are prescribed in the United States very rarely and only in exceptional cases. Schedule VI drugs are all drugs not otherwise included on Schedules I through V and are ordinarily controlled by local state licensure and/or regulation. Physicians must possess a DEA and state registration to prescribe Schedules I through V drugs but may prescribe Schedule VI drugs with only a state registration.

Dispensing without Prescription

DEA regulations define "dispense" as "means to deliver a controlled substance in some type of bottle, box or other container to the patient." Physi-

Table 12.1. ABBREVIATED SCHEDULE OF CONTROLLED SUBSTANCES

Schedule I

NARCOTIC ANALGESICS
Acetylmethadol (LAAM)
Heroin
STIMULANTS
Amphetamine variants
HALLUCINOGENS
Analogs of phencyclidine
Ibogaine
Lysergic acid-diethylamide
  (LSD)
Marijuana, Hashish
Mescaline
Peyote
Psilocybin, Psilosyn
Tetrahydro-cannabinois
  (except dronabinol)
DEPRESSANTS
Methaqualone

Schedule II

NARCOTIC ANALGESICS
Alphaprodine
Anileridine
Codeine
Dihydrocodeine
Ethymorphine
Etorphine (M99)
Fentanyl
Hydrocodone
Hydromorphone
Levorphanol
Meperidine (Pethidine)
Methadone
Morphine
Opium
Oxycodone
Oxymorphone
Phenazocine
DEPRESSANTS
Amobarbital
Pentobarbital
Secobarbital

Sufentanyl
STIMULANTS
Amphetamine
Cocaine
Methamphetamine
Methylphenidate
Phenmetrazine
HALLUCINOGENS
Phencyclidine
ANTIEMETICS
Dronabinol

Schedule III

NARCOTIC ANALGESICS
Acetaminophen + codeine
APC & Codeine
Aspirin + codeine
Nalorphine
Paregoric
DEPRESSANTS
Any compound containing
  an unscheduled drug and:
  Amobarbital
  Secobarbital
  Pentobarbital
Glutethimide
Methprylon
STIMULANTS
Benzphetamine
Clortermine
Phendimetrazine

Schedule IV

DEPRESSANTS
Alprazolam
Barbital
Bromazepam
Camazepam
Chloral Betaine
Chloral hydrate
Chlordiazepoxide
Clonazepam
Clorazepate

Diazepam
Ethchlorvynol
Ethinamate
Fenfluramine
Flurazepam
Halazepam
Meprobamate
Mephobarbital
Oxazepam
Paraldehyde
Pentazocine
Phenobarbital
Propxyphene
Prazepam
Triazolam
STIMULANTS
Diethylpropion
Mazindol
Phentermine
Pemoline

Schedule V

Mixtures containing
  limited quantities of
  narcotic drugs, with
  non-narcotic active
  medicinal ingredients.
  Less abuse potential
  than Schedule IV.
  Generally for anti-
  tussive and anti-
  diarrheal purposes.

Schedule VI*

All prescription drugs not
  in Schedules I–V.

This table is based on federal regulations. *Massachusetts only.

cians who deliver controlled substances in a quantity greater than one dose to be taken at the time it is delivered technically may be dispensing a controlled substance. This being the case, most states regulate the manner by which controlled substances are to be dispensed and usually require that the substances be placed in a container with the physician's name and address, patient's name, name of the drug, dosage, strength per dosage unit, and directions for use with any cautionary statements.[2] Accordingly, physicians' practices will typically fall outside of the dispensing definition under the federal act when they deliver more than one dose of medication, usually sample drugs, to a patient without complying with the labeling mandates under state law.

Prescriptions

There are three legally significant aspects of prescription writing to which physicians should be especially sensitive in order to avoid violations of applicable regulations. The three areas concern (1) issuing prescriptions for legitimate medical purposes, (2) self-prescribing, and (3) prescribing for members of one's immediate family.

PRESCRIBING FOR LEGITIMATE MEDICAL PURPOSES

The prescribing of a controlled substance must be for legitimate medical purposes by a practitioner acting in the usual course of his or her professional practice. Prescribing for legitimate medical purposes has been determined in most states to require, at the very least, the establishment of the following interconnected criteria:

1. There must be a physician-patient relationship which includes the maintenance of contact with the patient. In *United States v. Tran Trong Cuong,* the court found that the physician in question was criminally liable under federal law in that he prescribed drugs other than for legitimate medical purposes and not in the usual course of medical practice.[3] Specifically, it was found that Dr. Tran's cursory and superficial treatment, without the benefit of a proper diagnosis or exam, was insufficient to create the integral physician-patient relationship that would allow him to prescribe controlled substances.[4]

2. An appropriate medical history must be taken and a physical exam performed at the initial encounter. The importance of conducting a physical examination cannot be overemphasized, especially in the establishment of the baseline physician-patient relationship. Upon the first encounter with a patient, a physical exam is necessary, and mandated in some states, in order to stay within the minimum standard of care that all physicians must apply.[5] In *United States v. Moore*, the U.S. Supreme Court ruled that a physician did not operate within the boundaries of "professional practice" and therefore violated the federally enacted Comprehensive Drug Abuse Prevention and Control Act when he conducted inadequate physical examinations prior to prescribing methadone.[6] If the physical exam is not possible or clinically appropriate due to circumstances, reference to the family physician or primary care physician may be appropriate.

3. Medication prescribed by the physician should be warranted by and consistent with the physician's diagnosis of the patient. This criterion cannot be divorced from and must be followed in conjunction with the previous two criteria. In *U.S. v. Moore*, the physician, who was successfully prosecuted for a variety of violations concerning the wanton and random prescription of methadone, ostensibly covering all four of these interconnected guidelines, was found, in the end, to have operated outside the bounds of "professional practice."[7]

In *Tran Trong Cuong*, experts testified that the physician had inappropriately and excessively prescribed a variety of Schedule II, III, and IV painkillers for vague complaints of pain. Even if the physician's substandard physical exams and diagnoses were correct, his excessive and prolonged prescriptions of the narcotics would nullify any potentially useful effects and, more likely, lead to the addiction (as well as other harmful side effects) of his patients to the prescribed substances. Charging the jury which convicted Dr. Tran, the court indicated that a guilty verdict would be warranted if they found that the physician's practices fell "outside the usual course of medical practice."[8]

4. The physician is required to maintain accurate and complete treatment records with respect to each patient for whom he or she is prescribing controlled substances. Such records should contain, at a minimum, a complete identification of the patient, relevant dates of treatment, any medically significant events, a medical history, the results of the physical examination, any other test results, the diagnosis, a treatment plan, any past or present prescriptions, any "consents" or "waivers" provided by the patient, and any other recordable data or documentation that the context demands. Improper recordkeeping may result in substantial liability.[9]

Physicians found to have written prescriptions for patients without following these guidelines may be subject to disciplinary action by local boards and/or the DEA, and/or to criminal liability. Sanctions and penalties may include fines, loss of registration, loss of license, and imprisonment.

SELF-PRESCRIBING

Local regulations usually limit the extent to which physicians may prescribe medications for themselves. As a threshold matter, any prescription written by a physician for him- or herself must be in accordance with legitimate medical purposes (see above). Accordingly, those physicians who write prescriptions for themselves for a controlled substance and who have not followed the standard of prescribing for legitimate medical purposes may find themselves in violation of local and/or federal law.

There are additional levels of liability which may befall physicians who prescribe controlled substances for themselves for illicit purposes. In some states self-prescribing physicians have been determined to be in unlawful possession of those drugs, leading to criminal prosecution. In one Massachusetts case, *Commonwealth v. Perry,* the physician who prescribed controlled substances for himself without medical justification was determined not to have been dispensing or distributing within the confines of the law and, accordingly, it was determined that he knowingly possessed illegal drugs.[10]

PRESCRIBING FOR IMMEDIATE FAMILY

Again, most states restrict the prescription of medications to the physician's immediate family, usually to the drugs in Schedules II and III. Attention should be paid to state regulation with respect to this prohibition but, more important, if one is prescribing to one's immediate family it should be for legitimate medical purposes following the recommendations stated in the beginning of this chapter. Prescribing to family members for any other reason may be found to violate such standards.[11]

Recordkeeping Requirements

Physicians who dispense or administer medications are required by DEA regulations to maintain records of their transactions. Inventories of medications held by the physician must be taken every two years and must include their DEA registration number, date of inventory, and signature of the inventory taker. This inventory must be maintained for two years.

Likewise, physicians who order drugs through the mail for office use must maintain accurate records every time a unit dose is dispensed from those drugs. Often, the DEA and/or local authorities will access records of drug manufacturers and will call upon physicians and request to see the records that are required to be maintained for the possession of these drugs. If such records do not reflect where each dose has been administered, the DEA and/or local authorities are likely to charge the physician with personal use of these drugs, which can lead to severe penalties.

Physicians are also required, when keeping controlled substances in their offices, to maintain such substances in securely locked, substantially constructed cabinets or safes. DEA recommends that the stock/inventory of all controlled substances be kept in minimal amounts. In those cases where it is necessary to have a substantial quantity of controlled substances, DEA encourages maintaining a system of security which exceeds minimum requirements. Finally, any physician involved in the loss or theft of a controlled substance must notify the nearest DEA field office of the theft or significant loss upon discovery. Physicians are also required to notify the local police department of any such thefts.

Narcotic Treatment Programs (Methadone Clinics)

Federal and state laws are very strict with respect to the prescription of drugs to "drug-dependent persons." A drug-dependent person is defined as "a person who is unable to function effectively and whose inability to do so causes or results from the use of a drug other than alcohol, tobacco, or lawful beverages containing caffeine and other than from a medically-prescribed drug when such drug is medically indicated and the intake is in proportion to the medical need."[12] The danger for physicians in the area of prescribing to drug-dependent persons comes not when they are knowingly treating a drug-dependent person in a registered program but rather when they are prescribing medications for other medical purposes to patients who are drug-dependent.

The risk in such circumstances is that it appears the physician is treating the drug dependency without having met the applicable registration and reporting requirements under both federal and local law. Accordingly, physicians should pay special attention when prescribing drugs to drug-dependent patients, especially if such prescriptive drugs could be considered a treatment for or exacerbation of the drug dependency. By way of example, DEA regulations dictate that a physician who is not part of a narcotic treatment program and is not registered accordingly may administer narcotic substances to an addicted individual to relieve that individual's acute withdrawal symptoms while the physician makes arrangements to refer the individual to a narcotic treatment program. Not more than one day's medication may be administered at one time. This treatment cannot last more than three days and may not be renewed or extended. A hospital that has no program on the premises or a physician who is not part of a treatment program may administer narcotics to a drug-dependent individual for either detoxification or maintenance purposes if the individual is being treated for a condition other than the addiction.

Narcotics for Patients with Terminal Illness or Chronic Disorders

Controlled substances and, in particular, narcotic analgesics may be used in the treatment of pain experienced by a patient with a terminal illness or chronic disorder. As these drugs have a legitimate clinical purpose, the physician should not hesitate to prescribe, dispense, or administer them when they are indicated for a legitimate medical purpose.

Tips for Prescribers of Controlled Substances

The following are some guidelines to be used in the prescribing of controlled substances:

1. Keep prescription pads in a safe place where they cannot be easily stolen, and keep the number of pads to a minimum.
2. Prescriptions for Schedule II controlled substances should be written in ink or indelible pencil or typewriter, and the order must be signed by the physician.
3. The actual amount on the number of units should be written in Arabic number or Roman numeral to discourage alterations or, for added safety, should be both spelled out and written in numerals (e.g. "thirty (30)").
4. All prescriptions should be written for the minimum necessary dosages.
5. The stock of controlled substances that is maintained in a medical bag should be kept to a minimum.
6. Caution should be taken whenever a patient mentions that another physician has been prescribing a controlled substance for him or her. Consult the other physician or the hospital records or examine the patient thoroughly and decide if a controlled-drug product should be prescribed.

7. Prescription blanks should be used only for writing prescription orders and not for memo notes.

8. Never sign prescription blanks in advance.

9. Accurate records of controlled-substance products that are dispensed should be maintained at all times as required by the Controlled Substances Act and regulations. When in doubt about a patient's motive in requesting controlled substances, you should call the order in to the pharmacist to determine whether the patient is receiving similar medications from any other physician.

/ / /

Pitfalls in prescribing controlled substances can be avoided if a physician adheres to both the detailed regulatory and statutory restrictions and mandates and the general standard of care that governs all aspects of medical practice. The "dos and don'ts" which are delineated in the statutes and administrative regulations of state and federal government leave no room for ambiguity, and a physician should take great pains to comply with both state and federal mandates. Similarly, a physician, from the establishment of a physician-patient relationship, to the treatment of that patient, to the documentation of such treatment, must adhere to the standard of care which has evolved over time and which is applicable to all physicians in their chosen fields of practice.

Notes

1. 21 USCS §§ 811, et seq.; e.g. Massachusetts General Laws (M.G.L.), C. 94C, § 3; 105 Code of Massachusetts Regulations (CMR) 700.002.

2. E.g., M.G.L., C. 94C, §21; 105 CMR 722.070.

3. 18 F.3d 1132, 1137 (4th Cir. 1994).

4. Ibid. at 1389; *Oklahoma State Board of Medical Licensure and Supervision v. Ray,* 848 P.2d 46, 47 (Okl. App. 1992).

5. See, e.g., Commonwealth of Massachusetts Board of Registration in Medicine, *Prescribing Practices and Guidelines,* p. 15.

6. 423 U.S. 122, 142 (1975); see also *Tran Trong Cuong,* 18 F.3d at 1138–39; *U.S. v. Hooker,* 541 F.2d 300, 305 (1st Cir. 1976).

7. 423 U.S. at 141–143.

8. *Tran Trong Cuong,* 18 F.3d at 1135, 1138–39.

9. See *Nadell v. Ambach,* 523 N.Y.S.2d 637, 638 (A.D. 3rd. Dept. 1988).

10. 391 Mass. 808, 812 (1984).

11. See *Reid v. Axelrod,* 429 N.Y.S.2d 84 (A.D. 3rd. Dept. 1980) (prescriptions to family members so that physician could obtain drugs for his own illicit use).

12. E.g., M.G.L., C. 111E, § 1.

13

Boundary Violations in Psychotherapy

Robert I. Simon, M.D.

The concept of treatment boundaries was largely developed during the twentieth century from outpatient psychodynamic psychotherapy. Treatment boundaries have been a continuing issue since the beginning of psychoanalysis, reflected in Freud's disputes, for example, with Ferenczi and Reich. Ethical principles developed by the mental health professions and the legal duties imposed by courts and statutes have further defined treatment boundaries. For example, the clinician's duty to maintain confidentiality derives from three distinct origins: professional (clinical), ethical, and legal.

Treatment boundaries are set by the therapist and define the therapist's professional relationship with the patient for the purpose of promoting a trusting, working alliance. The boundary guidelines described in this chapter are generally applicable along a broad spectrum of psychiatric treatments. Nevertheless, considerable disagreement exists among therapists concerning what constitutes treatment-boundary violations. The therapy techniques of one therapist may be anathema to another who considers such practices as clear boundary violations.

Much variability in defining treatment boundaries appears to be a function of the nature of the patient, the therapist, the treatment, and the status of the therapeutic alliance. For example, notable boundary exceptions do occur in alcohol and drug abuse programs, in inpatient settings, and with certain cognitive-behaviorally based therapies. However, regardless of the therapy used, every therapist must maintain basic treatment boundaries with all patients. If boundary exceptions are made, they must be made for the benefit of the patient. Every effort must be exerted to therapeutically restore breached boundaries. Brief boundary crossings or even violations that are quickly recognized and rectified before harming the patient can provide important insights into conflictual issues for both the therapist and patient. Boundary crossings, in themselves, are not necessarily harmful (Gutheil and Gabbard, 1993). The danger to treatment arises when boundary violations increase in frequency and severity over time.

Since boundary guidelines maintain the integrity of therapy and safeguard both the therapist and the patient, proponents of therapies that breach generally accepted boundary guidelines risk harming the patient and suffering the legal consequences thereof (Simon, 1991a). Psychiatry continues to be highly receptive to innovative treatments that offer the hope of helping the mentally ill (Simon, 1993). The maintenance of basic treatment boundaries, by itself, should not be an impediment to therapeutic innovations. On the contrary, conducting innovative therapies in general in accordance with accepted treatment boundaries should provide added credibility.

Boundary Maintenance: An Impossible Task?

All psychiatric therapies, regardless of their philosophical or theoretical orientation, are based upon the fundamental premise that interaction with another human being can alleviate psychic distress, change behavior, and alter a person's perspective on the world (Simon and Sadoff, 1991). Psychotherapy can be defined as the application of clinical knowledge and skill to the dynamic psychological interaction between two people for the purpose of alleviating mental suffering. This definition of psychotherapy also applies to biological and behavioral therapies. But psychotherapy has been called an impossible task (Simon, 1990). There are no perfect therapists or perfect therapies.

Psychotherapy also has been defined as a mutually regressive relationship with shared tasks but different roles (Shapiro and Carr, 1991). Boundary violations are therapist role violations that inevitably occur to some degree in every therapy. Although maintaining boundaries is a major psychotherapeutic imperative, the competent psychotherapist must recognize when he or she has erred. Often the real work of psychotherapy involves the therapeutic restitution of breached boundaries. Treatment boundaries usually can be reestablished if the therapist raises the boundary violation as a treatment issue. Since therapists use themselves as a therapeutic tool, sensitivity to boundary violations must be maintained at a high level.

From a clinical perspective, the therapeutic alliance is considered by most practitioners to be the single most critical factor associated with successful treatment (Marziali et al., 1981). The maintenance of treatment boundaries sets the foundation for the development of the therapeutic alliance and the subsequent work of therapy. Trust is the essential basis for a secure therapeutic relationship that permits patients to reveal their innermost yearnings and fears. The patient's trust is based upon the belief that the therapist is acting professionally and using skills in a competent manner for the benefit of the patient. The maintenance of consistent, stable, and enabling treatment boundaries creates a safe therapeutic environment for the patient to risk self-revelation. The therapist's professional concern and respect for the patient ensures that treatment boundaries will be preserved.

Treatment-boundary violations usually occur along a continuum, interfering with the provision of competent clinical care to the patient. Boundary violations frequently are a consequence of the therapist's acting out personal conflicts. As a result, the patient's diagnosis may be missed. Inappropriate treatment may be rendered. Moreover, the patient's original psychiatric condition may be worsened. Boundary violations frequently represent deviations in the standard of care that are alleged to have harmed the patient, forming the basis of a malpractice claim. Boundary violations as an integral part of negligent psychotherapy are inevitably present in claims of therapist sexual misconduct as well as in other types of suits alleging exploitation of patients.

Boundary violations also encourage malpractice suits by creating a misalliance between therapist and patient. Boundary violations, usually reflecting the personal agenda of the therapist, set patient and therapist against each other. Langs (1990) notes that the failure to maintain treatment boundaries may lead to autistic, symbiotic, and parasitic relationships with patients. Langs observes that autistic relationships (severed link) between therapist and patient damage meaningful relatedness, symbiotic (fusional) relationships pathologically gratify the patient, and parasitic (destructive) relationships exploit the patient. As frequently happens, bad results combined with bad feelings set the stage for a malpractice suit (Gutheil, 1989).

Principles Underlying Boundary Guidelines

RULE OF ABSTINENCE

There are a number of basic, overlapping principles that form the underpinning for the establishment of boundary guidelines. One of the foremost principles is the rule of abstinence, which states that the therapist must refrain from obtaining personal gratification at the expense of the patient (Freud, 1959). Extra-therapeutic gratifications during the course of treatment must be avoided by both therapist and patient (Langs, 1990).

A corollary of the principle of abstinence states that the therapist's main source of professional gratification arises from the psychotherapeutic process and the satisfaction of helping the patient. The only material satisfaction directly received from the patient is the fee for the therapist's professional services. Treatment boundaries are violated when the therapist's gratification is primarily received *from* the patient directly rather than through engagement in the therapeutic process *with* the patient. The principle of abstinence underlies virtually all boundary guidelines.

DUTY OF NEUTRALITY

The rule of abstinence attempts to secure a position of relative neutrality for the therapist's interactions with the patient. Therapeutic neutrality is not defined here in the sense of equidistance between the patient's ego, superego, id, and reality. Rather, it means knowing one's place and staying out of the patient's personal life (Wachtel, 1987). Therapeutic neutrality allows for the patient's agenda to be given primary consideration. The relative anonymity of the therapist ensures that self-disclosures will be kept at a minimum, thus maintaining the therapist's neutrality. Also, the law independently recognizes the therapist's duty of neutrality toward patients (Furrow, 1980).

The concept of relative neutrality refers to the limitations imposed upon psychotherapists from interfering in the personal lives of their patients. Life choices such as marriage, occupation, where one lives, and with whom one associates, while grist for the therapeutic mill, are fundamentally the patient's final choice (Wachtel, 1987). Nor should the personal views of the therapist concerning politics, religion, abortion, or divorce, for example, be used to influence the treatment situation.

If an otherwise competent patient is contemplating making a decision that appears foolish or potentially destructive, the therapist's role is limited primarily to raising the questionable decision as a treatment issue. For example, the therapist can appropriately explore the psychological meaning of the decision as well as its potential adverse consequences on the patient's treatment and life situation. On the other hand, situations do arise with patients when the psychotherapist must intervene directly. If a patient's decisionmaking capacity is severely compromised by a mental disorder, the therapist may need to actively intervene to protect the patient or others (Simon, 1990). As an obvious example, a psychotically depressed, suicidal patient who refuses to enter a hospital voluntarily is likely to require involuntary hospitalization. Under these conditions, the therapist is intervening in the patient's life for valid clinical, not personal, reasons.

PATIENT AUTONOMY AND SELF-DETERMINATION

Fostering the autonomy and self-determination of the patient is another major principle underlying treatment-boundary guidelines. Maintaining patient separateness through the process of separation-individuation follows as a corollary. Of the over 450 different types of currently available psychotherapies, none have as their long-term treatment goal patient dependence and psychological fusion with their therapists or others. Obtaining informed consent for proposed procedures and treatments also preserves the autonomy of the patient (Simon, 1992).

Patient self-determination requires that the therapist's clinical posture toward the patient be expectant. That is, the patient basically determines the content of his or her sessions. Generally, this does not apply in cognitive behavioral therapies or even with some forms of interpersonal therapy. Moreover, the strictures that physical contact with patients be essentially avoided and that the therapist stay out of the patient's personal life (no past, current, or future personal relationships) derive in large measure from the principle of autonomy and self-determination.

Progressive boundary violations invariably limit the patient's freedom of exploration and choice. Properly maintained treatment boundaries foster the separateness of the patient from the therapist while also maintaining the psychological relatedness of the patient to others.

FIDUCIARY RELATIONSHIP

As a matter of law, the physician-patient relationship is fiducial. In *Omer v. Edgren* (1984), a lawsuit was brought against a psychiatrist for alleged sexual exploitation of a patient. The Washington Court of Appeals noted: "Washington also has characterized the relationship between physician and patient as fiduciary: 'The physician-patient relationship is of fiduciary nature. The inherent necessity for trust and confidence requires scrupulous good faith on the part of the physician.' "

The asymmetries of knowledge and power that exist between therapist and patient require the therapist not to use the patient for his or her personal advantage (Peterson, 1992). This responsibility is "implicit" in the therapist-patient relationship and is a fundamental aspect of the general "duty of care." The special vulnerabilities of the patient rather than the special powers of a profession give rise to a fiduciary duty (Simon, 1993).

A fiduciary relationship arises, therefore, whenever confidence, faith, and trust are reposed on one side and domination and influence on the other (Black, 1990). Not only psychiatrists but all mental health professionals have a fiduciary responsibility to their patients. The maintenance of confidentiality, privacy, a stable fee policy, and consistent time and treatment settings are derived in large measure from the fiduciary duties of the therapist.

RESPECT FOR HUMAN DIGNITY

Moral, ethical, and professional standards require that psychiatrists as well as nonmedical professionals treat their patients with compassion and respect. The dedication of physicians to their patients has a long and venerable tradition so artfully expressed in the Hippocratic oath. *The Principles of Medical Ethics with Annotations Especially Applicable to Psychiatry* (American Psychiatric Association, 1995, sec. 2, annotation 6) states: "A physician shall be dedicated to providing competent medical service with compassion and respect for human dignity." On clinical grounds alone, the competent therapist always strives to maintain the patient's healthy self-esteem during the course of therapy. Exploitative therapists, however, relate to patients in part as objects to be used for their own personal gratification. Often such therapists attack the self-esteem of their patients in order to gain control over them. All of the boundary guidelines are substantially based on the principle of respect for human dignity.

Boundary Guidelines

Treatment boundaries are set by the therapist according to accepted professional standards. It is the therapist's professional duty to establish and maintain appropriate treatment boundaries in the provision of good clinical care. This duty cannot be delegated to the patient. Once treatment boundaries are established, boundary *issues* inevitably arise in working with the patient that form an essential aspect of treatment.

Boundary crossings that arise from either the therapist or the patient or both are usually quickly addressed and rarely harm the patient (Gutheil and Gabbard, 1993). Boundary *violations,* on the other hand, arise solely from the therapist and are often inimical to treatment, particularly if unchecked and progressive. Therapists who establish idiosyncratic boundaries or set no boundaries at all are likely to provide negligent therapy that harms the patient and invites a malpractice suit. A major continuing task for therapists is the maintaining of constant vigilance against boundary violations and immediately repairing any breaches in a clinically supportive manner.

Generally, observing the following boundary guidelines for psychotherapy will help maintain the integrity of the treatment process:

Maintain relative therapist neutrality.
Foster psychological separateness of patient.
Protect confidentiality.
Obtain informed consent for treatments and procedures.
Interact verbally with patients.
Ensure no previous, current, or future personal relationship with the patient.
Minimize physical contact.
Preserve relative anonymity of therapist.
Establish a stable fee policy.
Provide consistent, private, and professional setting.
Define time and length of sessions.

Some of these guidelines have been considered by Langs (1990) to form a necessary treatment frame for the conducting of psychodynamic psychotherapy. Although additional boundary rules can be elaborated, a consensus generally exists among clinicians concerning the basic rules listed above. Other rules concerning the management of transference and countertransference could be included but might not find ready acceptance among behaviorists, biological psychiatrists, and "here and now" treatments such as Gestalt therapy. Nevertheless, regardless of theoretical orientation, all therapists must recognize that transference and countertransference play an important role in any therapy.

An absolutist position concerning treatment-boundary guidelines cannot be taken. Otherwise, boundary guidelines would be termed boundary standards. Effective treatment boundaries do not create walls that separate the therapist from the patient. Instead, they define a fluctuating, reasonably neutral, safe space that enables the dynamic, psychological interaction between therapist and patient to unfold. Although the mere listing of boundary guidelines serves an important heuristic purpose, clinicians must remain vigilant to the *process* of gradual, progressive violation of boundaries. Progressive boundary violations are almost invariably the consequence of an exploitative relationship established by the therapist with the patient early in the treatment.

Exigent Boundary Crossings

In the course of therapy, it may be necessary for the sake of the patient or the welfare of others for the psychiatrist to cross accepted treatment boundaries. Boundary excursions may be driven by crises in clinical care, and by intervening, superseding ethical or legal duties. For example, an agoraphobic patient may be incapacitated and unable to come to the psychiatrist's office. Home visits may be required initially. The potentially violent patient who threatens others puts the psychiatrist in a conflicting ethical position regarding maintaining confidentiality. Professional and legal duties to warn and protect endangered third persons may necessitate a breach of the patient's confidentiality. In the latter example, if the patient can be included in the process of issuing a warning, treatment boundaries may be stretched but not necessarily broken. Engaging patients in the decision to readjust treatment boundaries as a result of treatment exigencies may permit salutary boundary reshaping that actually facilitates the treatment process.

Managed care systems that impose limitations on treatments may lead therapists to take shortcuts. The need to obtain patient consent for a proposed treatment, for example, may be a casualty of managed care time pressures. Managed care will undoubtedly reshape treatment boundaries. The therapist must remain alert to the potential boundary excursions and violations endemic to managed care settings.

Sexual Exploitation

Invariably, in cases of therapist-patient sex, progressive boundary violations precede and accompany the eventual sexual acts (Simon, 1989a). Patients are psychologically damaged by the precursor boundary violations as well as by the eventual sexual exploitation (Simon, 1991b; Schoener, 1989). Even if the therapist and patient stop short of an overt sexual relationship, precursor boundary violations often interfere with the proper diagnosis and treatment of the patient. Therapists may be sued for negligent psychotherapy in addition to sexual misconduct. Under either circumstance, patients are not provided essential treatment. The patient's original mental disorder is often exacerbated and other mental disorders are iatrogenically induced.

Sexual misconduct cases usually demonstrate boundary violations in the extreme. Thus, their study can be very instructive. The following fictional though representative clinical vignette illustrates the progressive, increasingly flagrant violations of treatment boundaries that often precede therapist-patient sex.

VIGNETTE

A thirty-five-year-old single woman with previously diagnosed borderline personality disorder and drug abuse seeks treatment for severe depression following a spontaneous abortion. The psychiatrist is fifty-two years old, and recently divorced by his wife. His ex-wife is a very attractive, talented artist who had an affair with a concert pianist. The psychiatrist is increasingly relying on alcohol to deal with his feelings of loss and humiliation.

The patient is quite bright and attractive. She talks at length about her feelings of isolation and emptiness. Clear vegetative signs of depression are present. The patient had hoped for a child as a remedy for her feelings of emptiness and loneliness.

The psychiatrist notices that the patient bears a resemblance to his ex-wife but is inattentive to this association. He becomes quickly enamored of the patient, overlooking and minimizing her major depression. His clinical judgment is further impaired by the appearance of improvement in the patient's depression as the psychiatrist shows a personal interest in her. The psychiatrist looks forward to seeing the patient for her twice-a-week appointments, finding solace and relief from his own sense of desolation. For the first two months, treatment boundaries are maintained. Then gradually, the sessions take on a conversational, social tone.

Psychiatrist and patient begin to address each other by their first names. The psychiatrist discloses the facts surrounding his divorce, talking at length about his wife's infidelity and his feelings of betrayal and humiliation. He also confides in the patient intimate details about his other patients, treating her as a confidante. The patient feels special because of the psychiatrist's disclosures. However, she is distressed by the psychiatrist's unhappiness and feels guilty that she cannot be of more assistance. Initially the psychiatrist sits across from the patient, but gradually he moves his chair closer. Eventually, doctor and patient sit together on the sofa. The psychiatrist puts his arm around the patient when she tearfully describes extensive childhood physical and sexual abuse. Treatment sessions are extended, some lasting as long as three hours. The patient feels grateful that she is receiving special treatment.

Because the extended sessions disrupt the psychiatrist's other appointments, the patient is scheduled for the end of the day. Whenever possible, therapist and patient meet for brief periods of time at a nearby park or at a bar for a drink. When the patient complains of sleep problems, the psychiatrist prescribes diazepam. He has not kept up with developments in psychopharmacology, having used medications very sparingly in his practice over the years. The psychiatrist is unaware of her prior addiction to narcotics. He does not explain the risks of taking diazepam. The patient requires higher doses of diazepam over time that interfere with her ability to function independently. The psychiatrist begins to make day-to-day decisions for the patient, including balancing her checkbook. He settles a dispute between the patient and her landlord. When she loses her job as a broker, he finds her a job as a secretary. The patient drops the few friendships she has maintained and centers her life around the psychiatrist. The psychiatrist discourages her relationships with others. Much time is spent chatting with each other over the phone.

During sessions, therapist and patient begin to embrace and kiss. The psychiatrist finds the patient more compliant to his advances when she has had a few drinks. During one session when the patient drinks too much, sexual intercourse takes place. The psychiatrist stops billing the patient as their sexual relationship continues.

A few months later, the psychiatrist takes an extended vacation. While he is away, the patient learns from another patient that the psychiatrist has revealed details of her childhood sexual abuse. The patient becomes extremely depressed and takes an overdose of diazepam. While hospitalized, she is weaned from the diazepam. She discloses the fact of her sexual involvement with her outpatient psychiatrist. The patient is successfully treated for major depression with antidepressants. She is also diagnosed as having borderline personality disorder that is severely aggravated due to the sexual exploitation by her therapist. The exploiting psychiatrist attempts to see the patient upon his return. She refuses. One year later, the patient brings a $2 million malpractice suit against the psychiatrist for sexual misconduct.

DISCUSSION OF VIGNETTE

Neutrality and self-determination. The rule of abstinence and the relative neutrality of the therapist empower patient separateness, autonomy, and self-determination. In the vignette, the psychiatrist abandons a position of neutrality and undercuts the patient's separateness through numerous boundary violations that promote fusion between psychiatrist and patient. He gradually gains control over the patient's life, making basic decisions for her. As often occurs in cases of sexual exploitation, the therapist becomes the center of the patient's life, cutting her off from outside relationships. Whether intended or unintended, boundary violations cut short a patient's options for recovery and independent psychological functioning. The achievement of psychological independence is a goal of treatment. Maintaining patient separateness that permits pursuit of this goal is a boundary issue.

Confidentiality. The psychiatrist in the clinical vignette fails to maintain confidentiality. In order to gain the patient's trust, he shares intimate information about other patients. This creates the illusion that she is special.

The maintenance of confidentiality is an absolute boundary guideline that must be followed unless specific clinical, ethical, or legal exceptions arise (Simon, 1992). Confidentiality must be maintained unless release of information is competently authorized by the patient. Breaches of confidentiality typically occur when therapists are in double-agent roles (Simon, 1987). Such roles occur when the therapist must serve simultaneously the patient and a third party. For example, prison and military mental health professionals frequently find themselves in double-agent roles. Clinicians working in managed care settings also often find themselves struggling with dual roles.

Informed consent. Although the law requires informed consent for treatments and procedures, informing patients of the risks and benefits of a proposed treatment incidentally, but importantly, maintains patient autonomy and fosters the therapeutic alliance (Simon, 1989b). Informing patients about treatments and procedures is antithetical to exploitation agendas. In a number of sexual misconduct cases, drugs and even ECT have been used to gain control over patients (Simon, 1992). Boundary violations involving medication are particularly egregious in these cases. Obviously, no effort is made to inform the patients of the risks and benefits of prescribed medication. Frequently, large amounts of addictive medications are given, usually barbiturates and benzodiazapines. Lawyers defending therapists who become sexually involved with their patients raise the issue of patient consent. Patients are unable to provide a valid consent for therapist-patient sex for a variety of reasons (Simon, 1994).

In an effort to gain control over the patient, the psychiatrist in the vignette negligently plies her with increasing amounts of diazepam and alcohol. If the addictive risks of diazepam had been explained to the patient, her earlier history of narcotic addiction might have been revealed. The psychiatrist, however, is pursuing an exploitative rather than a clinical agenda. Thus, the patient's need for autonomy and self-determination is subjugated to the therapist's desire to make the patient dependent upon him.

Verbal interaction. The process of psychotherapy requires that the interaction between therapist and patient be basically verbal. Engaging the patient verbally tends to check acting out responses by the therapist. In psychotherapy, the therapist needs to be alert to the possibility of acting out his or her emotional conflicts with the patient. This can manifest itself either through the therapist's behavior or by inducing the patient to act out.

There is, however, a fundamental difference between active interventions undertaken by the therapist and the therapist's acting out. For example, when somatic therapies or behavioral modification techniques are used, active interventions are made in the service of the treatment, not for the purpose of exploiting the patient. Moreover, therapists frequently find it necessary to clinically intervene actively on behalf of patients in crisis. All therapies, even Rogerian therapy and psychoanalysis, employ active interventions and reinforcement approaches (Wachtel, 1987). The danger to patients and their therapy does not arise from therapists' activity per se, but from therapists' acting out. Managed care settings encourage active treatment and dispositional approaches toward patients. For some therapists, becoming more active may breed acting-out behaviors. Such an environment can be conducive to heightening the acting-out potential that exists, more or less, in every therapist. Boundary violations may be rationalized as acceptable treatment adaptation for managed care settings. Therapists, not entrepreneurs, determine appropriate treatment boundaries.

Bibring (1954) pointed out that all dynamic psychotherapies variously utilize catharsis, suggestion, manipulation, clarification, and insight in their therapeutic approaches to the patient. Regardless of the methods favored, the patient should be primarily engaged on a verbal rather than an action level. Although it is certainly possible for therapists to act out exclusively on a verbal level, behavioral acting out by therapists is much more common and damaging to patients. For example, in the clinical vignette, the psychiatrist induces the patient to engage in a host of acting-out behaviors including a sexual relationship.

Personal relationships. The specific boundary violations in the vignette are, unfortunately, all too common in reality. Even if sex had not taken place, the psychiatrist abandoned a neutral position and damaged the patient. The progressive precursor boundary violations prevented appropriate diagnosis and treatment of the patient's depression, inducing a benzodiazapine addiction and exacerbating a preexisting borderline personality disorder.

Most therapists accept the boundary-guideline principle of no previous, current, or future personal relations with the patient. For a number of sound clinical reasons, post-termination relationships with patients should be avoided (Simon, 1992). Past and current personal relationships with a patient hopelessly muddle treatment boundaries and doom therapeutic efforts. The social chit-chat that usually ensues is not psychotherapy. Transference can be timeless, raising serious concern about a former patient's ability for autonomous consent to a post-termination relationship.

Physical contact. The avoidance of physical contact with patients remains a controversial issue (Bancroft, 1981). Occasions may arise in treatment when a handshake or a hug by the therapist is an appropriate human response. Necessary clinical touching often occurs in the course of a procedure or treatment. Therapists who work with children, the elderly, and the physically ill frequently touch their patients in an appropriate, clinically supportive manner. An absolute prohibition against touching the patient would preclude such therapeutic human responses and supportive clinical interventions. Obviously, the psychiatrist in the vignette egregiously violates the guidelines against a personal relationship with the patient and the avoidance of most physical contact.

Therapists must be extremely wary of touching patients. Hugging may seem innocuous, but when closely considered, most hugs contain erotic messages. The practice of gratuitously touching the patient is clinically inappropriate and may be a prelude to sexual intimacies (Holub and Lee, 1990). Holroyd and Brodsky (1980) found that nonerotic hugging, kissing, and touching of opposite-sex patients but not same-sex patients by heterosexual therapists is a sex-biased therapy practice at high risk for leading to sexual intercourse with patients. Every patient has the right to the integrity and privacy of his or her own body.

Some psychiatrists still perform their own physical examinations of patients. The transference and countertransference complications associated with physically examining psychiatric patients are well known. It is very important that a physical examination not become the first step to progressive physical involvement with the patient. The presence of a chaperon will protect against false charges of sexual misconduct during the physical examination.

The issue of sex with a terminated patient is more complicated (Simon, 1992). An earlier proposal advanced by Appelbaum and Jorgenson (1991) of a one-year waiting period after termination that "should minimize problems and allow former patients and therapists to enter into intimate relationships" (p. 1466) would be likely to disrupt treatment boundaries from the outset. What deviations in treatment boundaries would occur if, during the course of therapy, the therapist considered the patient to be a potential sexual partner after termination? Would the therapy become a courtship? Would the therapy be prematurely ended so as to get to the sexual relationship? For the sake of the treatment, should not the patient be irrevocably and unequivocally renounced from the very beginning as a sexual partner for the therapist?

Ethically, post-termination sex is proscribed. The *Principles of Medical Ethics with Annotations Especially Applicable to Psychiatry* (American Psychiatric Association, 1995, sec. 1) clearly states: "Sexual activity with a current or former patient is unethical." Suffice it to say that the most credible clinical position for a therapist is to stay out of the patient's life after treatment ends. Some therapists sexualize the termination with the patient because they are unable to cope with feelings of separation, grief, and loss as the patient prepares to leave treatment. The patient should be allowed to go forward with his or her life, unencumbered by the therapist and the inevitable psychological baggage carried over from treatment.

Anonymity. In the vignette, the relative anonymity of the therapist is not maintained. The patient is burdened by the problems of the therapist, wasting valuable treatment time that the patient critically needs for her own care.

Therapist self-disclosure is also a complex topic (Stricker and Fisher, 1990). Self-disclosures that demonstrate the therapist's struggle with the problems of being human can be very supportive to some patients (Yalom, 1989). But they can trouble others. Patient and therapist sharing regression is one of the obvious dangers of therapist self-disclosure. Although some therapists have found that sharing a *past* personal experience may prove helpful to a patient, the self-disclosure of *current* conflicts and crises in the therapist's life may create a role reversal in the patient, who then attempts to rescue the therapist. Even if role reversal does not occur, therapist self-disclosures may burden the patient. Details of the therapist's personal life, particularly sexual fantasies and dreams, should not be shared with patients (Gutheil and Gabbard, 1993). Therapist self-disclosures appear to be highly correlated with the development of therapist-patient sex (Schoener, 1991; Borys and Pope, 1989). On the other hand, clinically appropriate self-disclosure may be necessary if the therapist is suffering from an illness that might negatively impact upon the treatment or may cause the therapist to be absent from therapy for a long period of time. Also, it has become standard practice for therapists providing substance-abuse treatment to reveal their own history of substance abuse.

The position of relative anonymity does not require that the therapist be a blank screen. The therapeutic relationship between therapist and patient is fundamentally interactive (Wachtel, 1987). For example, the therapist's overt and covert reactions to the patient can be therapeutically valuable. The therapist can point out to the patient the repetitive, maladaptive aspects of the patient-therapist interaction as they manifest themselves in other important relationships.

Fees. A fee policy that is mutually acceptable should be explained and established between the therapist and the patient at the beginning of treatment. Fees will change over time according to general economic exigencies and the personal circumstances of patients. Diminishing or discontinuing fees, however, must not be linked to boundary violations as a quid pro quo for the therapist to exploit the patient. The payment of the therapist's fee should be by money only. It emphasizes that therapy is work. Nonmonetary forms of payment should not be accepted (Simon, 1992).

Money-driven boundary violations are very common (Simon, 1992). Unless particularly egregious, money and insurance violations go unreported by comparison with spectacularly scandalous sexual misconduct cases. However, boundary violations involving money are a part of many other boundary problems in therapist-patient sex cases. Managed care settings where capitation systems or negative incentives exist may pressure therapists to exploit the patient's trust for financial gain. Therapists are penalized financially for providing more rather than less care.

As demonstrated in the vignette, therapists who become sexually involved with patients frequently discontinue billing. Will the patient who does not have to pay a bill be unlikely to discover the fact of his or her exploitation because of feeling special? Although this practice may have a number of meanings, the exploiting therapist often does so in the erroneous belief that not billing the patient terminates the treatment relationship and the possibility of being sued. The establishment and continuance of the doctor-patient relationship is not dependant on the payment of a fee (King, 1986).

Treatment setting. As Langs (1990) points out, a consistent, relatively neutral professional treatment setting provides a physical constant that helps to maintain an optimal degree of consistency, certainty, and stability for the treatment experience to unfold. In the vignette, the psychiatrist meets the patient in a park and a bar in addition to his office. Such practices tend to undercut the professional decorum of the therapist and trivialize the therapy. Since many patients have suffered from inconstancy and intrusiveness in their relationships and physical environments, maintaining privacy, stability, constancy, and professionalism of the treatment situation is of critical psychological importance. Therapists who see patients in their homes must be careful to maintain a private, professional setting distinct and separate from the living quarters. When patients must walk through and see or be seen by family members in the therapist's home, privacy and confidentiality may be compromised. Observing the domestic side of the therapist's life can cause patients a variety of problems and resistances in therapy. Such exposures to the therapist's domestic life can be the equivalent of intimate therapist self-disclosures.

Behavior therapists, however, do accompany phobic patients into threatening environments and situations as an appropriate part of their treatment regimen. Patients who have fears of using public bathrooms may be accompanied at some point by a therapist using behavior modification techniques. Therapists with religious orientations may attend services with their patients. Under exceptional circumstances or in an emergency, the therapist may need to make a house call. Thus an absolute prohibition cannot be issued against meeting patients outside the office because of clinical exigencies that arise with patients and the existence of reasonable variations in treatment approaches.

Psychotherapy usually cannot be conducted effectively over a telephone. Generally, the telephone is best used in making or breaking appointments or for patient emergencies. The patient should come to the therapist's office for treatment. The telephone or other technological devices (answering machines, beepers) should not be allowed to create barriers between the therapist and the patient (Canning et al., 1991).

On the other hand, therapists who treat patients suffering from multiple personality disorder may receive emergency calls from alters, requiring some sort of therapeutic intervention. Sometimes therapy may be temporarily conducted over the phone when patients cannot come to the office for reasons of work, travel, or physical illness. Medication adjustments between sessions may require use of the phone. If nonemergency telephone interviews are to be scheduled, they should be well structured, prearranged, time-limited therapeutic engagements, and paid for at the regular rates (Strasburger, 1991).

Time. Defined time and length of sessions also add stability to the treatment relationship. In addition, it is reassuring to the patient that psychic distress arising in therapy is time-limited. Generally, in sexual misconduct cases, sessions progressively lose time definition both in scheduling and in length with progressive boundary violations. The sessions take on a timeless id quality as therapist and patient appear to enter a time warp. Therapists must always question their rationale for lengthening or shortening sessions. Longer sessions may cause the patient to feel special and, thus, more vulnerable to exploitation. In the vignette, sessions went on for as long as three hours as boundary violations intensified.

On the other hand, the length of some sessions may need to be responsive to the exigent clinical needs of the patient. Patients in crisis may need additional time during a session. Patients with multiple personality disorder (MPD) often require flexibility in the length of sessions. Putnam (1989) recommends that MPD patients be seen for one-and-a-half-hour sessions. Prolonged sessions may be needed as various alters emerge (Treatment of Psychiatric Disorders, 1989). Patients with MPD, however, can exert inordinate pressure on the therapist to abandon conventional treatment boundaries.

Prevention

Treatment boundaries set by the therapist fluctuate in response to the dynamic, psychological interaction between therapist and patient. As a consequence, boundary excursions inevitably occur in almost every therapy. The boundary-sensitive therapist usually can reestablish treatment boundaries before the patient is psychologically harmed. Epstein and Simon (1990) have devised an Exploitation Index that provides therapists with early warning indicators of treatment-boundary violations. A survey of 532 psychiatrists who were administered the Exploitation Index revealed that 43 percent found that one or more questions alerted them to boundary violations, and 29 percent felt that the questionnaire stimulated them to make specific changes in future treatment practices (Epstein et al., 1992).

Prevention of progressive, damaging treatment-boundary violations has many facets. Education of psychiatric residents through tutorials and seminars about appropriate treatment boundaries should be undertaken. Psychiatric residents and other therapists in training should be familiar with the professional literature on setting treatment boundaries (Epstein, 1994). In a number of psychiatric residencies, this subject is scanted or totally ignored. Therapist-patient sex has a rather typical "natural history" that can aid early identification (Simon, 1995). Early consultation with a colleague should be undertaken if the therapist is able or willing to stop progressive boundary violations. Consultation may have a "Dutch Uncle" effect, banishing the transference and countertransference thrall that is beginning to endanger both the patient and therapist. Freida Fromm-Reichman, a renowned psychoanalyst, issued such a wake-up call when she warned, "Don't have sex with your patients, you will only disappoint them."

Damaging boundary violations begin insidiously and are progressive. During the segment of the therapy session that occurs "between the chair and the door," patients and therapists are more vulnerable to committing boundary excursions and violations. Inchoate boundary violations with a potential for damaging progression usually appear first within this interval. Both therapist and patient may cast off their respective roles prematurely, launching into social interaction before the patient actually leaves. This part of the session can be scrutinized for early warning of boundary violations and studied for its instructive value in risk management and the prevention of sexual misconduct (Gutheil and Simon, 1995).

Referral of the patient should not be reflexive when the therapist becomes aware of sexual feelings toward the patient. Countertransference has become a bad word to some therapists rather than an opportunity to use the therapist's feelings to further the therapeutic process. Pope and colleagues (1986) surveyed 575 psychotherapists and found that 87 percent (95 percent men, 76 percent women) felt sexually attracted to their clients but only 9.4 percent of men and 2.5 percent of women acted on those feelings. Sixty-three percent felt guilty, anxious, or confused about the attraction. The therapist should consider consultation and/or personal therapy if sexual feelings toward the patient are making the therapist too uncomfortable. If the therapist's feelings toward the patient threaten to lead to acting out, then the patient should be referred immediately.

Although "minor" boundary violations may initially appear innocuous, they may represent progression toward eventual exploitation of the patient. An instant "spot check" can be used to determine whether the therapist has committed a boundary violation. First, is the intervention in question done for the benefit of the therapist or for the sake of the patient's therapy? Second, is the intervention part of a series of progressive boundary violations? If the answer to either question is yes, the therapist is on notice to desist immediately and take corrective action. If basic treatment boundaries are violated and the patient is harmed, the therapist may be sued, charged with ethical violations, and deprived of his or her professional license and career.

References

American Psychiatric Association (1995). *The Principles of Medical Ethics with Annotations Especially Applicable to Psychiatry*. Washington.

Appelbaum, P., and L. Jorgenson (1991). "Psychotherapist-Patient Sexual Contact after Termination of Treatment: An Analysis and a Proposal." *American Journal of Psychiatry* 148: 1466–73.

Bancroft, J. (1981). "Ethical Aspects of Sexuality and Sex Therapy." In *Psychiatric Ethics,* ed. S. Block and P. Chodoff. New York: Oxford University Press.

Bibring, E. (1954). "Psychoanalysis and the Dynamic Psychotherapies." *Journal of the American Psychoanalytic Association* 2: 745–770.

Black, H. C. (1990). *Black's Law Dictionary,* 6th ed. St. Paul: West Publishing.

Borys, D., and K. Pope (1989). "Dual Relationships between Therapist and Client: A National Study of Psychologists, Psychiatrists, and Social Workers." *Professional Psychology: Research and Practice* 20: 287–293.

Canning, S., M. Hauser, and T. Gutheil (1991). "Communications in Psychiatric Practice: Decision Making and the Use of the Telephone." In *Decision Making in Psychiatry and the Law,* ed. T. Gutheil et al. Baltimore: Williams and Wilkins.

Epstein, R. S., and R. I. Simon (1990). "The Exploitation Index: An Early Warning Indicator of Boundary Violations in Psychotherapy." *Bulletin of the Menninger Clinic* 54: 450–464.

Epstein, R. S., R. I. Simon, and G. Kay (1992). "Assessing Boundary Violations in Psychotherapy: Survey Results with the Exploitation Index." *Bulletin of the Menninger Clinic* 56, no. 2: 1–17.

Epstein, R. S. (1994). *Keeping Boundaries.* Washington: American Psychiatric Press.

Freud, S. (1959). "Further Recommendations in the Technique of Psychoanalysis." In *Collected Papers,* vol. 2, ed. E. Jones and J. Riviere. New York: Basic Books.

Furrow, B. (1980). *Malpractice in Psychotherapy.* Lexington, Mass.: D. C. Heath.

Gutheil, T. G. (1989). "Borderline Personality Disorders, Boundary Violations, and Patient-Therapist Sex: Medicolegal Pitfalls." *American Journal of Psychiatry* 146: 597–602.

Gutheil, T. G. (1995). "Legal Issues in Psychiatry." In *Comprehensive Textbook of Psychiatry,* 6th ed., vol. 2, ed. H. I. Kaplan and B. J. Sadock. Baltimore: Williams and Wilkins.

Gutheil, T. G., and G. O. Gabbard (1993). "The Concept of Boundaries in Clinical Practice: Theoretical and Risk Management Dimensions." *American Journal of Psychiatry* 150: 188–196.

Gutheil, T. G., and R. I. Simon (1995). "Between the Chair and the Door: Boundary Issues in the Therapeutic 'Transition Zone.'" *Harvard Review of Psychiatry* 2: 336–340.

Holub, E., and S. Lee (1990). "Therapists' Use of Nonerotic Physical Contact: Ethical Concerns." *Professional Psychology: Research and Practice* 21: 115–117.

Holroyd, J., and A. Brodsky (1980). "Does Touching Patients Lead to Sexual Intercourse?" *Professional Psychology: Research and Practice* 11: 807–811.

In the Service of the State: The Psychiatrist as Double Agent (Special Supplement). (1978). Hastings-on-Hudson, The Hastings Center.

King, J. (1986). *The Law of Medical Malpractice*. St. Paul: West Publishing.

Langs, R. (1990). *Psychotherapy: A Basic Text*. Northvale, N.J.: Jason Aronson.

Marziali, E., C. Marmar, and J. Krupnick (1981). "Therapeutic Alliance Scales: Development and Relationship to Psychotherapy Outcome." *American Journal of Psychiatry* 138: 361–364.

Omer v. Edgren, 38 Wash. App. 376, 685 P.2d 635 (1984).

Peterson, M. (1992). *At Personal Risk: Boundary Violations in Professional-Client Relationships*. New York: Norton.

Pope, K. S., P. Keith-Spiegel, and B. G. Tabachnick (1986). "Sexual Attraction to Clients." *American Psychologist* 41: 147–158.

Putnam, F. W. (1989). *Diagnosis and Treatment of Multiple Personality Disorder*. New York: Guilford Press.

Schoener, G. (1989). "Assessment of Damages." In *Psychotherapists' Sexual Involvement with Clients: Intervention and Prevention,* ed. G. Schoener et al. Minneapolis, Walk-in Counseling Center.

Schoener, Gary, Director, Walk-in Counseling Center, Minneapolis, (1991). Personal communication, Oct. 15.

Shapiro, E., and W. Carr (1991). *Lost in Familiar Places: Creating New Connections between the Individual and Society*. New Haven: Yale University Press.

Simon, R. I. (1987). "The Psychiatrist as a Fiduciary: Avoiding the Double Agent Role." *Psychiatric Annals* 17: 622–626.

Simon, R. I. (1989a). "Sexual Exploitation of Patients: How It Begins before It Happens." *Psychiatric Annals* 19: 104–112.

Simon, R. I. (1989b). "Beyond the Doctrine of Informed Consent: A Clinician's Perspective." *Journal for the Expert Witness, the Trial Attorney, the Trial Judge* 4: 23–25.

Simon, R. I. (1990). "The Duty to Protect in Private Practice." In *Confidentiality versus the Duty to Protect: Foreseeable Harm in the Practice of Psychiatry,* ed. J. Beck. Washington: American Psychiatric Press.

Simon, R. I. (1991a). "The Practice of Psychotherapy: Legal Liabilities of an 'Impossible' Profession." In *American Psychiatric Press Review of Clinical Psychiatry and the Law,* vol. 2, ed. R. I. Simon. Washington: American Psychiatric Press.

Simon, R. I. (1991b). "Psychological Injury Caused by Boundary Violation Precursors to Therapist-Patient Sex." *Psychiatric Annals* 21: 614–619.

Simon, R. I. (1992). *Clinical Psychiatry and the Law,* vol. 2. Washington: American Psychiatric Press.

Simon, R. I. (1993). "Innovative Psychiatric Therapies and Legal Uncertainty: A Survival Guide for Clinicians." *Psychiatric Annals* 23: 473–479.

Simon, R. I. (1994). "Transference in Therapist-Patient Sex: The Illusion of Patient Improvement and Consent, Part 1 and 2." *Psychiatric Annals* 24, no. 10: 509–515; 24, no. 11: 561–565.

Simon, R. I. (1995). "The Natural History of Therapist Sexual Misconduct: Identification and Prevention." *Psychiatric Annals* 25: 90–94.

Simon, R., and R. Sadoff (1991). *Psychiatric Malpractice: Cases and Comments for Clinicians.* Washington: American Psychiatric Press.

Strasburger, Larry H., M.D. (1991). Personal communication, November 19.

Stricker, G., and M. Fisher (1990). *Self-Disclosure in the Therapeutic Relationship.* New York: Plenum Press.

Treatment of Psychiatric Disorders (1989). A Task Force Report of the American Psychiatric Association. Vol. 3. Washington: American Psychiatric Press.

Wachtel, P. (1987). *Action and Insight.* New York: Guilford Press.

Yalom, I. D. (1989). *Love's Executioner and Other Tales of Psychotherapy.* New York: Basic Books.

14

Termination of Treatment with Troublesome Patients

James Hilliard, J.D.

The question is often posed: How can I terminate treatment with a patient who may need continued care but with whom, for any one of a number of reasons, continued therapy is impossible? The answer to this question is crucial because a treating doctor may be held legally responsible for damages resulting from the "abandonment" of a patient.

Abandonment of a patient has been generally defined by the courts as a severance of the professional relationship between doctor and patient without reasonable notice and without adequate consideration for the patient's condition at a time when there is still a need for continuing medical attention. Once initiated, the relationship between a physician and a patient continues until it is ended by the consent of the parties, until it is revoked by the dismissal of the physician, or until the services of the physician are no longer needed.

First, it should be understood that, as a general principle, psychiatrists *are not* required to treat everyone and may, with the proper procedure, terminate with a patient prior to an end result being reached. Section 6 of the *Principles of Medical Ethics with Annotations Especially Applicable to Psychiatry*[1] states: "A physician shall, in the provision of appropriate patient care, except in emergencies, be free to choose whom to serve." Implicit in such a principle is the *duty* of the physician/psychiatrist to exercise due care when terminating a relationship with a patient.

Second, an understanding of what constitutes abandonment from a practical point of view is necessary in order to avoid such a claim when termination is appropriate. Abandonment is a legal conclusion reached after examining the process of termination and determining that it substantially departed from accepted professional standards to the detriment of the patient. In other words, abandonment occurs when a psychiatrist terminates treatment with a patient without regard for the patient's condition or needs, or without the formation of an adequate plan for follow-up treatment. Abandonment can occur through neglect (for example, the psychiatrist ignores calls for appointments or misses appointments without appropriate notice) or through intentional conduct (for example, the psychiatrist affirmatively terminates treatment with the patient during a course of therapy and without a proper referral to another psychiatrist). Often abandonment will be precipitated by a falling-out between patient and psychiatrist caused by the patient's behavior (for example, threatening the psychiatrist, refusing to cooperate with medication, making undue demands or intrusive behavior, refusing to pay bill) which makes continued therapy difficult and sometimes impossible.

Additionally, several recent celebrated cases have involved, at least tangentially, allegations of abandonment spurred by the misconduct of psychiatrists or therapists (sexual improprieties, monetary abuses, boundary violations). However, in light of the fact that sexual misconduct is an intentional act that is universally excluded from a physician's liability insurance, a claimant will generally include an allegation of sexual misconduct as a subsidiary claim to the more substantial and insurable claim of abandonment.

The specter of abandonment does not preclude the ability of a physician to withdraw from an established relationship with a patient before the need for the physician's services has ended. Rather, regardless of the particular justification for withdrawal, a physician may terminate a relationship with a patient but is bound to give due notice to the patient and afford the patient ample opportunity to secure other medical attendance of his or her own choice.

Failure to properly withdraw from or terminate a physician-patient relationship may expose the physician to substantial liability. Damages to an affected patient may warrant awards for wrongful death, permanent physical incapacity, pain and suffering, mental anguish, an unnecessary hospital stay, and/or excessive hospital bills.

A review of the small but vital body of case law regarding abandonment may aid in the practical determination of the parameters of a physician's duties as well as potential liabilities. However, while a survey of the relevant case law provides perspective, the several states which have visited this issue have viewed the concept of abandonment in a variety of ways, and the corresponding variety of legal conclusions are not necessarily reconcilable.

Coddington v. Robertson,[2] a Michigan case, involved the termination by a psychologist of a relationship with a patient who routinely communicated death threats to the psychologist. In the psychologist's professional opinion, a respite from treatment was warranted, although further eventual treatment was not ruled out in the event that the patient ceased making threats. The psychologist provided proper notice to the patient of the cessation of the relationship. Due to the fact that the patient continued to make threatening telephone calls and write threatening letters, the psychologist refused to reinstitute the relationship. Two years after the cessation of the relationship, the patient filed suit against the psychologist, alleging abandonment.

Utilizing the date that the psychologist withdrew from the relationship, the court ruled that Michigan's two-year statute of limitations for malpractice actions was applicable to bar the patient's cause of action. Concurrent with this finding was the conclusion that the two-year gap in the relationship could not constitute "treatment" for the purpose of either establishing liability or staving off a defense that the complaint was time-barred. While the court's reasoning focused on the statute of limitations issue, the opinion it wrote scrutinized and found no fault in the psychologist's withdrawal in the face of physical threats by his patient.

In *Miller v. Greater Southeast Community Hospital*,[3] the Court of Appeals in the District of Columbia held that a patient who was refused the advice of her treating physician could not maintain an action for abandonment where she was provided with a suitable substitute physician. Prior to withdrawing from their relationship, the physician in this case provided the patient, whose condition did not require immediate attention from a physician, with a list of other capable physicians. The patient chose a new physician from the list, and in the interim her previous doctor arranged for continuous medical attention from the hospital and personally consulted with the physician who was replacing him. The initial physician's withdrawal was found to be "within accepted standards of medical care."

A South Carolina Appeals Court took a more expansive, albeit similar, view on the issue of a substitute physician in *Johnston v. Ward*.[4] In this case, a treating psychiatrist was informed by an emergency room physician that his patient, whom he had been treating for depression and anxiety, had been admitted to the hospital after an apparent overdose of her prescribed medication. While the patient's treating psychiatrist never actually traveled to the hospital to attend to his patient, he assumed responsibility and arranged for another physician to provide treatment. The substitute physician provided persistent medical attention to the patient and remained in contact with the original treating psychiatrist. However, because of an error in judgment by the emergency room physician, the patient lapsed into a coma and died. The court found no evidence of abandonment by the treating psychiatrist owing to the fact that the substitution was proper and that through his constant direction, consistent and proper medical attention was provided to the patient.

In so finding, the court implicitly opined that a treating physician need not always be present during the treatment of a patient. Rather, if a treating physician delegates treatment to another physician and directs said treatment, liability may only be premised upon the failure of the treating physician to appoint a competent substitute, or if any eventual negligence is perpetrated by a substitute who is also an employee of the treating physician. A non-negligent delegation to an otherwise competent substitute physician cannot form the basis of liability even if the substitute subsequently treats the patient negligently.

In *Brandt v. Grubin*,[5] a New Jersey court found that a family doctor who was not a specialist in mental disorders did not abandon his patient when, after a brief course of treatment, he referred the patient to more appropriate and specialized avenues of treatment and then withdrew from the relationship. The patient committed suicide while under the care of the subsequent treating professional.

Crucial to the court's reasoning were the findings that the patient sought out the doctor for a specific purpose, the doctor was unable to provide the necessary treatment, the doctor informed the patient of his inability to render proper treatment, and the doctor provided the patient with more appropriate alternatives for proper treatment. After the doctor withdrew from the relationship with the patient, he no longer possessed a duty to treat, despite repeated attempts by the patient's family to contact him.

Brief reference must also be made to *Knapp v. Eppright*,[6] a Texas case which held that no claim for abandonment may lie where a patient voluntarily and unilaterally chooses to terminate the relationship. An important caveat to this holding, and one that is virtually limited to the treatment of mental illness, is that of a patient's competence when making such a unilateral decision to terminate treatment. A psychiatrist, of course, owes a duty to care for an incompetent patient, and this duty may be modified by a number of factors, including the severity of the patient's illness and the risk of harm that a patient may pose either to him- or herself or to others. Depending on such variables, a psychiatrist may not pay heed to a patient's unilateral decision to terminate and, rather, may make arrangements for further treatment or even petition for hospitalization of the patient.

While abandonment is rooted in the overarching duty that a psychiatrist owes to the patient, the advent of managed care has created additional avenues whereby an injured patient may levy a claim of abandonment. In *Wickline v. California,*[7] the court reasoned that, despite the state's managed care system's patent denial of the services that were recommended by the treating physician, the physician could not absolve himself from the ultimate duty to care for the patient. The court found that "the physician who complies without protest with the limitation imposed by a third-party payor when his medical judgment dictates otherwise cannot avoid his ultimate responsibility for his patient's care." Although an allegation of abandonment against the physician was not made in *Wickline,* it is certainly plausible that the continued evolution of "abandonment theory" may include situations where a physician provides substandard or incomplete care in blind and unreasonable adherence to a managed care company's cost-conscious directives.

What, therefore, are the acceptable procedures for proper termination, and under what circumstances should termination be employed?

First, termination should *never* be precipitated by the anger of the psychiatrist. Nor should it occur while the patient is in a serious crisis. Termination should be a process that is employed in the severance of the professional relationship with a patient, and the use of this process must be properly documented by the psychiatrist. The following is an outline of a recommended termination process:

1. Honestly discuss with the patient your intention to terminate and the specific reasons for it. For example, if you have been threatened by your patient, tell him or her that this is the basis for your decision and how you feel about the problem. You should give your patient the opportunity to correct the situation in order to evaluate whether or not further treatment is possible.

2. Offer the patient one to three "termination" sessions (if appropriate, depending upon the reasons for termination). If this is not feasible in light of the reasons for termination (such as the patient threatening the psychiatrist), be sure to *properly document* your reasons.

3. Provide the patient with the names and phone numbers of available therapists suitable for his or her care *and* the address and phone number of the nearest hospital for emergency care if needed. If a patient needs immediate care and there is a concern that there may be a delay in treatment by a successor-therapist, it is recommended that you either delay termination or arrange for another therapist to assume care immediately upon your termination of the patient's treatment. However, absent overriding justifica-

tion for a ban on all further treatments (such as severe threats), it may be unreasonable to proscribe further treatments that may arise in an emergency or when alternative treatment is not available. Additionally, although hospitalization may not serve as a means of termination, in severe cases the hospitalization of a seriously ill patient may be a viable consideration and may operate to safeguard the patient's condition until the patient is stabilized and/or appropriate successor treatment can be arranged.

4. Your adherence to the protocol suggested above should then be put in writing in the form of memoranda to the patient's file and a letter to the patient (where appropriate) to be sure there has been no misunderstanding of the reasons for termination, the recommendation for continued treatment, the offer of termination sessions, and your willingness to cooperate with the subsequent treater. Additionally, you must be sensitive to the patient's right to confidentiality in his or her records, and such records should be transferred to successor physicians only after the patient has expressly waived privilege or has otherwise provided written permission for such a transfer.

In psychiatry, unlike other medical specialties, termination, even when proper, often leads to a complaint to either the professional society or the Board of Medicine, and if damages are alleged to have resulted from the termination it may lead to a malpractice claim. Accordingly, any termination should be given serious advance consideration and should then be handled and documented very carefully.

Notes

1. *The Principles of Medical Ethics with Annotations Especially Applicable to Psychiatry* (American Psychiatric Association, 1995).
2. 160 Mich. App. 460, 407 N.E.2d 666 (1987).
3. 508 A.2d 927 (D.C. App. 1986).
4. 344 S.E.2d 166 (S.C. App. 1986).
5. 131 N.J. Super. 182, 329 A.2d 82 (1974).
6. 783 S.W.2d 293 (Tex. App.-Houston, 14th Dist., 1989).
7. 228 Cal. Rptr. 661 (Cal. App. 2d Dist. 1986).

The Clinician
in Court

/ / /

15

Witnesses, Depositions, and Trials

Thomas G. Gutheil, M.D.

In this chapter I clarify the different roles the psychiatrist can play in court, and I discuss the two major contexts in which some form of testimony will occur, namely, the deposition and the trial itself. While, for completeness, one might also indicate various forms of hearings, administrative law reviews, ethics committee transactions for local professional organizations, and proceedings before Boards of Registration in Medicine or similar licensing agencies, the fundamental principles here addressed will either apply broadly or will require only slight modifications to fit the requirements of those situations.[1]

There are, of course, a number of situations in which a largely clinically based assessment enters into the legal system. Examples include the treatment or evaluation of substance abuse problems, the assessment of a contested case of disability claim, and treatment of offenders; these largely clinical activities will not be reviewed here.

Also not addressed here is a role which attorneys commonly fill, but which psychiatrists on a number of occasions, may also fill[2] known as the "guardian ad litem" (GAL). The word "litem," from the Latin, is etymologically related to the word "litigation." The GAL is a complex and flexible role played by individuals who broadly perform investigative functions for the court. To choose one example out of many, a patient might be the subject of a dispute around his or her right to refuse antipsychotic treatment during hospitalization. A GAL might be appointed by the court to visit the patient in the hospital and make preliminary determinations in a neutral and objective manner about the appropriateness of the diagnosis, the treatment plan, the situation, and any extenuating factors that the court wishes to know before placing the matter into the adversarial process with testimony on both sides. This function could be performed by an attorney with some knowledge of health law issues, by a psychiatrist, or—perhaps ideally—by an attorney/psychiatrist team. This role is addressed elsewhere.[1,2]

Kinds of Witnesses

There are many different varieties of witness that may be defined in terms of the legal strategy in accordance with which the witness's testimony is employed. For example, a witness may serve as an *alibi witness* in relation to a person involved in a legal proceeding; if the defendant, say, is alleged to have committed a crime at a particular time, the witness may provide an alibi by having seen the defendant in a place other than the crime scene at that time.

A *character witness* provides evidence from a history of acquaintance, observation, or other context that speaks to the character of an individual connected with the proceedings; thus, in an ambiguous case, testimony as to the character of, say, the defendant may be relevant to the legal decisionmaking.

A *rebuttal witness* is brought in solely to challenge, contradict, or refute—that is, to rebut—the testimony of another witness to the proceedings. Rebuttal witnesses may be used to attempt to refute the testimony of experts on either side, of alibi witnesses, of character witnesses, or of any other witness to the proceeding.

As noted, these categories of witnesses are defined in terms of their role within the broad legal strategy of the attorney managing that side of the case. Each of these roles is relatively straightforward and would be no different for a clinician serving these functions than for any other kind of witness. However, in terms of the clinician in court, the critical role usually takes one of two forms: the fact witness and the expert witness.

THE FACT WITNESS
The fact witness, in general, testifies to those phenomena legally identified as "facts." This is almost always limited to matters of direct observation and direct performance. The witness testifies to what he or she "heard, saw, thought and did myself." The overall principle here is that such witnesses testify only to those facts that dwell within their realm of personal knowledge obtained via the senses, as opposed to information told them by someone else. While ordinarily the latter situation would be dismissed as "hearsay," we must remember that for every mental health professional,

the entire history plays an essential role, and the history, indeed, is material reported by the patient or others, that is, hearsay. This sometimes raises questions of admissibility that are basically not the clinician's problem; the attorneys will be offering guidance in this area.

Two important distinctions must be addressed that sharply distinguish the fact witness from the expert witness. First, special expertise in a particular field is not required to testify regarding facts within one's personal knowledge. Second, unlike experts, fact witnesses are not permitted to draw conclusions from the facts being put forward in the testimony. For example, a fact witness may describe the symptoms and go so far as to offer the diagnosis that he or she applied to the patient in question. However, the fact witness, under most circumstances, is not permitted to testify as to whether certain treatments met the standard of care or whether the assessment of the patient was consistent with criminal nonresponsibility in an insanity case. Table 15.1 outlines the critical differences between fact witnesses and expert witnesses (the latter sometimes referred to as forensic witnesses to convey their connection with the legal process). Finally, note that in some jurisdictions, a judge may convert a fact witness into an expert witness.

Just as in the case of the treating clinician, the fundamental duty of the fact witness is generally to the patient in question. That is, the obligation to function as a clinician in the courtroom context does not alter the basic responsibility to consider the patient's welfare, even though the only official constraint is the taking of the oath. Finally, fact witnesses are generally not paid for their time in the courtroom, although under rare circumstances a patient or family may be billed for this time. A number of states offer a pittance as a fact witness fee when the subpoena is delivered.

Fact witnesses may appear in two legally determined roles and two clini-

Table 15.1. CHARACTERISTICS OF FACT WITNESSES AND EXPERT WITNESSES

Treater (fact witness)	*Expert witness*
Client = patient	Client = attorney
Goal = clinical care	Goal = assist the attorney
Confidential	Not confidential
Written note mandatory	Attorney decides
Patient as informant	Corroborating sources
Record review varies	Detailed record review
Insurance covers	No coverage
Patient pays	Attorney pays

cally determined ones. First, the psychiatrist as a fact witness may be the plaintiff in a case, although this would not be a common role; presumably, clinicians may under some circumstances find themselves in the position of bringing suit against someone and, here, the role of plaintiff is a function of the fact witness. As plaintiff, the clinician would testify as to the manner in which he or she was aggrieved and the incidents that led to the litigation.

Conversely, the clinician may serve as defendant in a malpractice suit or in any other kind of litigation (for example, litigation arising out of an auto accident or a similar event). Here, again, simple reporting of what happened defines the role function of the witness.

In a more clinical context, the clinician may be a fact witness in the purest form; that is, as the simple observer of events. The clinician may be neither diagnostician, treater, nor evaluator, but may have been standing by when legally relevant events occurred. One simple example of this is in a so-called hospital-slip-and-fall case; a clinician may have fortuitously observed an accidental fall and may be able to offer testimony about the context that would be useful to the court's deliberations.

Finally, the clinician may be the treater of a patient or of a defendant in a piece of litigation, the latter conceivably extending to criminal defendants as well as civil. It is fairly common for such treating clinicians to offer testimony as to a patient's condition before a contested event (an accident, a fall, alleged mistreatment by physicians) or the condition after an alleged event. These "bookend" roles are usually intended to assist the court in determination of the tension between such factors as preexisting conditions that may have to be subtracted, as it were, from the alleged impact of the particular events in question; and assessment of the patient *post facto* may provide substance in clinical terms to the claim of damages or harms resulting from the incidents in question.

THE EXPERT WITNESS

The expert witness plays a very different role. The expert, if qualified by the court, is permitted to testify (like a fact witness) to issues of direct observation. However, there are two areas where experts may testify that are closed to the fact witness. First, experts are permitted to testify to matters that are not accessible to lay knowledge. Examples include what constitutes the standard of medical care against which a particular course of treatment is measured, and the fit of a particular person to explicit criteria such as insanity, testamentary capacity, and the like. Second, unlike the fact witness, the expert may draw conclusions from the data at a second level of abstraction. The data involved may, indeed, include hearsay and the observations of others, as well as or even instead of direct examination.

An example of the latter issue might be whether the standard of care was met in relation to a patient who has committed suicide. Obviously, direct examination of that individual is foreclosed. Yet the expert is entitled to bring together the available data and offer testimony as to whether the standard of care was met.

The rules of confidentiality are also different for expert witnesses. An expert witness may be submitting reports or offering testimony in open court, so that the content becomes a matter of public record. Further comments on this issue are found below.

The expert witness has many other functions and roles which are addressed elsewhere and will not be rehearsed here.[1,3] Note for the present that the expert is paid for his or her time (and not, as plaintiffs' attorneys sometimes suggest, for testimony), in part as a reflection of the fact that the expert's responsibility is to the retaining attorneys, courts, or other third parties, rather than to the patient or client directly. A review of Table 15.1 will remind the reader of some other relevant differences. In the malpractice context, of course, the expert's primary role is to address the medical/legal bases for the four critical elements of malpractice litigation: the alleged deviation from the standard of care, the presence and validity of the duty from treater to patient, the extent of damages present, and the critical link between negligence and damages by way of causation in its legal sense.[1]

On a more sophisticated level, the expert may function to define (or, for that matter, to refute) additional theories of the case, to aid the attorney to define areas for recovery, and to assess the extent of damages. The expert can also offer the attorney advice about the management of the problematic client and his or her response to the various stresses of litigation, and may offer various forms of litigation support. This support might include education of the attorney as to the clinical issues in the case, assessment of the strength of the case, participation in the selection of other experts, and critique of expert testimony on the other side. An expert may also perform other consultative functions in relation to the preparation of direct and cross-examination of various witnesses and development of trial strategies, including sitting at counsel's table during the trial and offering relevant advice.

The Treater as Expert

A question that comes up frequently is whether a treating therapist who is working with a patient subsequent to an alleged harm may appropriately serve as the expert witness on the legal case. The short answer is that usually he or she should not do so. This answer rests upon clinical, legal, and ethical bases.

The clinical basis derives first from the fact that the clinician is the patient's ally and advocate. While these are both laudable and probably essential treatment considerations, they represent a profound and disqualifying degree of bias for the objectivity required of the expert. More significantly, the clinician is charged with seeing the world essentially through the patient's eyes. This is in contrast to the expert's role in obtaining a comprehensive database consisting of all the available information in the case, including data that contradict one's patient's claims.

Legally, there is a potential conflict of interest. If the patient has indeed been damaged, these damages provide both the incentive and the reason for the clinician to be treating this very patient. However, an award for damages also provides a financial incentive to continue treating the patient and a possible temptation to extend that treatment, not as far as the patient needs, but as far as the patient's financial award from the trial will stretch. Thus, the treater as expert is testifying about damages in a context which funnels the compensation for those damages into the treater's pocket.

Finally, on ethical grounds, the clinician's ethical mandate as treater is "first, do no harm" and then to act in all contexts in the service of the patient's welfare. This function contrasts with that of the expert, some of whose testimony may not be helpful—indeed, may be overtly harmful— to the patient's case and, hence, the patient's welfare.[4] Note that in the testimony function of the expert witness, the expert warns the examinee (since experts do not have a doctor-patient relationship, the person being interviewed is an examinee, not a patient) that the testimony is not confidential and that it may have positive, negative, or no particular impact on the case. These warnings permit the examinee's participation with a modicum of informed consent.

Attorneys surprisingly often attempt to get the treater to serve the expert role. In some cases it's a matter of simple economy: the treater is already involved in the case and the lawyer is disinclined to hire an additional clinician as expert witness because of the additional expense. Equally striking is the number of attorneys who fail to appreciate the distinction between treater and expert in regard to the various conflicts outlined above. And some attorneys argue that the value of "treater as expert" lies, as in other specialties, in the degree to which the treater "knows the patient best"; thus, the treater's testimony—not the least by being uncompensated financially—is intrinsically more credible than that of the expert, who may be suspected of testifying as a "hired gun." These attorneys tend to minimize the credibility-damaging effect of the treater's bias on behalf of the patient and the fact that some of the ultimate damage compensation may be destined for the treater's coffers.

Taking all of the foregoing into account, I must recommend that the roles of treater and expert be played by two different individuals. In my view, the validity, the credibility, the objectivity, and the accuracy of the testimony are all enhanced by this separation.[5]

The Deposition

For the average individual, a sufficient definition of a deposition might be the following: "A deposition is an oral examination under oath taken of a witness in a legal proceeding with relevant attorneys present and usually serving an information-gathering function in early or discovery phases of trial preparation in a piece of litigation."

This definition—though plausible and, in a limited sense, accurate on its face—fails to capture an essential reality: the actual deposition is the *written transcript* of the "oral examination under oath, etc." It is the written record that will be used to challenge, check, and, indeed, impeach the testimony of the witness at a later trial. This fact has several important implications.

First, it is extremely important in a deposition to think through one's answers carefully. As will be noted later, in a trial, a seeming spontaneity of answering is desirable. The reverse of this is true in the deposition context. The witness should pause to replay the question in his or her mind, to think through the response, to look for possible pitfalls or apparent contradictions, and—only then—should speak. Note that the transcript does not record pauses.

Second, the witness should not worry about sounding stiff, awkward, or pedantic, since such considerations would only have relevance for a live jury where they might be off-putting. Third, a witness's answers should have the self-sufficient, free-standing quality that comes from finding a way to include the question within the answer when a brief narrative response is called for. (The five classic deposition answers are "Yes," "No," "I don't know," "I don't recall," and a brief narrative response.) The brief narrative response should strive to encapsulate the question so that the answer can never be lifted out of context. For example, if the question is "What did you observe on your first meeting with the patient?" a possible brief answer would be "Anxiety symptoms." A preferable answer would be "On my first meeting with this patient on June 5, 1992, I observed a number of symptoms including but not limited to the following," and then one supplies whatever recollection or documented phenomena one has available.

Finally, it is critical to understand that—while the audience at a trial is the judge or jury—the audience at the deposition is *not* the examining or questioning attorney(s), but the stenographer, since the stenographer's accurate and verbatim transcribed record is the essence of the deposition. Experienced witnesses often directly face the stenographer and make every effort to speak slowly, while also spelling out names, bits of jargon, and technical terms that the stenographer might not be expected to know. The witness should overcome the concern that to speak to the stenographer is some form of rudeness to the attorney(s) asking the questions. The attorney who protests, "Look at me while I'm talking to you," may be politely informed that he or she is nowhere nearly as important to the process in which you are all involved as the stenographer, whose record will be binding upon all parties.

To summarize, common misconceptions concerning depositions can be grouped under the witness thinking the deposition *is* like a trial and the witness thinking the deposition is *not* like a trial. Both these views are in error.

The deposition *is* like a trial in that the testimony is given under oath and thus is vulnerable to the charge of perjury if conscious misstatements or deceptions are practiced. As with a trial, it is essential that the witness be sure about what is being said. Remember that "I don't know" and "I don't recall" are perfectly acceptable answers in this context. A deposition is also like a trial in that testimony at one point may be used to impeach or contradict testimony at another. This is true within different parts of a deposition as well as between the deposition and the trial. Finally, a deposition is like a trial in that it requires preparation as careful as that for testifying in court. Many a witness has gotten into serious difficulty by taking a cavalier attitude toward preparation before a deposition by reasoning falsely, "It's not as if I were actually going to court, after all." Deposition testimony can also be used in *other* trials to impeach the expert.

A deposition is *not* like a trial in the manner of speech. While the statements to the stenographer are to be made in a highly formal and careful manner, a more relaxed, spontaneous manner is preferred in the courtroom. Similarly, deposition answers must be free-standing, as opposed to the greater possibility of colloquialism in the jury context.

One variation must be addressed: the videotaped deposition. Videotaped depositions may be taken when it is impossible for a witness to arrive at trial because of various conflicts or obstacles, or when a witness's physical condition or illness makes it impossible for him or her to travel to the trial in a distant location. A videotaped deposition in this context more closely resembles a trial before a jury than an ordinary deposition. Indeed, the testifying witness should address the camera as though it were a jury box and communicate in the same spontaneous, alert, and interested manner as would be the case at trial. The expert should look directly into the camera. Otherwise darting eyes give the appearance of shiftiness.

Another difference between depositions and trials is the length of the answers supplied by the witness. While the brief narrative element may be similar in both situations, as a rule deposition answers should be short and crisp so as not to offer too much material for potential impeachment. An answer during trial testimony should be as long as it takes fully to answer the question being posed. Note that the limit on this discursiveness is the same as it would be with an audience, say, of medical students being addressed on some important point. That is, if the jury's eyes begin to glaze over, it's time to stop.

A witness going to trial or deposition should wear conservative business attire, since anything less formal may be distracting or interpreted as a lack of seriousness by the attorneys or jury.

In a number of witness roles, including that of defendant, the deposition may be taken by the opposing attorney. It may be helpful to the future witness to be alert to certain common deposition tactics. First, if you are the defendant, it is worth noting that senior attorneys set, as a specific goal, obtaining from the defendant doctor some self-defeating admission of negligence through some sort of concession in the course of the deposition. This covert agenda should place the defendant doctor on notice and encourage great vigilance and caution in responding to queries. To achieve this goal, opposing attorneys have a number of tricks up their sleeves, only some of which can be outlined here.

First, attorneys can play with the sequence of questions. Even inexperienced witnesses acknowledge having a certain mental map of how they expect the inquiry to go, beginning with basic demographic identifying data ("Please provide us with and spell your name, Doctor; your address, social security number . . .") and moving on to historical material and qualifications ("Where did you go to medical school, Doctor? Where did you train after that? When did you first take on Mr. Jones as a patient?"). In order to challenge these expectations and shake up the witness, some attorneys begin by saying, "Do you have any idea what damages Mr. Jones suffered?" or "Tell me everything that you think you did wrong, looking back on your care of Mr. Jones." By bringing up the conclusion at the very beginning of the examination, the attorney may succeed in rattling the witness.

The attorneys can also attempt to prevent the witness from thinking carefully before responding to questions. When a witness who follows the advice given earlier in this chapter is asked a question by the attorney, there is a brief silence in which the witness mentally replays the question, attempts to select and phrase the appropriate response, turns to the stenographer, and offers that answer. One strategy attorneys may use to break this defense is to fire questions at a high rate of speed in an attempt to both rattle the witness and draw the witness into answering at the same high speed. This can be quite effective in eliciting thoughtless responses. Even though a rapid question followed by a slow response with a long pause may sound a little strange to the ear, it is important to recall that it is the written transcript which defines the deposition; the speed of the questions and answers is unrecorded in the transcript.

A related strategy might be called "Let's chat." Here, the attorney attempts to ingratiate him- or herself with the witness and to lull the witness into having a casual and informal, unselfconscious, free-flowing conversation as though this were not a formal legal proceeding. Attorneys may express admiration for the witness ("Thank you, Doctor, that was an extremely clear answer"), make casual comments ("You sure had a lot of snow around here this week, I see"), use self-disclosure ("I never could handle going to medical school with all those big words, Doctor, so I'll ask you to define them"), and similar ploys. The witness should maintain a judicious degree of vigilance against lapsing into the chatty style. Again, it is not the witness's task to worry about conversational niceties in this context. Beware of discussions with opposing counsel during breaks or in the bathroom.

Even with the most articulate and slow-speaking witness and the most highly skilled stenographer, errors do creep into deposition transcripts. I strongly recommend that every witness for a deposition elect to read and sign the deposition transcript after it is completed. Traditionally, the recording service provides an errata sheet on which errors and typos can be corrected. It is considered ill-advised and potentially damaging to one's credibility to attempt to make extensive changes in one's testimony through this mechanism; substantive changes should be announced to the other side in an affidavit. Rather, misspellings and homophones can be corrected and distinguished to solidify the accuracy of the written report. Commonly, the errata sheet and a separate page attesting that the transcript is a true and accurate copy are notarized by the witness after reviewing the text.

Trial

Many a case is settled or dropped after a deposition; that is, when the discovery reveals to either party that the case is not what they thought it was. However, approximately 6 percent of cases do go on to trial. In the event that your case is among that 6 percent, let us now address the distinguishing features of trial testimony.

First, recall that the legal system grinds slowly. If you are called for a particular time to testify at trial, I strongly recommend clearing the entire day and being prepared to clear the following morning at least on short notice. It will certainly be worthwhile to bring materials relevant to the case along to review while waiting. If there is little substantive material of this sort to review, consider bringing along a book to occupy your time while waiting and to prevent impatience.

Attire should be conservative. Men should avoid casual clothing such as turtlenecks, unusual or flamboyant neckwear, and the like. Women should avoid dresses, pants, and either high heels or flat shoes (the first being too dressy and the second too informal). In short, both men and women should dress like the lawyers of their respective genders in suits appropriate to business wear. Ostentation in accessories, jewelry, wristwatches, and the like should also be eschewed.

Language, too, should be modified. After a question is asked, the witness in court should pause momentarily. In addition to allowing a quick replay of the question in one's own mind, this pause allows the relevant attorney to object if this is indicated. This may obviate the need to answer the question at all and, therefore, is worth this slight investment of the clinician's time. In contrast to the deposition, it is absolutely essential that the clinician in court speak in basic, jargon-free English, avoiding complicated sentence structure, technical terms, and excessively academic language. The educational level of the average jury, with certain exceptions, ranges from ninth to twelfth grade in many parts of the country. Those individuals are also likely to be available for jury pools without competing obligations. On the other hand, juries are rapidly turned off if the clinician appears to be speaking down to them; hence, the desired approach is basic English which does not sound as though you are making an effort to speak basic English. The difficulty of hewing to this line justifies some rehearsal sessions with partners, spouses, or trusted colleagues, since—short of teaching first-year medical students—most clinicians do not encounter this dilemma.

Experts on courtroom demeanor underscore the value of using graphics and blackboard or flip-chart aids in communicating with the jury. Besides permitting a jury to visualize complex data, such courtroom illustrative aids have two advantages over spoken testimony. The first is the fact that the doctor is obviously putting effort into making an issue clear to the jury. Even if the jury does not fully understand the substance of the demonstration, the doctor's effort to be clear will be perceived and appreciated. Second, in using such demonstrative evidence, the doctor is slipping into the most trusted role in modern society, that of the teacher.[3] If we look at this from the transference perspective, a juror may have hated the teacher or loved the teacher, but there is no question that the teacher knew the field, whether it may have been the capital of Arkansas or the number of free electrons in the oxygen atom. This transference aids in the conviction behind the expert's testimony. However, one must be careful not to seem to lecture the jury.

Later chapters will address the details of handling cross-examination on the witness stand. Here I will only note again that witnesses going to court should keep in mind that "I don't know" is a perfectly acceptable answer. Note also that attorneys can be astonishingly maladroit at phrasing questions even though they do this for a living; the witness should feel free to indicate inability to understand or to follow the question. It is the lawyer's obligation to get the question into an answerable form—that is not the witness's problem.

Notes

The author gratefully acknowledges the assistance of Ronald Schouten, J.D., M.D., in the preparation of this chapter.

1. Appelbaum, P. S., and T. G. Gutheil (1991). *Clinical Handbook of Psychiatry and the Law*. Baltimore: Williams and Wilkins.
2. Gutheil, T. G. (in press). *The Psychiatrist as Expert Witness*. Washington: American Psychiatric Press.
3. Gutheil, T. G., et al. (1987). "Participation in Competency Assessment and Treatment Decisions: The Role of a Psychiatrist-Attorney Team." *Mental and Physical Disability Law Reporter* 11: 446–449.
4. Strasburger, L. H. (1987). " 'Crudely, without Any Finesse': The Defendant Hears His Psychiatric Evaluation." *Bulletin of the American Academy of Psychiatry and the Law* 15: 229–233.
5. Strasburger, L. H., T. G. Gutheil, and A. Brodsky (1997). "On Wearing Two Hats: Role Conflict in Serving as Both Psychotherapist and Expert Witness." *American Journal of Psychiatry* 154: 448–456.

16

Patients Who Sue and Clinicians Who Get Sued in the Managed Care Era

Harold J. Bursztajn, M.D.

Archie Brodsky, B.A.

Managed care, by superimposing nonclinical decisionmaking imperatives on the traditional clinician-patient-family relationship, is creating new ethical dilemmas and, in turn, additional liability risks for psychiatrists and other mental health clinicians already well aware of the need for malpractice prevention.[1-5] The time and financial pressures introduced by managed care can exacerbate both the clinician's narcissism and the patient's (or family's) sense of abandonment and betrayal—two combustible ingredients in the tinderbox of litigation. These pressures are especially acute in psychiatry.

Under these stressful conditions it is essential for clinicians to use enlightened risk management principles while maintaining the integrity of the clinical decisionmaking process. To help the clinician identify and manage patient encounters that carry a high risk for malpractice litigation, some characteristics of the high-risk patient, family, clinician, and clinician-patient-family relationship are summarized here. In identifying the risk factors presented below, care must be taken not to stereotype or stigmatize. An awareness of such risk factors is, however, an essential first step to their containment.

Managed Care

Managed care, whether in the current private-sector environment or in proposed public/private health-care-financing plans overseen by the government, is profoundly changing the ground rules by which clinicians, patients, and families relate to one another.[6,7] Instead of simply a clinician-patient-family relationship, the relationship is now among clinician, managed care peer review, patient, and family. As the structure of decisionmaking becomes more complex, decisions increasingly are taken out of the hands of both the clinician and patient. In place of a dialogue in which the patient makes an informed choice with the aid of the clinician's best judgment, rulings by third parties far removed from the scene approve or deny funding for treatments recommended by the clinician and chosen by the patient.

Yet while the legal liabilities of those third parties are only beginning to be defined,[1,4] clinicians are still held to a standard of care that, for the most part, does not take into account the constraints imposed on medical decisionmaking by limited resources. As a result, the patient may feel compelled to sue the accessible second party, the clinician, in response to real or perceived abandonment by the inaccessible third party, the insurer or managed care agency. In other words, managed care will strengthen the tendency of some patients and families to scapegoat the clinician. For the clinician, this is a clear and alarming case of responsibility without authority.[3]

The disruptive effects of managed care on the communication, trust, empathy, and informed choice that are at the core of liability prevention— let alone the core of psychotherapy—are only beginning to be fathomed. For example, long-term, labor-intensive treatments, such as psychoanalysis for some personality disorders, are rarely funded and often called "medically unnecessary" by third-party reviewers. Such treatments, therefore, are rarely mentioned as a treatment choice by front-line clinicians. The patient, finding out about them anyway, may then ask, "Doctor, why didn't you tell me about these treatments?"

More routinely, patient confidentiality is compromised by the mandated divulging of medical records to third-party reviewers. As patients learn how third-party administrators (especially those associated with employers or the government) are gaining access to highly personal diagnostic information, they are likely to become less reliable informants. Such intrusions, together with ever-present uncertainties about reimbursement for long-term treatment, are believed by some observers to make the practice of psychotherapy impossible.[8,9]

As long as managed care is a reality, principles of fairness and accountability (and, indeed, the very viability of the health care system) demand that those who actually control the allocation of resources—*not* the clinicians whose requests for resources on behalf of their patients are denied— be held liable for the consequences of that denial. A Georgia federal court's ruling may herald a trend in this direction in the mental health field as well as in medicine. The court ruled that a health insurer could be held liable for its failure to respond to a hospital's repeated requests for confirmation of coverage of cardiac bypass surgery that had been ordered for a patient.[10]

Pending the systemic reform that such legal precedents may inspire, information and advocacy have become primary foci of clinician ethics under managed care.[1,3,5] Clinicians can best serve patients' interests as well as protect themselves from liability by informing patients as to what the limitations on coverage are and when those limits prevent implementation of the clinician's best judgment. In an extension of a traditional role to the new context of economic resource allocation, the clinician should then be a partner to advocate vigorously with the patient, or else (where possible) to help the patient find a better source of coverage.

The High-Risk Patient

Not all patients are equally likely to sue. A useful heuristic rule is that one-third of litigants are likely to sue if given any reason to do so; one-third are extremely unlikely to sue no matter what happens; and one-third may or may not sue depending on a variety of factors, including the outcome, the attendant feelings, the strength of the treatment alliance, and circumstantial pressures such as instigation by relatives, friends, or attorneys' advertisements. Whereas the first third include those motivated by pure greed or simple hate, patients in the final third are often those who will sue their treating clinician if they feel abandoned. A patient who feels abandoned may go to court to force the clinician to continue the relationship, albeit now an adversarial one. Denial of benefits by managed care is particularly devastating to such patients, especially when they feel that the treating clinician could have advocated more vigorously for the benefits that have been denied, or even when the clinician has advocated strenuously but unsuccessfully.

The following categories of patients do not represent psychiatric diagnoses; nor are they hard and fast schemata. Clinicians working with different patient populations or within different health care systems may find different sets of categories useful in predicting which patients are at especially high risk for acting out various feelings in lawsuits directed at physicians or mental health professionals:

THE ''HYPOCHONDRIACAL'' PATIENT
Patients who are considered hypochondriacal may also be depressed and desperately fear being alone. They may suffer from a mental illness ex-

pressed through chronic physical complaints and/or a medical illness whose true nature is lost in the background noise of those complaints. It is important not to abandon these patients. Their suffering needs to be heard through the complaints they articulate. Otherwise, in the absence of discriminating therapeutic support and exploration, the patient who repeatedly "cries wolf" may finally develop a serious medical condition that goes unnoticed amid the patient's incomplete, imprecise reports, the clinician's skepticism and fatigue, and the prior experience of managed care denial of benefits as "medically unnecessary." The patient, whose fantasies of being dismissed and abandoned are thereby confirmed, then takes the clinician to court.

THE PATIENT WHO HAS SUFFERED PRIOR TRAUMA

People who have experienced threats to survival, pain, abuse, abandonment, and helplessness at some point in their lives are at prime risk for the emotional reactions that lead to litigation. These include abused or neglected children, torture victims, combat veterans, and others who suffer from some variant of post-traumatic stress disorder (PTSD).[11] When a bad outcome of illness leaves the patient in pain, the patient's anger toward those who inflicted the earlier pain may be transferred to the clinician, the human agent who is associated with the present pain and on whom the patient feels dependent. At the least sign that the clinician is not totally devoted, the patient is likely to think, "You're doing to me what my parents [the Nazis, the North Vietnamese] did to me." Insurance laws intended to protect abuse victims may be useful to patients who have been denied benefits because of prior abuse.[12] If such laws are not available in a given state, the clinician and patient may form an "advocacy alliance," strengthening their therapeutic alliance as they oppose injustice together.

THE NARCISSISTIC PATIENT

People who can be characterized as narcissistic with respect to health are individuals who fend off feelings of insecurity and mortality through "body/mind worship" and incessant pursuit of perfection—eating wholesome food, lifting weights, jogging ten miles a day, working long hours at full capacity. Often high-achieving professionals, they tend to be chronically dissatisfied with their interpersonal relationships and intolerant of the natural physical processes associated with illness and aging. "My body/mind is my temple" is their motto. But when something goes wrong in the temple, the temptation to blame the messenger is strongly felt. "Surely there isn't anything wrong, Doctor, or if there is, it's something you can quickly fix." Such individuals tend to seek compensation for their suffering. Moreover, a lawsuit vindicates the narcissist's belief that the imperfection lies not in his or her body or mind, but in the clinician.[13]

THE LITIGIOUS PATIENT

A patient who is already suing somebody else is more likely to sue the treating clinician as well. It is useful, therefore, to take a legal as well as a medical history, especially when a suspicion of litigiousness has arisen. Under such conditions it is appropriate to ask a new patient, "Are there any stressful things going on in your life? For example, are you involved in any lawsuits?" If the patient replies, "Well, right now I'm involved in half a dozen lawsuits, but no, I don't think there are any special stresses in my life," that, too, is of diagnostic and risk management significance. Patients with paranoid personality disorders or manic depressive illness may occasionally present in this manner. For such patients, litigation can be a way of denying psychotic exacerbations of major mental illness. During such exacerbations, such patients can provoke abandonment even among the most dedicated care providers.

The clinician should also be alert for specific circumstantial indicators (and triggers) of a litigious outlook. People who are receiving workers' compensation or social security disability income for a chronic disability may expect compensation for any untoward outcome regardless of negligence. Likewise, those who have received compensation for motor-vehicle-accident injuries or other civil damages may, in the face of losses suffered through illness, return to the courts for compensation. Once such a pattern is established (to the point where several generations of family members may have received workers' compensation), litigation can become the alternative of first resort in response to suffering. In a particularly malignant variation of this pattern, patients with a history of criminal activity may malinger illness or fabricate damage from clinical treatment in order to receive compensation and/or to avoid criminal responsibility.

Finally, ongoing or unsatisfactorily resolved prior disputes with managed care can often be displaced onto the clinician. This is a major reason why psychiatrists now face greatly increased exposure to malpractice suits, with one source reporting a near doubling of psychiatric malpractice claims in the early 1990s.[14] Frank discussion of previous experiences is helpful by way of marking the boundaries between third parties (such as managed care) and the clinician-patient relationship.

THE THERAPIST-SHOPPER

Why should a patient who has pronounced six previous clinicians inadequate feel any differently about the seventh? With just a bit of bad luck, the current clinician will be the last one this patient sees before calling 1-800-LAWSUIT. Be especially alert for therapist-shopping around multiple somatic complaints for which no known cause has been identified. Suspicion should also be aroused by a history of therapist-shopping in the context of chronic physical or mental illness, where the degree of disability manifested is disproportionate to the organic or clinical configuration. Often, therapist-shopping and the need to cut one's clinician "down to size" are symptoms of an underlying sense of being defective, which the patient defends against by saying either "I don't need you" or "It's not me; it's you."

The High-Risk Family

When the patient either dies or becomes too disabled to take action, the patient's family becomes the moving party in any litigation that results. Some family characteristics that typically prompt litigation are as follows:

FAMILIES THAT HAVE TAKEN CARE OF SOMEONE WITH A CHRONIC, DEBILITATING ILLNESS

The burden of taking care of chronically ill patients has been made heavier by managed care policies which tend to shift the burden of care from inpatient to outpatient services without adequate provision for supportive home care. When a person dies after a long, disabling illness that drained the family's resources, family members often experience exhaustion combined with relief that the patient finally has died. These feelings, while entirely normal and understandable, engender discomfort and guilt. All too often, family members displace the guilt onto the deceased relative's other caretaker, the clinician. "I'm not guilty," they think. "You, the doctor, are guilty. You're the one who killed her." Feelings of resentment also may surface at this time, such as "Aunt Sally has finally died, and what do we have to show for it except painful memories of taking care of her?" How much easier it is to blame the doctor than to live with one's mixed feelings toward the long-dependent family member.

FAMILIES THAT HAVE TAKEN CARE OF A "DIFFICULT" OR ABUSIVE PATIENT

The risk of litigation by the survivors of a chronically mentally ill patient is magnified if the patient's condition entailed mistreatment of the caretaking relatives. For example, those who have lived with a chronically alcoholic family member have paid a tremendous emotional cost. What they feel toward the deceased, such as anger at the abuse they have endured but kept silent about, is correspondingly intensified and projected by blaming a clinician—perhaps the one who is identified as having kept the patient alive, but never cured, during all those years, or even the one who saw the patient last, such as the one who happened to be on duty when the patient came in for the twentieth time after a drunken brawl, only this time with a fatal subdural hematoma.

FAMILIES OF PATIENTS WITH SOMATOFORM DISORDER
The patient who "cries wolf," expressing an underlying depression with vague somatic concerns, presents a high risk not only of patient-initiated litigation, as noted above, but of family-initiated litigation as well. For instance, aroused and alarmed repeatedly by the patient's complaints, the family takes the patient to the health professional, who cannot find any identifiable condition. Particularly in managed care settings, where referral to a specialist such as a psychiatrist is discouraged, the potential for tragedy increases. After countless such false alarms, the exhausted clinician performs yet another routine examination based on the patient's standard complaint: "Doctor, I have a headache." This time, with no additional data from the patient, the headache is caused by a subdural hematoma. In the aftermath, the family is furious at the physician's failure to diagnose what many diligent clinicians might have overlooked under the circumstances.

FAMILIES THAT HAVE EXPERIENCED UNEXPECTED CLINICALLY
RELATED DEATHS OR OTHER DISASTROUS OUTCOMES
A family that has in the past experienced an unanticipated psychiatric catastrophe, especially a suicide by a family member while in treatment, is more likely to seek legal redress when another family member suffers even a minor untoward clinical event. Such predisposing psychiatric events are analogous to typical predisposing medical events such as a congenital anomaly resulting from birth trauma or an unexpected death following a minor surgical procedure. Reinforcing the family's sense of alienation and betrayal, the new event may serve as a lightning rod for unresolved feelings of grief, rage, and entitlement. Moreover, it may be seen as an opportunity to gain compensation for the uncompensated earlier loss.

The High-Risk Clinician

Psychiatrists, like other physicians, understandably find it easier to think about what makes a patient or family likely to sue than about what makes a clinician likely to be sued. Yet it is our own suit-vulnerable traits, not those of the patient or family, that (once identified) we can most readily correct and change. The following risk factors for clinicians are most usefully understood not as representing character traits (although they sometimes do), but as highlighting tendencies which all of us in the mental health professions are susceptible to expressing under stress.

THE CLINICIAN AS GOD

Anxiety about a patient's well-being, as well as denial of one's own mortality, all too often prompts the clinician to make sweeping reassurances and unrealistic promises. This narcissistic streak can come out in any of us under sufficient stress, especially as a kind of reaction formation in compensation for the feelings of frustration and helplessness induced by managed care. In high-anxiety situations, feeling under fire, we seek to exert control by playing God, denying the natural course of physical or mental illness and invoking the spurious certainties offered by an uncritical reliance on medical technology and prescription drugs.[10] The managed care notion of the primary care physician and mental health care provider as gatekeepers, guarding access to specialists such as psychiatrists, is particularly likely to evoke such unintegrated character edges in the course of professional practice. This is a temptation to be resisted; people love to sue sham gods for breach of promise.

THE CLINICIAN AS TECHNICIAN

The time and practice-pattern profiling of managed care mandates has left many psychiatrists feeling that, to survive, their practice must be reduced to time-limited psychopharmacology. Like some physicians in other specialties, the psychiatrist who acts as such a technician may use detachment to defend against the possibility of error and the grief and potential liability attendant upon a tragic outcome. Beginning with pro forma informed consent,[16] the clinician takes the necessary task of documentation (made especially burdensome by managed care) to an extreme, even to the point of appearing to treat the chart rather than the patient.

Managed care time pressures on the encounter between clinician and patient often evoke such a technical stance, as when, because of time constraints, the "psycho" gets omitted from psychopharmacology, or nonpsychiatrists are put in the role of dispensing medication scripts written by a psychiatrist who has not recently (or ever) examined the patient. A psychiatrist's responses can become so routinized by having to "point and click"[17] on programs for meeting managed care requirements that, in effect, the program becomes the patient. If the outcome is disappointing, the clinician withdraws further into the attitude, "If I can't cure you, then I can't treat you, and no one else can, either." This stance is counterproductive, since the patient may well conclude, "It looks to me as if this doctor is just protecting herself. The doctor seems worried that I might sue, so maybe I will."

Disregard of the importance of patient autonomy and authenticity[18] in managed care restriction of various treatments can also contribute to tragic outcomes, such as suicides, and subsequent litigation. Although some of the grosser limitations (on inpatient treatment, for example) have been addressed by "best practice" guidelines of professional organizations,[19] the subtler effects (such as favoring psychopharmacology over psychotherapy) can lead to severe restrictions on patient autonomy and authenticity. Such restrictions can result in a range of outcomes, from the depressed patient's simply dropping out of treatment and giving up on psychiatry to stopping medications because of relatively minor side effects, with the patient subsequently deteriorating to the point of suicide or even homicide within the family.

THE GUILT- OR SHAME-RIDDEN CLINICIAN

The clinician who is involved in a tragic outcome naturally asks, "Could I have done something differently? Is there anything else I could have done?" The guilt and shame many clinicians feel about having compromised professional standards by acquiescing to managed care requirements are one emerging variant of this reaction. Such self-questioning is appropriate in the context of continuing education and peer review. However, clinicians who obsess and browbeat themselves over what they did not see and did not do become suit-vulnerable clinicians. Patients and families sense the clinician's guilt or shame and draw their own conclusions: "If the doctor is feeling guilty, he must *be* guilty. Where there's smoke, there's fire."

THE DEFENSIVE CLINICIAN

At the opposite extreme from the guilt-obsessed clinician, the defensive clinician raises the banner of defiance: "I never make mistakes, and I never apologize." For example, a clinician who reacts to managed care intrusion into professional practice by defensive denial of such intrusion ("There is no problem") is asking that the patient join the clinician to the source of the problem, managed care, as codefendants in a lawsuit.

Contrary to this rigid reaction, there are ways of acknowledging error that do not reek of guilt and do not amount to an admission of negligence. "I made a mistake here, and I did my best to remedy it" is the message one wants to give. By clearing the air and expressing an empathic bond, this kind of statement can contribute to preserving and even strengthening the treatment alliance.[20,21] If the clinician accurately acknowledges an error, the patient does not need to go to court to force such an acknowledgment. It is important to distinguish, in one's attitude, the acknowledgment of an error from an admission of negligence.

The High-Risk Relationship

Vulnerability to litigation resides not only in the clinician, patient, and family members individually but in the relationships they form with one another. A relationship tends to be suit-vulnerable to the extent that it has the following characteristics, which themselves are typical of the practice environment fostered by the more odious intrusions of managed care:

1. The first encounter occurs under stress or duress, as in a psychiatric or medical emergency.
2. There is no continuing care or ongoing relationship, so that treatment is conducted as a series of encounters between strangers.
3. Informed consent is at best pro forma, with no attempt to share uncertainty or to reach a deep understanding of the implications of the decisions to be made.
4. There is no attempt to assess and, if necessary, to enhance the patient's decisionmaking competence at the affective as well as cognitive level.[22,23]
5. No attempt is made to involve the family in decisionmaking.
6. Care agreed to by patient and clinician as treatment of choice is subsequently termed "medically unnecessary" by a relatively uninformed, pro forma third-party review, followed by unduly burdensome and often unsuccessful appeals.

With the limitations imposed by managed care, such encounters are occurring ever more frequently, even in psychiatric settings. For psychiatrists who want something better than this kind of toxic relationship, the literature of forensic psychiatry[16,24] as well as of general medicine[25] provides a model of clinician-patient alliance-building through the empathic sharing of uncertainty. This model has been extended to the clinician-patient-family alliance as well.[15]

Containing High-Risk Factors

Identification of risk factors for litigation allows for thoughtful intervention. High-risk patients are those who come to the clinician with an unspoken, unexamined agenda, a weight of preexisting bad feelings focused on the clinician in the form of unrealistic expectations, demands, and resentments. With the exception of a few malingerers, their suffering is real. Rather than reject these suffering patients as troublemakers, the clinician (with appropriate supervision and consultation) should help them work through the issues that otherwise drive malpractice litigation.

Similarly, identification of the litigation-prone family is the first step toward detoxifying the unbearable feelings with which such families live. This is best done through careful alliance-building, beginning with listening closely while taking a family history to learn what the family's experience with medical or psychiatric care has been. A referral for brief family counseling can be offered in a manner sensitive to the family's distress.

For the clinician, self-examination is an invaluable tool in identifying suit-vulnerable traits. However, one does not always see what one is not looking for. Therefore, feedback from colleagues or from one's own therapist can be helpful as well.

In a high-risk situation created by third-party denial of benefits, the clinician must take care not to overidentify with the managed care position. A common pitfall is to deny either the existence or the value of the proposed treatment in the face of the anticipated denial of benefits. Under such circumstances, the patient may well identify the clinician with the controlling third party.

The Forensic Psychiatric Consultation
as a Risk-Management Tool

When one or more risk factors for malpractice litigation exist, a forensic psychiatric consultation can be a useful precaution for the treating clinician even as it enhances patient care. From the clinician's point of view, the consultation can be used to document that the patient was fully informed and that the patient's competence to consent to treatment (as well as to follow treatment recommendations) was assessed. Indeed, in cases in which competence may be subtly impaired by the effects of past and present illnesses, the consultation itself may furnish the most effective forum both for assessing and for enhancing competence.[18] The consultant can also document how the denial of third-party benefits exacerbates the patient's suffering by interacting with the pain, fear, and helplessness. In the context of life- or function-threatening illness, denial of treatment benefits can create or rekindle chronic post-traumatic stress disorder.

By giving the patient an additional supportive relationship, the consultation reduces the risk that the patient will use the treating clinician as a lightning rod for feelings of helplessness, hopelessness, disappointment, frustration, or vulnerability. The consultation can also give the family of a chronically ill patient relief from the feelings of guilt and shame that might otherwise be translated into rage. Finally, when a tragic outcome has occurred, a consultation can help the patient or the family communicate their bad feelings in some other manner than via a lawsuit. Even when a lawsuit seems inevitable, a "psychological autopsy" consultation on both the clinician's decisionmaking process and the patient's competence to consent can lay the foundation for a successful defense. Although the conditions of medical and especially psychiatric practice today may appear to overwhelm any and all efforts at patient-sensitive risk management, the informed clinician (with consultation as needed) is not without strategic resources in this effort.

Notes

1. P. S. Appelbaum, "Legal Liability and Managed Care." *American Psychologist* 48 (1993): 251–257.
2. M. A. Hall, "The Malpractice Standard under Health Care Cost Containment." *Law, Medicine, and Health Care* 17 (1989): 347–355.
3. E. H. Morreim, "Stratified Scarcity: Redefining the Standard of Care." *Law, Medicine, and Health Care* 17 (1989): 356–367.
4. L. I. Sederer, "Judicial and Legislative Responses to Cost Containment." *American Journal of Psychiatry* 149 (1992): 1157–61.
5. S. M. Wolf, "Health Care Reform and the Future of Physician Ethics." *Hastings Center Report* 24, no. 2 (1994): 28–41.
6. P. S. Appelbaum, "Managed Care and the Next Generation of Mental Health Law." *Psychiatric Services* 47, no. 1 (1996): 27–28, 34.
7. M. F. Shore and A. Beigel, "The Challenges Posed by Managed Behavioral Health Care." *New England Journal of Medicine* 334 (1996): 116–118.
8. A. A. Stone, "Psychotherapy and Managed Care: The Bigger Picture." *Harvard Mental Health Letter* 11, no. 8 (1995): 5–7.
9. R. L. Zuckerman, "Iatrogenic Factors in "Managed" Psychotherapy." *American Journal of Psychotherapy* 443 (1989): 118–131.
10. *Mimbs v. Commercial Life Insurance Co.*, 832 F. Supp. 354 (S.D. Ga. 1993).
11. A. A. Stone, "Post-Traumatic Stress Disorder and the Law: Critical Review

of the New Frontier." *Bulletin of the American Academy of Psychiatry and the Law* 21 (1993): 23–36.

12. A. Gerlin, "Insurer Laws Aim to Protect Abuse Victims." *Wall Street Journal,* Feb. 8, 1996, p. B1.

13. D. Bakan, *Disease, Pain, and Sacrifice: Toward a Psychology of Suffering* (Boston: Beacon Press, 1971).

14. A. I. Levenson, "Re: 1996–97 Professional Liability Policy Renewal" (letter) (Washington: Psychiatrists' Purchasing Group, 1996).

15. H. J. Bursztajn et al., *Medical Choices, Medical Chances: How Patients, Families, and Physicians Can Cope with Uncertainty* (New York: Routledge, 1990).

16. T. G. Gutheil, H. J. Bursztajn, and A. Brodsky, "Malpractice Prevention through the Sharing of Uncertainty: Informed Consent and the Therapeutic Alliance." *New England Journal of Medicine* 311 (1984): 49–51.

17. L. MacFarquhar, "Point and Click," *New Republic,* April 8, 1996, pp. 14–16.

18. H. J. Bursztajn and A. Brodsky, "Authenticity and Autonomy in the Managed-Care Era: Forensic Psychiatric Perspectives." *Journal of Clinical Ethics* 5 (1994): 237–242.

19. "Manderscheid Discusses Key Managed Care Trends." *Mental Health Report,* April 3, 1996, p. 60.

20. A. Goldberg, "The Place of Apology in Psychoanalysis and Psychotherapy," *International Review of Psycho-Analysis* 14 (1987): 409–417.

21. T. G. Gutheil, "On Apologizing to Patients." *Risk Management Foundation Forum* 8, no. 6 (1987): 3–4.

22. H. J. Bursztajn, "From PSDA to PTSD: The Patient Self-determination Act and Post-traumatic Stress Disorder," *Journal of Clinical Ethics* 4 (1993): 71–74.

23. H. J. Bursztajn et al., "Beyond Cognition: The Role of Disordered Affective States in Impairing Competence to Consent to Treatment," *Bulletin of the American Academy of Psychiatry and the Law* 19 (1991): 383–388.

24. T. G. Gutheil and H. J. Bursztajn, "Clinicians' Guidelines for Assessing and Presenting Subtle Forms of Patient Incompetence in Legal Settings," *American Journal of Psychiatry* 143 (1986): 1020–23.

25. J. D. Stoeckle, "On Looking Risk in the Eye," *American Journal of Public Health* 80 (1990): 1170–71.

17

The Wellsprings of Litigation

Thomas G. Gutheil, M.D.

In the old days, it would seem, nobody sued anybody. Most people had long-term relationships with their physicians and treaters and viewed them in a positive light, incompatible with bringing suit. Nowadays the situation is significantly different. We now face a torrent of litigation from the serious to the trivial fed by a number of different forces. This chapter will address some of the forces relevant to the clinician.

Media and Social Factors

A cartoon in a weekly comic strip portrays a little boy who is ill during a vacation and thus fails to miss any school time as a "reward" for being ill. His response to this happenstance in the final panel is "Somebody owes me big for this." This amusing illustration captures a more serious underlying question of wide-scale narcissistic entitlement which links any insult, injury, or frustration to the need to obtain some form of compensation. Indeed, the evidence suggests far beyond Lasch's "culture of narcissism"[1] that this assumption of entitlement is surprisingly widespread.

Any such feelings of entitlement are clearly fed by lawyer advertising. Printed material from television schedule newspaper inserts to telephone directory yellow pages is replete with full-page advertisements: "*Injured?* You may have a case. Call the law offices of so-and-so for a free consultation," after which an 800 telephone number is supplied. Daytime television, as well, is punctuated with law firm advertisements. They typically feature an authoritative-looking male figure in a three-piece suit standing against a wall of putative law books and discussing the concept of "big cash awards" as a direct result of retaining that particular firm to aid in your litigation. Such advertisements enhance the public perception of the link between injury or difficulty and litigation. In the therapeutic model, popular decades ago, setbacks and traumata were phenomena to "work on in therapy" with the idea of rising above, going beyond them and getting on with your life. It has now been replaced with the idea that you sue to obtain compensation because it is what you are entitled to do.

The chilling effect of this climate on all kinds of activities is clear: many a small town simply cannot afford to have a Little League because of the fear of injury-related litigation. Schools voluntarily surrender or restrict athletics and other programs; playgrounds shut down; companies providing valuable and worthwhile goods are forced to discontinue production of a particular item or face bankruptcy. The realm of medical and clinical practice is far from exempt from these permissive social forces.

The Role of Technology

The science fiction author Arthur C. Clarke is said to have posited "Clarke's Law," which states that sufficiently advanced technology is indistinguishable from magic. The rapid advance in all phases of medical and clinical practice, and the increase in ever more miraculous treatments for the variety of human ills, have created a somewhat magical atmosphere around medicine. This reasoning holds: "Medicine can do practically anything. If something happens, it must be a result of some failure meriting compensation." To understand how this operates, we must first touch briefly on the psychological underpinnings of litigation in the context of the legal requirements that apply.

The core criteria for malpractice litigation can be mnemonically summarized as the "4 D's": *dereliction* of a *duty directly* causing *damages*. That is, the plaintiff or former patient must establish, first, that the clinician owed a duty of care to a particular patient because that patient was under treatment with that clinician. Next, it must be established that the level of care delivered by the clinician to the patient fell below the standard of care of the average reasonable practitioner in a comparable situation. The complexities of determining the standard of care and presenting it to the legal process are discussed elsewhere[2] and earlier in this book. Next, it must be claimed and demonstrated that certain damages occurred as a result of the alleged negligence and departure from the standard of care. Finally, the plaintiff must establish that the link between the alleged negligence and the resulting harms was that of direct causation. In law school professors speak of the "but for" test: "But for this negligence, the harm would not have occurred."

Like many things learned in law school, this formula has almost nothing to do with the real world. In the real world, malpractice litigation results from the malignant synergy of a bad outcome for any reason and what my colleagues and I have elsewhere called "bad feelings."[3] These two factors combine in a kind of emotional "critical mass"—the wellsprings of litigation.

A simple thought experiment can probe the validity of this model. Most individuals are familiar with the delivery of perfectly sound care where someone has nevertheless brought litigation, and alternatively, the provision of horrible care where no one has brought litigation. Hence, plaintiffs' attorneys' strident claims to the contrary, bad care alone is not the steam that drives the malpractice engine. Rather, it is the two criteria noted above: a bad outcome and bad feelings.

A law scholar has described malpractice as occurring at the intersection of patient injury and patient anger.[4] Similarly, a survey performed by the Risk Management Foundation of a number of plaintiffs in malpractice cases revealed that the number-one response when plaintiffs were asked why they sued in a particular instance was "anger and fears."[5] These findings clearly suggest the importance of the emotional component in the decision to bring suit.

Bad Feelings

What are some of these bad feelings? Examples include the following common emotional states:

GUILT

Guilt in the form of survivor guilt is a very common emotional wellspring to the litigation process. The survivors lament, "If only we had done more or acted sooner on behalf of our injured loved one." This form of guilt may easily be transferred to the treaters: "It was not we ourselves who weren't attentive enough, prompt enough in obtaining care, and responsive enough to the needs of our loved one; rather, it was the treaters." In this situation the tort system, ostensibly a form of compensation for injury, is used for the psychological purpose of displacement of guilt. This mechanism is extremely common in cases of a tragic outcome. These dynamic issues also explain why suicide is the first-rank claim against mental health clinicians. This tragic outcome almost invariably leaves a residue of guilt—a variant of survivor guilt—in its wake.

RAGE

The role of patient anger in litigation is both well recognized and easy to grasp. One particularly common form of this emotion is some form of outrage at the clinician's arrogance, inaccessibility, or insensitivity in the face of the bad outcome. In one famous example, a physician whose patient committed suicide sent the widow a quite touching condolence card in the same envelope with the final bill for clinical services. It appeared to the expert witness on the case that this detail was a prime mover in the widow's decision to bring litigation and to refuse to settle before the case had gone to the highest court in the state.

One clinician (Ronald Schouten, M.D., personal communication) refers to a principle whereby the likelihood of suit is directly proportional to the ratio of the physician's arrogance to his or her competence; by this model, as the arrogance approaches infinity, it doesn't matter how great the competence is, since the likelihood of suit remains solidly greater than one. Clinicians who repeatedly fail to keep appointments without notification, leave confusing coverage during absences, and manifest other irritating practice patterns are prime candidates for promoting patient rage and its consequences should there be a bad outcome.

GRIEF

All civilized societies have grief rituals, for restoring the individual's connection with the community, healing and coping with loss, and, in some cases, distracting the individual from the sorrow of the loss. For some individuals, severe grief reactions around loss or injury of a loved one may be staved off by a process of distraction through litigation itself; that is, a lawsuit provides a form of activity which takes everyone's attention away from the necessary process of mourning. Observations of persons who attempt this defense against natural affect reveal that they are prone to severe depressions after the litigation is over, regardless of which side wins.

SURPRISE

Surprise can be one of the most powerful fomenters of litigation in the emotional spectrum. Certain kinds of surprise, in particular those which engender feelings of helplessness and anxiety, metamorphose rapidly into anger, then into paranoid views of the treaters, and finally into litigation. To test the validity of this claim, consider the following situations in which two patients experience an unfortunate side effect, where one of them has been prepared by the physician to expect it and the other is surprised.

> *Patient A:* Oh yes, there's that muscle stiffness the doctor warned me that I might expect with this medication. Clearly the doctor knows what she is doing to predict this outcome. I will mention this to the doctor at my next appointment.
>
> *Patient B:* My God, what is this strange feeling? What is the doctor doing to my body and without even telling me? Did the doctor even know this was going to happen?

Note that although the side effect may be unpleasant or uncomfortable, the absence of surprise allows even a negative side effect to strengthen the doctor-patient alliance. The doctor gets the credit for being a correct forecaster. Indeed, clinical experience reveals that patients, if sufficiently forewarned and mentally prepared, can tolerate astonishing levels of pain and distress.

In contrast, even mild dysphoria, when taking the patient by surprise, may lead to a loss of faith in the doctor's candor, honesty, and sensitivity to the patient's concerns. This response captures the capacity of surprise to demoralize. Thus, even the mild side effect, in the context of surprise, may disrupt the treatment alliance; while the major side effect, if sufficiently prepared for, may not. The complaint "No one told me to expect this" precedes many a lawsuit against health care providers.

BETRAYAL OF TRUST

This more subtle affective connection (or disconnection) with the treating clinician represents the classic point at which defensive medicine not only fails to prevent litigation but may actually foment a suit where none was originally intended. The betrayal of trust arises from the patient's feeling that the clinician does not have the patient's best interests at heart. Clearly, because of its adversarial nature, defensive practice represents a typical and dramatic example of this misalliance. The patient reasons: "The doctor is not striving to help me but to protect her own interests." The following example may illustrate this point.

> A woman went to a gynecologist for an examination and discovered that a minor procedure was indicated. In the course of informing her about the planned procedure and its consequences, the gynecologist initially stated, "The law requires me to inform you of certain facts."
>
> He then began to chant in a ritualized monotone: "There is a 30 percent

chance of blah, blah complications blah, blah hemorrhage blah, blah post operative consequences . . . etc. . . . ." As the patient later described it, "A steel shutter descended over the front of my mind. Whatever else was going on, this doctor was not talking to me. He appeared to be performing some arcane religious ritual, so I waited patiently until he had finished, as one might do when someone you're speaking with undergoes a burst of sneezing. Needless to say, I remembered practically nothing of the interchange except the fact that, at the point when he was supposed to tell me about the procedure, he stopped talking to me as a person."

This vignette perfectly illustrates the way in which an attempt to practice defensively—that is, by engaging in a virtual parody of informed consent, where one emits a bolus of facts relevant to the procedure without any attempt to achieve some communication with the patient—can actually further adversarialize the relationship and make it paradoxically *more* likely that litigation will occur if a bad outcome supervenes. The indifference to communication revealed in the vignette constitutes the thin end of the wedge, as it were, of adversarialization, which may then expand into the full-fledged lawsuit.

ABANDONMENT

Formal abandonment is itself a cause of action within malpractice, whereby a physician fails to provide or arrange for alternative services to a patient in need or terminates with a patient without making provision for future care. The abandonment we speak of here, however, is more psychological than legal. In this situation, let us say, some bad outcome occurs and suddenly the nurses will not meet the patient's eyes and the doctor will not return the patient's phone calls. Left in the lurch in this manner, the patient feels "left out in the cold" with the bad outcome, in an extremely dysphoric, threatening, anxiety-producing, and paranoia-engendering state. Many a patient, feeling thus outcast, attempts to return to the fray through litigation.

One could describe the situation as one in which the patient, deprived of the relationship in a clinical sense, forges the hostile dependent relationship of a lawsuit in exchange or compensation. The clinician's risk management guidance from this common factor would come in the form of the need to help patients work through bad outcomes, even those caused directly by the provision of medical care. This means outreach to the patient and, in some cases, to the family, in the event of a bad outcome. Many patients whose anxiety and anger make them think of litigation find these impulses dissipating when the clinician "hangs in there" with them through the aftermath of a bad outcome and remains available and attentive even though the situation has become strained.

Emotion-Based Risk Management

One of the most valuable studies about the wellsprings of litigation is the Harvard study of New York hospitals,[6] which revealed that the ratio of negligent events to actual claims was 7.6:1. That is, there were approximately eight instances of clearly negligent care in the treatment of a patient for every one situation in which a patient filed suit. This leaves a large number of cases in which actual negligence has occurred and has resulted in injury, but litigation has not occurred. These are the cases in which the presence or absence of bad feelings is most likely to determine whether or not a patient will sue. And these are the cases in which various risk management interventions by the clinician may lessen his or her chances of being sued.

The bad feelings listed above carry within themselves predictable guidance for the clinician interested in risk management. The proper management of familial *guilt* is an important area of clinician outreach after a bad outcome: reassuring families that they behaved in a reasonable manner, that they were appropriately responsive to the needs of the patient, and the like. After a patient's death, holding a meeting for interested family members to explain what happened may be emotionally stressful for clinicians, but extremely valuable for the family's peace of mind and for malpractice prevention. Families have been known to bring suit simply to find out what happened. The inability to get a straight answer from clinical staff drives families into the hands of lawyers and the juggernaut of litigation begins to roll. The clinician's supportive efforts, explanations of the relevant psychology or physiology, and the like may go a long way toward helping the family appreciate the uncertainties of the clinician's task, and may counter the family's "magical thinking" that the only possible reason for a bad outcome must be clinician negligence.

At the Program in Psychiatry and the Law, Harvard Medical School, we recommend that clinicians not only reach out to families after a bad outcome but arrange to attend the funeral or memorial service. While some clinicians find this emotionally daunting, the rewards are considerable; while the rare family may turn on the doctor, most families are grateful for the thoughtfulness of the gesture.

Avoidance of *outrage* is similarly direct. The maintenance of good manners in situations of stress or even in the context of the patient's abusive manner toward the clinician, attention to issues of availability, and sensitivity in portraying the issue to the patient are all important features of the management of outrage. Being supportive to the patient and the family in the context of grief and occasionally recommending clinical support in the grief work may help.

The power of *surprise* in moving families and patients in the direction of litigation suggests that careful and particular attention be paid to this element. From a practical viewpoint, this frequently means deciding to disclose certain risks and problems to the patient even when the clinician would prefer not to. Almost any negative outcome is worsened by occurring in the context of patient surprise; this fact should encourage the clinician, when in doubt, to disclose "the bad news" in the interest of avoiding surprise.

In regard to *betrayal of trust*, it is important not to practice defensive medicine. Defensive practice adversarializes the relationship even before the patient necessarily feels adversarial toward the clinician—that is, before the bad outcome has supervened. Clinicians who behave in a defensive or "lawyeristic" manner toward their patients have only themselves to blame if the patients enter into the spirit of the thing and hire their own lawyers. It is far better to enter into an open, collaborative position with the patient in order to support an alliance-based atmosphere.

Finally, the best response to psychological *abandonment* is outreach and follow-through. One of the most important articles published in recent years is one entitled "Facing our Mistakes,"[7] which articulates the challenge for clinicians of acknowledging errors in judgment or practice. This is an art form well worth mastering for all clinicians in the modern era.

General Risk Management Principles

While prevailing in a malpractice suit is a wonderful experience, it is still inferior to avoiding litigation in the first place. Hence, while reading other chapters in this book will aid the clinician in *winning* a malpractice suit, attention should be paid to the much more sanguine prospect of avoiding litigation from the outset.

In order to do this, it is important to grasp "Gutheil's principle" of medical care: "No patient in the history of medicine ever sought out a doctor for medical care." Though counterintuitive, this statement captures an important point. As noted at the beginning of this chapter, when patients come to a doctor they are instinctively seeking magic. In this context, magic is defined as reversing the irreversible, cheating death, overcoming years of loose living, breaking bad and destructive habits with no personal effort on the part of the patient.

What is the poor clinician to do? In the very best of circumstances, the clinician can only provide top-level clinical care. Magic, alas, is beyond any of us. Just for perspective, I recall an incident in which I was giving a presentation on risk management at a internationally famous hospital. During the question period, one of the physicians argued that, at this particular hospital, magic was indeed being supplied, in that people came from all over the world seeking that very commodity and left the hospital apparently satisfied with their care. (I could not say it then, but in this hospital the previously mentioned ratio of arrogance to competence may well have been relevant.)

The cognitive dissonance between the wish for magic and the availability only of good clinical care can be somewhat resolved by an approach elsewhere described as "malpractice prevention through the sharing of uncertainty."[8] This approach has four elements.

First, it is necessary to understand and empathize with the wishes of patients for certainty. Psychiatric practice provides the understanding that patients who are ill become regressed; they become more infantile and thus more prone to believe in and wish for magic. This is a universal trait: if we were sick, we would want magic too.

One next empathizes with the patient's unrealistic wishes. This may appear to be barking up the wrong tree, since the clinician is ordinarily supposed to "reality test" the patient's fantasies or even delusions and serve as the representative of the reality principle. How then is this empathy with the unrealistic side to be achieved? Note the purpose of this intervention, which is to wean the patient from the fantasies of certainty. This "weaning" is a deliberately chosen verb to address the regressed level at which these interactions occur. The point of empathizing with the patient's unrealistic wishes is to avoid entering into an oppositional dialogue with the patient along these lines: "Dammit, I am not a witch doctor or a magician, I'm only a [fill in your specialty]!" Such a response, in addition to being adversarial, dashes the patient's hopes in an absolute and insensitive manner. Instead, responses like the following may be more appropriate:

> I wish the good Lord in his wisdom had designed a drug that was guaranteed entirely free of side effects.
>
> I sure wish I had an iron-clad guarantee that you were going to survive this surgical procedure.

I wish this couples therapy could be guaranteed to save your marriage.

I wish this course of psychotherapy could be guaranteed to keep you alive despite your long history of suicidal tendencies.

I wish this course of treatment were guaranteed of success.

Note that all of these responses, in different clinical contexts, have one factor in common: the clinician is on the side of the patient wishing for magic. The physician, too, wishes that there were guarantees available, that certainty could be obtained, and that perfect treatment actually existed. By beginning the dialogue on the same side as the patient (by also wishing for magic), the physician reasserts the alliance and validates the patient's longing for magic instead of humiliating the patient for having such regressive feelings. Simultaneously, by casting the communication in rueful tones, the clinician gently and tactfully disabuses the patient of the likelihood of certainty and titrates the degree of disillusionment to the patient's expectations: this "lets the patient down easy" in the context of the uncertainty of treatment. Note that all of the above sample responses also stand for whole universes of discourse between doctor and patient, tailored to the particular considerations at hand.

The final result of these efforts is that the alliance with the patient is not based on the certainty of magic—you either deliver magic or you don't, and if you don't, you are at fault—but on the fact that the intrinsic uncertainty of the treatment is faced frankly and squarely by both parties together. Hence the alliance is based on the *sharing* of uncertainty, with the implicit message that the clinician will remain available in spite of a bad outcome. The patient who is experiencing some side effect or complication is spared the additional anxiety of somehow letting the clinician's expectations down by being a "bad patient."

The Role of Apology

There is an additional intervention that may be needed: the apology. Clinicians are as reluctant to apologize after a bad outcome as they are to acknowledge the possibility of failure before the procedure has been attempted. Apology is, however, a means of repairing the alliance even after the strain of a bad outcome. There is, moreover, a "technology of apology" that permits the apology to serve its alliance-healing function without either adversarialization or acknowledgment of guilt and, hence, culpability.

To address the worst-case scenario immediately, let us agree that if the clinician were to say: "I'm sorry I deviated from the standard of care so as proximately to cause you these damages," the insurance company would feel that was infelicitously phrased, to say the least, since it is the technical definition of malpractice. Without going nearly that far, however, the clinician can acknowledge certain regrets and sorrows without jeopardizing a potential case. Many a plaintiff has indicated that, if the clinician had apologized or had even acknowledged hurting the patient, the patient would have felt that the doctor was at least taking responsibility for the consequences of his or her actions and would not have fallen into a litigious mood. Though these are hindsight estimations, they are nevertheless worthy of serious consideration in the context of the value of apology in staving off litigation.

First, one can and arguably should always apologize for what might be termed simple error. A misscheduled appointment, a lab slip ending up in the wrong chart, the missing of a particular administrative deadline, and the like merit a straightforward apology and the offer to remedy the slight, for example by rescheduling the appointment, perhaps at no charge. Many clinicians paint themselves into interpersonally adversarial and indefensible corners by the refusal to apologize even for such minor slips.

The second form of apology is somewhat more problematic. This is the apology for choosing the wrong course of action. This may occur when one's preliminary working diagnosis proves to have been wrong or when a particular treatment turns out to be either ineffective or unacceptable because of side effects. Here, one strikes a delicate balance between self-castigating laments and a reasonable assessment of the erroneous decision along the following lines: "By hindsight I guess we can see that that was the wrong way to go. I will now try to remedy this error and go in the right direction and I'll be with you every step of the way."

Finally, regret for a bad outcome is a critical component of the clinician's empathy. Any clinician who does not regret a bad outcome arguably has no business being in the field. The way in which this is phrased may be critical to its impact. A comment like "I regret that my colleague, Dr. Smith, botched your case" or "I'm really sorry the respirator blew up in your face" would be an infelicitously phrased example of the recommended approach. What is important to communicate is the clinician's regret for the patient's *distress:* "I'm sorry you're feeling so bad, and I'm sorry things haven't worked out in the way we hoped." In this form, apologies support and encourage the patient while leaving the alliance intact.

Some states, Massachusetts included, have apology statutes that can be enormously valuable in allowing clinicians to express appropriate regrets without feeling they are slipping the noose of liability around their own necks. Here is the Massachusetts apology statute:

> Statements, writings or benevolent gestures expressing sympathy or a general sense of benevolence relating to the pain, suffering or death of a person involved in an accident and made to such person or to the family of such person shall be inadmissible as evidence of an admission of liability in a civil action. (Mass. General Laws, ch. 233, sec. 23D, 1986.)

Clinicians practicing in other states may wish to borrow this phraseology and attempt to propose it as a bill for their own state legislatures.

/ / /

To practice well in one's specialty should alone stave off liability litigation; but it does not always do so. Instead, malpractice prevention flows from understanding and dealing with the wellsprings of litigation, as this chapter has explained. Such an approach offers the significant advantages of a clinical basis, respect for the patient, and focus on the critical decision modes of malpractice litigation.

Notes

1. C. Lasch, *The Culture of Narcissism* (New York: Norton, 1978).
2. P. S. Appelbaum and T. G. Gutheil, *Clinical Handbook of Psychiatry and the Law* (Baltimore: Williams and Wilkins, 1991).
3. T. G. Gutheil et al., *Decision Making in Psychiatry and Law* (Baltimore: Williams and Wilkins, 1991).
4. Anna Stern, personal communication.
5. J. Holzer, Risk Management Foundation, personal communication.
6. T. A. Brennan et al., "Incidence of Adverse Events and Negligence in Hospitalized Patients: Results of the Harvard Medical Practice Study, I," *New England Journal of Medicine* 324 (1991): 370–376.
7. D. Hilfiker, "Facing Our Mistakes," *New England Journal of Medicine* 310 (1984): 118–122.
8. T. G. Gutheil, H. J. Bursztajn, and A. Brodsky, "Malpractice Prevention through the Sharing of Uncertainty: Informed Consent and the Therapeutic Alliance," *New England Journal of Medicine* 311 (1984): 49–51.

18

Ethical and Effective Testimony after *Daubert*

Harold J. Bursztajn, M.D.

Archie Brodsky, B.A.

The professional expertise, ethics, and objectivity a witness brings to the courtroom are the best tools for communicating effectively with a judge and jury. Some attorneys advise professionals testifying in court to consider the courtroom a stage for a theatrical performance calculated to elicit a desired response. That is bad advice. Likewise, a common mistake is to think that the way to communicate in the courtroom is to act like a lawyer. Although it is important to understand how lawyers work and how to communicate with them, the witness has a different responsibility from the lawyer. The witness's duty is best done by maintaining the highest ethical standards of one's own chosen profession.

Professionals may appear in court either as fact witnesses, who testify to events within their own personal observation or knowledge, or as expert witnesses, who are retained by one side or the other to provide an informed opinion on matters beyond the scope of the layperson's knowledge, such as the standard of care in a medical specialty. The defendant in a medical malpractice case, for example, would testify as a fact witness, while expert witnesses would be retained to testify for either the plaintiff or the defendant. Although the duties of a professional who is a fact witness and one who is an expert witness are quite different, certain principles apply to both.

Increased scrutiny of expert professional testimony has been brought about by the U.S. Supreme Court's much-discussed *Daubert* decision in 1993.[1] In *Daubert*, which concerned the admissibility of expert testimony about the birth defects allegedly caused by the prescription drug Bendectin, the Court responded to the growing importance of advanced science and technology in courtroom testimony. Ruling that the Federal Rules of Evidence had set appropriate (but not rigid) limits on the admissibility of purportedly scientific evidence, the Court affirmed that the trial judge must make the determination of admissibility so as to ensure that an expert's testimony is both *reliable* and *relevant*.

When a psychiatrist's expert testimony fails to meet these criteria, as when the methodology used to support the opinion is found by the trial judge to be unreliable, such testimony is disallowed with explicit reference to *Daubert*. For example, in *Gier v. Educational Serv. Unit No. 16*,[2] the U.S. Eighth Circuit Court affirmed a federal district court's decision to prevent a psychiatrist and two psychologists from testifying that seven mentally retarded students in a state school had been sexually, physically, and emotionally abused. The district court had found that the methodology the experts had used to reach this conclusion lacked sufficient reliability because the Child Behavior Checklist (CBC) on which they had relied had not been validated for use with mentally retarded children and was insufficient to establish that a child had been abused. Similarly, the *Daubert* language of reliability is being used to disallow testimony on the basis of well-established clinical and forensic standards.[3] Thus, in the *Daubert* atmosphere, professional standards become legal standards.

Although the *Daubert* ruling applies only to expert testimony, professionals who testify as fact witnesses, such as defendant physicians in malpractice cases, should be aware of it as well. In the first place, defendants who are professionals can work more effectively with colleagues who are retained as expert witnesses on their behalf if they understand what an expert needs to do. Second, even defendant physicians testifying as fact witnesses increasingly will be held to the standards of expertise and objectivity that *Daubert* has set, at least by association, for all professionals testifying on complex matters.

The impact of *Daubert* on the evaluation of not only expert-witness but also fact-witness testimony was made explicit by the Second Circuit Court in 1995 in *Borawick v. Shay*.[4] The court, using a case-by-case or "totality of the circumstances" standard, ruled that a plaintiff's testimony about childhood sexual abuse, based on memories allegedly recovered through hypnosis, was inadmissible because her hypnotist lacked adequate academic qualifications and had not kept sufficient records of her hypnosis to corroborate her testimony credibly. Moreover, the plaintiff's allegations of abuse were inherently incredible. The court noted that although the *Daubert* ruling on admissibility did not apply to fact witnesses' testimony, if it *were* applicable it would allow for the totality-of-the-circumstances approach used by the court to rule the plaintiff's testimony inadmissible. In the words of one commentator, "Lawyers and trial courts must now think as scientists do."[5] By extension, so must testifying clinicians, as applied scientists.

Foundations of Effective Testimony

The witness's responsibility begins long before entering the courtroom. In addition to gaining a thorough understanding of the issues specific to the case, there is a more general type of preparation for being an effective witness. This preparation involves mastering the principles of ethical and effective testimony, beginning the dialogue with the attorney that will continue throughout the case (and will be enlarged to include the jury or judge), and confronting unspoken emotional dynamics that might interfere with clear communication. If these foundations are in place, the witness can approach both direct and cross-examination more confidently.

BASIC PRINCIPLES

Ethical, effective testimony is an application of certain fundamental principles, which may be summarized as follows:

At its best, a trial can be an extended "continuing education" dialogue for all concerned: the witness, the attorney, the judge, and the jury. Learning and teaching are ongoing. If you listen and keep your own mind open, you will be in a good position to educate your attorney, the finders of fact (judge or jury), and even a good cross-examining attorney.

The primary goals of a witness testifying on matters of professional expertise are as follows:

To communicate the truth to the jury in an ethical, objective, and effective way.

To maintain your autonomy, authenticity, and integrity.

To uphold the values of your profession.

To interact with attorneys and with the judge and jury in an atmosphere of mutual respect.

To engage in an ongoing dialogue with your attorney so that, together, you can educate as well as learn from the judge and jury as to what questions each may have.

To speak directly to the issues.

To make complex matters understandable without oversimplifying.

Tricks and formulas are no substitute for a thorough and deep understanding of the facts of the case and their interrelationships. Resist any attempts to portray you as a performer or magician, whether these come from an opposing attorney's adversarial projections or your own attorney's well-intentioned projections. Instead, you want to present yourself as just what you are—an authentic, compassionate, but objective seeker of understanding. Whether as a fact witness (treater) or an expert witness (evaluator), you first use your deep knowledge of the case to arrive at your understanding, and then you communicate it as a professional.

The pitfalls for a witness to avoid include the following:

Grandiosity or false humility.
Verbosity or uncommunicativeness.
Adversarial partisanship or complacent detachment.
Overcomplexity or oversimplicity.

UNDERSTANDING PROJECTED AFFECTS

Psychiatrists and other practicing clinicians who testify either as expert witnesses or as fact witnesses need not and should not leave their understanding of human beings behind at the courtroom door. A case may well be influenced by unspoken witness attitudes which are nonetheless apparent to the observing jurors. Particularly for a defendant accused of negligence, it is all too easy to project feelings of guilt or shame that may be taken as confirming the jury's suspicions. Other projected affects that can undermine a witness's credibility are fear of the process or outcome, anger at one's accuser or the opposing attorney, arrogance (perhaps in compensation for guilt or fear), and false humility and condescension toward the jury.

If you are the defendant, it is best to deal with feelings of pain resulting from the tragic outcome before you enter the courtroom. If you feel guilty or ashamed about anything related to the case, talk about it with your attorney and/or expert witness or with your own therapist before testifying. (Your attorney may not be able to help you deal with your feelings, but he or she needs to know how they may affect your testimony.) If, on reflection, you conclude that you have been negligent, leading to the negative outcome in question, direct your attorney to settle the case. Do not allow false pride to get in the way of a just settlement. On the other hand, if you conclude that you have not been negligent, allow yourself to feel regret over the outcome without assuming unjustified blame on the witness stand.

Another type of emotional dynamic to take into account is the typical fantasies of perfection encouraged by plaintiffs' attorneys in malpractice cases, which the defendant may pick up and reflect to his or her disadvantage. Among these fantasies are:

Omniscience: "Didn't you know that . . . ?"
Omnipotence: "Couldn't you have saved the patient by . . . ?"
Omnipresence: "Weren't you there when . . . ?"

These fantasies are to be countered by clear testimony by both the defendant and expert witness delineating the real standard of care and the limits on a physician's knowledge, power, and presence under actual conditions of prospective uncertainty.

In claims of physical and/or emotional trauma,[6] it is possible that the judge and jury will feel some identification with the plaintiff's alleged trauma and therefore will, in varying degrees, process the testimony they hear as if they themselves had been injured. Or they may avoid such identification by taking the attitude that "it could never happen to me." The professionally informed witness avoids both theatrics and superficial detachment by creating and maintaining an atmosphere of calm, reasoned deliberation in the face of heightened emotional pressure.

Direct Examination

A common mistake of both witnesses and attorneys is to focus on cross-examination to the point of underpreparing for direct examination. It seems natural to take the direct examination for granted, since the questions are coming from a friendly source. This approach is shortsighted, however, since direct examination is your only chance to present your case in an accurate, clear, and convincing narrative.

One of the shorthand decision strategies that people use to process and act on information[7,8] is called *anchoring and adjustment.* As applied to jury decisionmaking, this means that the juror makes a provisional judgment on the basis of earlier testimony and then adjusts that judgment on the basis of later testimony. Jurors may also use other, counterbalancing heuristics that give greater weight to the testimony heard more recently. Nonetheless, the likelihood that some jurors "anchor" their opinions on the direct examination of a witness, thus reducing the potential impact of cross-examination, suggests that those who do not prepare carefully for direct examination do so at their own peril.

PREPARATION

Your role as a witness differs from a stage performance in being guided by the ethical imperatives of honesty and objectivity. These standards have been articulated most explicitly for forensic psychiatrists.[9] They can be especially difficult to implement in cases where there is a blurring of boundaries between clinical and forensic goals—for example, when a treating clinician testifies even as a fact witness for a patient involved in third-party litigation. The clinician, whose task is to alleviate suffering, should disqualify himself or herself from serving as an expert witness, whose duty is to be objective and to serve the goals of justice.[10]

Preparation for direct examination is just one pivotal stage in a dialogue with your attorney (or, in the case of an expert witness, the retaining attorney) that should begin early and continue to influence the conduct of the case right down to the closing arguments. Just as testifying is not a performance, preparation for testimony is not a rehearsal. Rather, it means achieving a deep understanding whereby you can communicate effectively both with your attorney and with the judge and jury. If the case is justly settled or dropped, then this deep understanding will have achieved its purpose without your having to testify. If you do go to court, your attorney will be communicating with the jury a good deal more than you will. Therefore, you will convey your understanding far more effectively if your attorney shares it in sufficient depth.

One purpose of this dialogue is to make sure your attorney has a sufficiently firm understanding of issues pertaining to complex scientific evidence to ask focused and relevant questions. To foster this understanding in complex cases, it can be useful to have an expert consultant in the presentation of scientific evidence available to you and your lawyer—a decided asset in satisfying the *Daubert* criteria.[11] Sometimes this expert consultant can also serve as the expert witness. Such a consultant not only can strengthen your preparation for direct examination but also can help you withstand misleading cross-examination.

The pretrial phase also gives you an opportunity to confront any problems that arise in communicating with your attorney. On your side, beware of projecting arrogance or superiority when educating the attorney on scientific matters. The imperial witness may find his grandiosity handed back to him on the witness stand. As in medical school or any other setting, the best way to educate is to support honestly the self-esteem of your student. If your attorney appears not to respect your professional knowledge, try to move the attorney away from such a narcissistic position by modeling a climate of mutual respect. If that fails, raise the issue directly and without delay as a matter to be discussed and worked through. Otherwise, you need to withdraw from the case (as an expert) or change attorneys (as the defendant).

COORDINATION WITH OPENING AND CLOSING STATEMENTS

An additional benefit to be gained from close communication between witness and attorney is the achievement of thematic continuity from the beginning to the end of the trial. If the burden of the case rests largely on your testimony on medical and scientific issues, it will be advantageous to have the themes of your testimony reflected in your attorney's opening and closing statements. At the same time, you must balance the need for coherence between your testimony and the overall narrative presented to the finders of fact with the imperative of authenticity.

CREDENTIALING

The credentialing of a witness should be completed quickly and efficiently at the beginning of the direct examination. Credentials most relevant to the case should be highlighted. In a medical malpractice case, these credentials include any documented expertise in medical decisionmaking. Your professional fees, either as an expert witness or as a clinician, should be stated matter-of-factly. Make clear that you are paid for responsibly exercising your professional judgment, not for your testimony, opinions, or clinical outcomes, as the case may be. More important than anything said in the credentialing phase, however, is your overall demeanor and that of your attorney. If your attorney treats you as a stage prop, a hired gun, or a guilty party, so will the jury.

NARRATIVE STRUCTURE

A witness's testimony can be heard as a narrative that weaves together many details into a coherent structure of meaning.[12] An expert witness's narrative consists of a clearly and convincingly stated opinion, followed by the basis of the opinion—that is, the data and reasoning by which it was reached. The expert reviews both supporting and opposing evidence, acknowledges gaps in documentation and difficulties in assessment, and shows how it was still possible to reach an opinion with reasonable medical certainty. A fact witness's narrative takes a different form, that of a chronological, "once upon a time and place" sequence of observations and decisions made in the course of treatment. Thus, as explained in the next section, both kinds of witnesses are testifying as to the decisionmaking process in the case. The difference is that the treating physician as fact witness testifies from the perspective of memory, whereas the expert witness reconstructs the same sequence of events by applying a general understanding of decisionmaking processes to the specific context at issue.

Whether you are testifying as a fact witness or as an expert witness, of course, be truthful and thorough in laying out your narrative. Admit when you don't know or need to think about something. By the same token, apparent contradictions need to be acknowledged, since it is not apparent paradox that undermines a witness's effectiveness, but glib superficiality or unnecessary abstruseness. Finally, while you do need to avoid boring the judge and jury, don't be afraid of repetition. You are trying to create a dialogue with people who are less informed and may even be more anxious than you. People who are anxious may not hear, understand, or remember everything the first time around.

RECONSTRUCTING DECISIONMAKING UNDER UNCERTAINTY

One key to a successful defense in a medical malpractice case is to free the jury's attention from exclusive focus on the tragic outcome (and the overwhelming feelings associated with it), so that the jury can also consider the decisionmaking process that occurred before the outcome could be known. Absolute certainty is a luxury of hindsight. On the other hand, the exercise of professional judgment requires reasonable and prudent decisionmaking under some degree of uncertainty. Before the fact, all decisionmaking in medicine,[13] including psychiatry,[14] requires working with degrees of uncertainty and turning them into estimates of probability. Since it is impossible to eliminate risk entirely, the communication of risk (both prospectively, to the patient, and retrospectively, to the jury) becomes an essential skill requiring subtle, in-depth understanding of context-sensitive professional decisionmaking processes.[15]

If the defense does not lay out the process of decisionmaking and risk assessment from the prospective viewpoint, involving some degree of uncertainty, the jury may be left only with the plaintiff's hindsight perspective. It is advisable, therefore, that the defendant physician remember accurately his or her own decisionmaking process in the course of treatment. That will enable an expert in decisionmaking to reconstruct the process by an assessment of both physician and patient decisionmaking embedded in the informed-consent dialogue and the clinical context.

An example of such a successful defense, against unfavorable odds, is the case of *Drewry v. Harwell*.[16] A young woman who had suffered chronic pelvic pain sued her obstetrician/gynecologist following a hysterectomy during which an embryo of one month's gestation was discovered and, as a necessary consequence of the surgery, aborted. The plaintiff alleged that the physician had performed an unwanted procedure, causing an unwanted abortion. An additional charge of sexual misconduct was dropped before trial, subsequent to a court-ordered forensic psychiatric examination of the plaintiff for her claims of emotional and physical damages. The examining forensic psychiatrist was nonetheless able to use the results of the examination in testifying at trial as to the informed-consent and decisionmaking processes engaged in by the physician and patient.

This case had the potential for a major damage award based on the jury's sympathy for the plaintiff, a woman who had lost her baby and could never have another. The defense, however, presented a forensic psychiatric evaluation which relied on the testifying psychiatrist's analysis of the processes of medical decisionmaking and informed consent. This analysis was based on his expertise in the area as well as on the data gathered in the court-ordered examination.

In his direct examination, this witness drew a decision tree on the courtroom blackboard to represent the choices made by the physician and patient at each stage of the process. He was thus able to help the jury move from a "hot" (emotional) to a "cool" (reflective) consideration of the issues in the case.[17] Having established that framework, he testified that the physician and patient had appropriately considered the risks and benefits of four possible courses of action: medical treatment, psychiatric treatment, surgery, and no treatment. The patient had been competent to give informed consent and had in fact done so, both formally and in the course of the informed-consent dialogue. On the basis of these facts, the witness concluded that the physician's actions met the standard of care in the areas of medical decisionmaking and informed consent. This testimony was reinforced by a psychological analysis of why the plaintiff might, in retrospect, have unwittingly revised her memory of the choices she had actually made.

ANTICIPATING CROSS-EXAMINATION

The dialogue you have with your attorney on direct examination should include anything that, on cross-examination, might confuse your testimony as either a fact witness or an expert witness. To make sure you have a complete understanding of the basis of your testimony, it is important to consider alternative, especially adversarial perspectives. Your direct examination should anticipate most of the significant issues the cross-examining attorney will raise.

Cross-Examination

In our adversarial system, cross-examination has several legitimate functions: (1) to expose weaknesses in the opponent's case, as reflected in the testimony of the opposing witnesses; (2) to bring out the strengths of the cross-examining attorney's own case; (3) to expose any problems reflecting on the credibility of an opposing witness's testimony, such as bias, lack of opportunity to perceive the facts at issue (for a fact witness), or inadequate professional training and experience (for an expert witness). The attorney who vigorously pursues these goals is providing effective advocacy in keeping with the ethical standards of the legal profession. Unfortunately, in the heat of a trial, even an ethical attorney may stray from this model of effective cross-examination and resort to tactics designed to mislead and confuse. These tactics usually prove ineffective against a witness who is thoroughly grounded in the issues of the case and is honest and straightforward in testimony.

You must prepare for cross-examination before you take the stand. Cross-examination is a continuation of direct examination in more than a temporal sense, since you will want to maintain in cross-examination the basic themes you have laid out in response to your attorney's questions. Typically, the cross-examining attorney is not trying to argue you out of your position, but rather to break the narrative flow of reasoning, or of time and space, that you have established. Your job is to maintain that flow in the face of challenges to your character, your credibility, and the content of your testimony.

PRINCIPLES FOR RESPONDING TO CROSS-EXAMINATION
The following are principles of effective testimony applied specifically to cross-examination:

Avoid the natural tendency to identify with the aggressor. You can protect yourself from the aggression of some cross-examiners without being aggressive yourself. You may, however, need to set limits on the cross-examiner who is verbally abusive. As explained in a later section, you do this by stating exactly what the cross-examiner is doing.

Maintain mutual respect. Follow the Golden Rule when you take the stand.

Maintain a spirit of inquiry. Your mission is still to seek understanding of the relevant issues in the pursuit of justice. Your cross-examination testimony should continue the inquiry begun in direct examination.

Maintain professional ethics. Stay on the high road (without being holier-than-thou) even if the cross-examining attorney tries to bring you down to the low road.

Listen and learn. Listen carefully and respectfully, whether it is your own or the other side's attorney who is questioning you. The following nine ways of *not* listening[18] are more likely to occur in an adversarial atmosphere. Indeed, some cross-examining attorneys may try to provoke these various forms of inattention in a witness to reduce the effectiveness of testimony:

Mind Readers wonder, "What is this person really thinking?"

Rehearsers think about what they're going to say after the speaker stops talking.

Filterers hear only what they want to hear.

Dreamers drift off and may ask for repetition.

Identifiers relate what is said to their own experiences.

Comparers are provoked by the messenger to respond personally to being insulted and thereby neglect the message.

Derailers change subjects too soon or too often due to lack of interest.

Sparrers belittle the value of what is said.

Placaters agree with everything to avoid conflict.

Don't be led into overcomplexity or oversimplicity. A cross-examining attorney may try to portray you as someone who obfuscates the issues or talks over the heads of the jury. At the other extreme, the attorney may lead you into the trap of oversimplification so as to expose your inadequate understanding of the complexity of the case. You need to keep your balance, steering a course between the Scylla of overcomplexity and the Charybdis of oversimplicity.

THE CROSS-EXAMINER'S TECHNIQUES

Attorneys are taught specific techniques of effective cross-examination. As an example of what you can expect to face, here are the law professor Irving Younger's Ten Commandments of Cross-Examination:[19]

1. Be brief.
2. Ask short questions using plain words.
3. Ask only leading questions.
4. Do not ask a question if you do not know the answer.
5. Listen to the answer.
6. Do not quarrel with the witness.

7. Do not allow the witness to repeat his or her direct testimony.
8. Do not permit the witness to explain.
9. Avoid asking one question too many.
10. Save the explanation for summation.

You must also be prepared for the possibility that a cross-examiner will go beyond these standard prescriptions and engage in diversionary tactics that run counter to ethical and effective courtroom practice. You should be aware of the tricks a cross-examining attorney may use to distort your testimony, but you should not respond in kind. In many instances, such tricks will elicit sustainable objections from your attorney. When you are left to respond on your own, the suggestions that follow will help you do so.

THE WITNESS'S BILL OF RIGHTS

You can continue to be an effective and ethical witness when responding to cross-examination. You can protect yourself while upholding your professional dignity and ethics by employing the remedies listed in what we call a Bill of Rights for witnesses, which is actually a list of standard courtroom procedures. As a witness you have the right . . .

1. To give and expect mutual respect.
2. To ask the cross-examiner to rephrase ambiguous or misleading questions.
3. To ask the judge whether the material asked for is privileged.
4. To refuse to answer questions you do not understand (instead, ask the attorney to repeat or clarify).
5. To say you don't know when you don't know.
6. To ask the judge whether you can qualify or expand on your answer when a simple yes or no won't do.
7. To ask to complete your answer when interrupted.
8. To refer to written records or notes (which the other side will then have the right to examine).

CHARACTER AND CREDIBILITY

Many attorneys begin by questioning the character and credibility of the witness they are cross-examining. They may home in on your fees, motives, training, or experience in relevant areas, the presence or absence of academic credentials, and how much or how little you have treated or testified about this type of case. Part of the purpose of this opening phase is to point out to the jury any weaknesses in your professional training and qualifications.

Fees. With an expert witness, a cross-examining attorney may give the impression that getting paid for your professional work makes you a hired gun. Testify truthfully as to how much you are being paid, but make clear that you are paid for time spent exercising professional judgment, not for your testimony.

A fact witness can expect questions about clinical fees, such as "Is it not correct that you were paid about $20,000 by Mr. G. for the care you provided him, and now he's dead?" This question is designed to make you look mercenary as well as incompetent. You must put these innuendos in perspective, showing that you are not paid for the outcome, but, again, for the exercise of professional judgment in clinical care. Otherwise, no one could treat very sick people. You can make these general points while bringing in specific reminders of your direct narrative testimony by answering, "Over the past four years, during which Mr. G. had three hospitalizations and three suicide attempts, I saw him for about 200 visits, and my average fee is $100 an hour." This shows that you have expended time to gain a deep understanding.

Writings and public appearances. Anything you have written or said in medical textbooks, journal articles, or taped lectures to colleagues or attorneys is fair game. If, as an expert witness, you teach your colleagues about testifying in court (as in this chapter), you may be defamed as a hired gun. Again, you respond by placing any quotes in context and straightforwardly (not defensively) demonstrating that your work is grounded in the ethics of your profession.

CONTENT

In the next phase of cross-examination, the cross-examiner turns to the content of your testimony. As the interchange draws to a close, an attorney who believes that his or her case is weak may shift into damage control, resorting increasingly to diversions to make the whole cross-examination, and your testimony, appear to have been a contest or debate. In this way the attorney hopes to undercut the meaningfulness of your testimony. Here are some of the many tricks you can expect in this phase, along with some suggested ways of answering them. Note that the latter do not involve answering one trick with another, but simply continuing to seek honestly an objective understanding in the pursuit of justice, in keeping with the ethical guidelines of the American Academy of Psychiatry and the Law.[9]

The "shell game" (misleading facts or inferences). A trick question may appear in the guise of a simple statement of chronology: "Isn't it true that you saw Mr. G. on March 20, 1995?" When you say that you did, the attorney smugly reveals that it was March 21. You can avoid this trap by answering, "I saw Mr. G. on or about March 20, 1995," or "I'm not sure I can remember the exact date, but it was in March 1995."

What is true for dates is also true for quotations of things you have said or written. If you don't have your original statement in front of you, don't agree that the wording is accurate without checking. Your job is not a recitation of facts, but the communication of a reasoned opinion. You can put irrelevant memorization into the perspective of "I'm here to present my understanding of what I did and why" by saying as much when called for.

Out-of-context quotes. Anything you have said or written before (from teaching manuals to depositions) may be brought up as a challenge to your statements or actions in the case at hand. This is true both for the fact witness who has taught or written about relevant medical diagnoses or treatments and for the expert witness who has written about relevant medicolegal issues. "In 1986, in a case similar to this one, you said such and such. And yet now you say thus and so. Which is your true position, Doctor?" If the quote sounds unfamiliar, answer that you would like to see it in context. If the quotation is clearly misleading out of context, feel free to say so. Then your attorney can allude to such opposition tactics in closing argument.

An apparent contradiction between your past and present views can, when appropriate, be addressed by saying, "Thank you for reminding me of what I said ten years ago. As I recall, I said that because of the following circumstances in that particular case . . . Now *this* particular case is different because . . ." This also demonstrates that you have scrupulously paid attention to each individual patient/evaluee.

Imprecise characterizations. Don't give overly simplistic yes-or-no answers to questions phrased in vague generalities, such as "Isn't it true that you've been seeing Mr. G. for a very short (or very long) time?" When you answer this kind of question without qualification, you buy into what may be a mischaracterization of the situation. Just stick to the facts: "I saw Mr. G. for 200 hours over four years."

Compound questions. Questions like the following simultaneously raise doubts about both your character and the content of your testimony: "Doctor, you direct the mental health program in New York City. And isn't it true, Doctor, that Mr. G. is now dead?" Here the attorney wants to make you look self-important while implying that the patient's death is your responsibility.

You should never be compelled to answer such compound questions. While you are pausing to process the question (which you should always do before answering), your attorney should object, and the judge should sustain the objection. If this does not happen, repeat the question silently to yourself. Can you really answer the question "yes" or "no" as worded, or do you need to clarify it? If it is a compound question, break it down and answer each part separately: "Yes, I have been medical director of the program for the past six years, during which I've treated over 600 patients. Of course, it is a tragedy that Mr. G., whom I also treated, is now dead."

"When did you stop beating your wife?" Here a question of chronology is reduced to an accusation: "When was it that you finally figured out that Mr. G. was suicidal? Was it only after he committed suicide?" You can answer by reframing the question as follows: "From hindsight it's easy to see that Mr. G. was suicidal. But when I assessed him for two hours, I checked for the following symptoms and signs . . ." Instead of damaging you, such questions can highlight a series of details that the jury might not have remembered from your direct examination.

Double-negative questions. A simple way of trying to confuse you—and the jury—is to pile on the negatives: "Isn't it true that you didn't . . . ?" Again, a question that is unnecessarily complicated should be disallowed by the judge. If it is not disallowed, by pausing before answering you can take apart the question and either answer it correctly or ask for a clarification: "Is this what you mean?" or "I don't understand." In other words, if the attorney is inviting you to play such verbal tennis, don't be afraid to decline the invitation and stick to ethical and effective testimony.

"Yes, yes, yes, no" questions. In what resembles a children's word game, a cross-examiner may hit you with a rapid-fire series of questions, all of them to be answered "yes," until the one that requires a "no" answer goes right by you. You end up saying, "Yes, yes, yes, yes—oops, what did I say?" Some cross-examining attorneys see the professional who is testifying as a master chess player and themselves as novices who can beat the

master only in a speed game. By pausing to reflect before answering each question, you won't get caught up in the momentum of mindlessness.

The silent treatment. In Zen this is called "the question of no question." You answer one question, and the attorney says nothing. You can respond by looking with the jury at the attorney. Or ask, "Is there any other way I can help you?"

Interruption. If the cross-examiner tries to cut you off before you have finished answering, say, "May I explain?" If the attorney will not let you do so, the jury may well take away an accurate impression that the attorney's tactics are not in keeping with the search for truth and justice.

Sarcasm. If you maintain your professional demeanor, any sarcasm directed at you will cause the cross-examining attorney to suffer by contrast with your effort to formulate thoughtful answers. If the sarcasm is persistent or seriously out of line, your attorney can object, or you can just ask the judge, who may admonish the offending attorney. Finally, you yourself can call attention to the attorney's behavior: "Well, if I can separate the content of your question from the sarcastic language in which it was couched . . ."

Irrelevant, intrusive questions. Pause for your attorney to object.

Redirect Examination

In some complex cases the decisive testimony is given in redirect examination. Often, the questions asked on redirect are in response to what transpired in cross-examination. You can always respond on cross-examination to a question requiring a complex answer by saying, "There is no simple way of answering this question yes or no." If you do not or are not allowed by the cross-examining attorney to clarify, your attorney can, on redirect, ask you to complete your answer in your own way.

With or without such collaboration, it is the attorney's responsibility to listen to the cross-examination with a view toward redirect. Cases have been lost unfairly because an attorney was not sufficiently attentive to a witness's testimony on cross-examination to be able to clarify or build on it on redirect.

Recommendations for Testifying

The following recommendations—some of which have appeared in other sources[20]—distill some of the principles and concepts discussed above into practical guidelines for defendant clinicians as well as for expert witnesses. Keep in mind that, in line with the *Daubert* framework, the judge who sets the tone for courtroom proceedings will be assessing the relevance and reliability of all testimony in terms of the professionalism with which that testimony is presented.

1. Don't lose the forest for the trees. For example, don't be afraid to admit an oversight such as the failure to record something you (or the treating physician) did. It's not how you treated the record; it's how you treated the patient.

2. Don't lose trees for the forest. Although any particular detail usually will not by itself trip you up, you do need to lay out and explain a whole framework of details that constitutes your (or the treating physician's) handling of the case. It is essential to break down the components of the decisionmaking process to show whether the treating physician met the standard of care and acted in an ethically and professionally responsible manner. Familiarity with the use and presentation of medical decision trees can be particularly helpful in this area.[13]

3. Don't deny or overemphasize uncertainty. Distinguish clearly between uncertainty and confusion, and communicate awareness of uncertainty in a manner that is not confusing. Any effort by the plaintiff to hold up a standard of absolute certainty must be met with a clear demonstration that a degree of uncertainty is a condition of all medical decisionmaking.[13] By the same token, avoid the temptation to take refuge in the extreme relativism of "it is all uncertainty" or "it is all judgment," which denies the real knowledge and responsibility professionals are expected to exercise.

4. Use common sense, but don't be a slave to it. When commonsense reasoning and analogies will help you communicate effectively, by all means use them. However, when common sense would lead the jury astray in understanding complex scientific or technical matters, feel free to address the paradoxes that put some subjects outside the boundaries of ordinary everyday thinking.

5. Speak to the jury and "listen" to their feedback. Professional expertise is beneficially applied in monitoring the dialogue you have with the jury. By speaking directly with the jurors and avoiding obfuscations such as engaging in a meaningless debate with an aggressive cross-examiner, you can observe jurors' nonverbal reactions and make educated guesses about what the jury seems to be understanding or not understanding. Do you sense that the jurors are puzzled, skeptical, or inattentive when it comes to specific areas of testimony? Share these observations with your attorney, who should be watching for the same things. The attorney can then decide what points need to be clarified in redirect examination and/or closing argument.

If you believe that you are at a disadvantage because the other side is persistently oversimplifying complex matters, your attorney can file a motion to allow jurors to question witnesses directly under the judge's supervision. This procedure, which moves jurors' reactions from the nonverbal to the verbal realm, is vastly underutilized.[11,21] Some of the most useful questions a witness can be asked come from the finder of fact (judge or jury), precisely because the finder of fact does not operate out of an adversarial position, as do the attorneys for the contending parties.

/ / /

In conclusion, courtroom testimony by a professional is best understood not as a debate, but as a dialogue, informed by a deep understanding and a striving for meaningful truth. In the end, the most ethical testimony is also the most effective.

Notes

1. *Daubert v. Merrell Dow Pharmaceuticals, Inc.,* 113 S. Ct. 2786 (1993).

2. *Gier v. Educational Serv. Unit No. 16,* 66 F.3d 940 (8th Cir. 1995).

3. *Rodriguez Cirilo v. Garcia,* 908 F.Supp. 85 (D.P.R. 1995).

4. *Borawick v. Shay,* 68 F.3d 597 (2d Cir. 1995).

5. D. M. Levy, "Scientific Evidence after *Daubert,*" *Litigation* 22, no. 1 (1995): 48–52.

6. G. C. Read, "Defending against the Emotional Distress Claim," *The Brief,* Winter 1996, pp. 14–19, 42–49.

7. R. M. Hogarth, *Judgment and Choice: The Psychology of Decision* (Chichester, U.K.: John Wiley, 1980).

8. D. Kahneman, P. Slovic, and A. Tversky, eds., *Judgment under Uncertainty: Heuristics and Biases* (Cambridge: Cambridge University Press, 1982).

9. American Academy of Psychiatry and the Law, *Ethical Guidelines for the Practice of Forensic Psychiatry,* 1991.

10. H. J. Bursztajn, A. E. Scherr, and A. Brodsky, "The Rebirth of Forensic Psychiatry in Light of Recent Historical Trends in Criminal Responsibility," *Psychiatric Clinics of North America* 17 (1994): 611–635.

11. H. J. Bursztajn, L. S. Saunders, and A. Brodsky, "*Daubert* without Prejudice:

Achieving Relevance and Reliability without Randomness," *Journal of the Massachusetts Academy of Trial Attorneys* 4, no. 1 (1996): 54–58.

12. N. Pennington and R. Hastie, "The Story Model for Juror Decision Making," in R. Hastie, ed., *Inside the Juror: The Psychology of Juror Decision Making* (Cambridge: Cambridge University Press, 1993).

13. H. J. Bursztajn et al., *Medical Choices, Medical Chances: How Patients, Families, and Physicians Can Cope with Uncertainty* (New York: Routledge, 1990).

14. R. M. Hamm, J. A. Clark, and H. J. Bursztajn, "Psychiatrists' Thorny Judgments: Describing and Improving Decision Making Processes," *Medical Decision Making* 4 (1984): 425–447.

15. B. Fischhoff, "Risk Perception and Communication Unplugged: Twenty Years of Process," *Risk Analysis* 15 (1995): 137–145.

16. *Drewry v. Harwell et al.,* no. CIV-94-1600-T U.S.D.C. W.D. (Okla. 1995).

17. I. L. Janis and L. Mann, *Decision Making: A Psychological Analysis of Conflict, Choice, and Commitment* (New York: Free Press, 1977).

18. The Writing Lab, Department of English, Purdue University, manuscript.

19. H. W. Asbill, "The Ten Commandments of Cross-examination Revisited," *Criminal Justice,* Winter 1994, pp. 2–6, 51–54.

20. S. L. Brodsky, *Testifying in Court: Guidelines and Maxims for the Expert Witness* (Washington: American Psychological Association, 1991).

21. C. Shrallow, "Expanding Jury Participation: Is It a Good Idea?" *University of Bridgeport Law Review* 12 (1991): 209–246.

19

Suggestions for Expert Witnesses

Larry H. Strasburger, M.D.

The American appetite for litigation has grown to astonishing proportions. Lawsuits against individuals and institutions have become commonplace; criminal trials attract major media coverage. Psychiatry has had a long and at times troubled relationship with the legal system. Controversy over such events as the insanity defense of would-be presidential assassin John Hinckley has prompted repeated efforts to banish psychiatrists from the courtroom, or at least to limit their input. However, as Alan Stone, the distinguished professor of law and psychiatry at Harvard Law School, has pointed out, the greater the efforts to remove psychiatrists from the courtroom, the more they seem to be needed.[1] Yet there can be many hazards for the inexperienced clinician who provides this type of consultation. This chapter deals with the role of the expert witness and offers practical suggestions about avoiding some of the pitfalls encountered in doing this work.

Law and Psychiatry: Common Ground and Incongruities

The clinician entering the legal world for the first time is likely to be dismayed at confronting language, concepts, and world view substantially different from the ambience of the psychiatric consulting room.[2] Although law and psychiatry are primarily concerned with human behavior and both strive to maximize human freedom and responsibility, fundamental differences exist between the legal and clinical approaches to these goals. Both psychiatry and the law grapple with the inherent tensions between individual good and social good, yet there are pronounced incongruities in purpose, types of relationships, views of the nature of humankind, causation, and proof.

The purpose of psychiatry, like clinical medicine, is healing and relief of suffering, whereas the purpose of the law is dispute resolution. The relationships which characterize the work of psychiatry are based on alliances, while the law depends on adversarial positions to achieve justice. The law views man as a rational, fully conscious creature, paying little attention to the hidden forces of the unconscious. The law has little tolerance for the ambiguity and ambivalence which the clinician confronts on a daily basis. Issues in court are resolved in an either/or manner with one side winning and the other losing. This zero-sum game differs radically from successful clinical interventions, from which everyone benefits.

Causation for the psychiatrist is often viewed as the result of complex interacting systems. The law's "proximate cause" can be simply the final straw that broke the camel's back. Standards of proof in psychiatry, as in the empirical sciences, are statistical standards. Legal standards of proof for a jury's decisionmaking are formulas such as "a preponderance of the evidence" or "beyond reasonable doubt." "Reasonable medical certainty," the standard for a psychiatric expert's opinion, may simply mean "more likely than not."

Contexts

CIVIL LITIGATION

Psychiatrists are called upon to lend their expertise to the legal system in a wide variety of case types. The most common area of psychiatric involvement is in civil litigation. In this area of the law one party (the plaintiff) sues another party (the defendant) to recover the monetary value of damages alleged to have been caused by the defendant. A civil suit may be brought to resolve all types of disputes between individuals, or between corporate and governmental entities. The area of civil litigation with the highest profile, however, is personal injury law. In these cases the plaintiff brings a suit alleging that the defendant has been negligent in certain activities and that this negligent behavior has injured the plaintiff in some demonstrable way.

In medical or psychiatric malpractice suits, psychiatrists functioning as expert witnesses may be asked to review the treatment in question and give an opinion as to whether or not the defendant doctor's performance met the standard of care, whether departure from the standard of care caused any harm, and the nature and extent of any harm which occurred. In addition to malpractice cases, psychiatric opinions may also be sought, for example, in regard to psychological damages following all types of accidents, violent crime, and physical and sexual abuse.

Psychiatrists frequently receive requests to perform competency evaluations. While most of these requests concern the issue of competency to consent to treatment, psychiatrists may be asked to consult on other specific competencies, such as an individual's capacity to execute a will (either before it is made or as part of a post mortem will contest), to enter into a contract to buy or sell property, or to marry.

Treatment of the mentally ill gives rise to a number of medical-legal issues and requests for forensic consultation. Independent evaluation of a patient's dangerousness or capacity to make treatment decisions (especially those involving antipsychotic medications) may be requested as part of civil commitment or probate proceedings. Child custody, abuse, and adoption, as well as divorce, are also common areas for forensic consultants. These family-related disputes can be among the most heated, prolonged, and challenging for the consultant.

CRIMINAL LITIGATION

Psychiatric involvement in the evaluation of criminal defendants is both frequently requested and controversial. It is here that psychiatrists and other mental health professionals come under the most intensive public scrutiny and receive the greatest criticism.[3] Psychiatric opinion is required by the criminal justice system on a range of specific questions, including competence to stand trial, criminal responsibility, pretrial bail evaluations, juvenile transfer, competence to plead, competence to be a witness, aid to sentencing, ability to serve time in a penal setting, and competence to be executed. Assessments of dangerousness are also requested by some governmental authorities with protective responsibilities, such as the Secret Service. Each of these referral questions has specific criteria of which the consultant must be aware in order to perform an adequate evaluation.

ADMINISTRATIVE PROCEEDINGS

The courts cannot be used to resolve every dispute or enforce every governmental regulation because of the expense and time requirements of judicial proceedings. In response to this problem, a quasi-judicial system has been established in all jurisdictions to handle a range of problems, with the courts available as a last stage of appeal. Workers' compensation, Social Security disability, and other pension-related disability questions are all handled through administrative processes. Psychiatrists are asked to testify not only about the existence and extent of disability but about whether the disability is the result of a work-related incident. Disciplinary bodies, such as boards of licensure for physicians or attorneys, may request opinions about mental status and fitness to practice of individual professionals under investigation. These evaluations pose special problems because of the degree of identification the consultant is likely to feel with the person being evaluated.

Definitions

CLINICAL PSYCHIATRY VERSUS FORENSIC PSYCHIATRY

Clinical psychiatry involves the application of psychiatric expertise to the goals of diagnosis and treatment of mental disorders. Forensic psychiatry is "a subspecialty of psychiatry in which scientific and clinical expertise is applied to legal issues in legal contexts embracing civil, criminal, correctional or legislative matters."[4] Practicing at the interface of two professions, each with its own rules and procedures, each with its own values, ethics, and vocabulary, the forensic psychiatrist must give careful attention to the potential for conflict and misunderstanding. For example, in the practice of forensic psychiatry no doctor-patient relationship is formed. The forensic psychiatrist refers to the individuals evaluated as examinees or evaluees rather than patients. The concept of *primum non nocere,* the time-honored admonition to physicians of the importance of doing no harm, does not apply to a forensic evaluation. The evaluee may lose money, liberty, or even life as a result of the forensic examination.

THE FORENSIC PSYCHIATRIC MODEL

Richard Rosner's model for the organization of both forensic psychiatric data and processes provides an invaluable conceptual framework for the potential expert witness.[5] First, the model asks what is the specific psychiatric-legal issue or question to be addressed. Is it, for example, a matter of competence to stand trial or competence to serve a sentence in a penal institution? Second, what are the specific legal criteria and legal definitions which are used in that jurisdiction to resolve the issue? These will be found in statutes, the precedents of prior court decisions, or administrative rules. Third, what information is relevant to the determination? These will be the medical or psychiatric data, such as clinical history, physical findings, laboratory studies, and mental status which relate to the question. Finally, the model outlines the reasoning process by which the clinical data are applied to the legal criteria in order to answer the legal question. What is the logic behind the expert opinion?

This model provides a clear approach to the multiplicity of entry points into the judicial system. Using it facilitates communication and understanding, as well as illuminating the basis for differences of opinion when forensic psychiatrists, as they often do, disagree.

FACT WITNESS VERSUS EXPERT WITNESS

A witness to fact is someone who has observed something and testifies about that observation during a court proceeding. The fact witness's testimony is confined to "just the facts" and may not include personal opinions or the opinions or reports of others about their observations. A reluctant fact witness may be compelled by court order to testify. For example, a treating psychiatrist may be called to testify about a patient who came for treatment of personal distress following an allegedly traumatic incident. The psychiatrist may be asked what observations were made, what diagnosis was established, and what treatment was prescribed, but may not be allowed to offer an opinion as to the causal connection between the incident and the diagnosis. (This ideal is occasionally breached when expert opinions are coerced from a psychiatric fact witness.)

By contrast, an expert witness is someone who has some knowledge of a science or profession that is beyond the ken of the average layperson. There are three critical differences between an expert witness and a witness to fact. The first difference is that an expert witness may offer an opinion to the court based on a conclusion. Indeed, that is the primary function of an expert witness—to inform the court about matters which special education and experience can clarify. Second, the expert witness appears voluntarily. Third, the expert is paid for the time required to form his opinion and appear in court.

What makes a good expert witness? An aura of trustworthiness appears to be the single most important factor.[6] A reputation for trustworthiness derives from manifest honesty and objectivity,[7] a lack of partisanship, and sincerity. The good expert balances his cases, not always appearing for plaintiffs, not always testifying on the side of defendants, not always working for the prosecution.[8] Avoiding the position of an ideological salesperson adds to credibility. Other important attributes are depth of education, clinical experience, and scholarship. Some attorneys place a high value on using as an expert a clinician who has never previously testified, as though being untainted by the judicial process ensures objectivity. Other attorneys value the authority which may come from substantial courtroom experience. Having written original work in the field enhances credibility. Finally, one's clarity and persuasiveness in court add to effectiveness. The best expert is an effective teacher (if he or she does not lecture the jury).[9]

Initial Consultation with Attorney

Upon receiving a forensic referral, clinicians with no prior forensic experience often have very mixed reactions. On the one hand, many are flattered by the request for their input, interested in the possibility of extra income, or excited by the chance to appear in court. On the other hand, there are often feelings of anxiety at the idea of working within an alien system and fear of unseen pitfalls which may lie ahead. This reaction[10] should be worked through at the outset, just as in the clinical context. It can be as influential in court as in the consulting room. If you do not like or cannot respect the attorney, these feelings may interfere with your work. If you are frightened by the opposing attorney, you may be inhibited on the witness stand. If you have some ideological alliance with the plaintiff or the defendant, you may be an overzealous advocate. Positive or negative feelings toward an evaluee (particularly problematic when evaluating other professionals) should not be allowed to detract from the objectivity of the evaluation.

No consultation, of any type, can be maximally effective unless the consultant knows the question he or she is being asked to answer. This is particularly true in forensic work. As in other areas of consultative work, the consultee may not understand the issue either. Lawyers, like doctors, emerge from the classroom in need of further training. They may not have the experience or knowledge necessary to articulate the issue to be addressed by the consultant. Therefore, the consultant may need to press the attorney who requested the consultation to define the issue clearly. If the consultant does not understand the question, it may be that the attorney is unable to explain it. This is a formula for disaster, and the consultation should not proceed unless the attorney can provide sufficient information or engage in a constructive dialogue to better define the issue.

Once the issue is defined, the potential expert witness must decide whether or not the matter in question is within his or her area of expertise. The general psychiatrist may not be the appropriate person to consult on a complex issue of neuropsychopharmacology. The pharmacologist is probably not the best consultant for a case involving negligent psychotherapy. The consultant must be objective and realistic about his or her limitations and explain these in the initial discussions with the retaining attorney.

The attorney who is considering retaining a psychiatrist as an expert witness will inquire about qualifications and will probably ask to be sent a current curriculum vitae outlining the psychiatrist's education and experience. There will be questions about skeletons in the closet. If the case involves a suicide, has the psychiatrist ever had a patient commit suicide? If the case involves child custody, has the psychiatrist ever been divorced and involved in custody litigation? Has the psychiatrist ever been sued in a malpractice action? Skeletons often take the form of past writings that are contradictory or compromising.

After the first contact with an attorney, a conference should be arranged in which ground rules and boundaries for the work are established. It should be established at the outset that the job of the ethical forensic expert involves arriving at an objective opinion. After that, the chips fall where they may. Avoiding the posture of the "hired gun," one whose opinion is for sale, means making sure that the retaining attorney is aware that he may not find the conclusions of the expert helpful to his client. The attorney then may settle or drop the case or find another expert.

Issues of time, money, access to information, and access to counsel need to be spelled out. This is a good time to find out if any fiscal, time, or examinational constraints or any conflicts of interest exist. An estimate should be made of the amount of time required to evaluate the matter at issue. Will clinical interviews with the plaintiff be supplemented by interviews with others who may have corroborative information? Are there medical records, depositions, or police reports to be reviewed? Will travel be required?

Agreement about fees must be established at the outset. Charges for time at all phases of the work need to be made clear—interviewing, review of records, conferences with counsel, report preparation, testimony at deposition or trial, travel time. Will work be done pro bono? Physicians, by and large, are uncomfortable with written fee agreements and retainers. Lawyers, however, are quite familiar with them in their own practices. Unlike an attorney, the expert witness may not take a contingency fee which is dependent on the outcome of the case. It is, however, ethical to ask for and to accept a retainer. Indeed, being paid up front can help you avoid the difficulty of collecting from disgruntled unsuccessful litigants.

Attorneys may attempt to refer clients for "treatment" with the expectation of later using the psychiatrist as an expert witness. This should be avoided. It is essential to refrain from giving expert testimony on behalf of treated patients because of irreconcilable role conflict and inherent bias due to differing concepts of truth and causation, differing forms of alliance, different types of assessment, and differing ethical guidelines.[11] The consultant must make a decision as to which role, if any, he or she is willing to play and remain strictly in that role. The distinction between clinician and expert witness should be explained to the attorney and, if necessary, other referral sources suggested. While later treatment of a former forensic evaluee has considerable risks, expert testimony on behalf of a current patient almost always portends disaster for the treatment. It is the rare psychotherapy that can survive the experience of having the psychiatrist objectively spell out the details of the litigant's history and emotional turmoils in court in the presence of the patient.[12]

As a rule, all contracts for forensic consultation should be made between the consultant and the attorney or court. This serves several purposes. First, it defines the psychiatrist's role as being that of consultant to the attorney or court and not treater of a patient. Second, it creates an arm's-length relationship with the attorney's client, thus allowing for objectivity in evaluation. Third, establishment of the relationship between doctor and attorney, with the attorney responsible for payment, increases the likelihood of being paid.

Individuals without attorneys may seek forensic evaluations, often in anticipation of litigation or workers' compensation claims. These individuals should be asked about their legal representation, informed that evaluations are performed only at the request of counsel, and instructed to have their attorney call. A prospective plaintiff's inability to obtain legal representation usually speaks to the potential merits of the case (or lack thereof) and low likelihood of success. The involvement of another professional, in most cases, allows for some rational discussion of the merits of the case, a discussion which may be unlikely to occur with a totally biased, and perhaps mentally ill, potential litigant. All this having been said, it is possible for a meritorious, even groundbreaking case to be filed *pro se* (without counsel) because the issues in the case fall outside the patterns with which attorneys are familiar, and the plaintiff gets an attorney only after she finds an expert. In such cases it might be appropriate to do a preliminary evaluation for the benefit of prospective attorneys for this client.

Evaluation and Subsequent Consultation with Attorney

Clinical evaluations of individuals should follow standard procedures, which will not be addressed here, except to emphasize the importance of a carefully detailed mental-status examination. The expert's job is to evaluate each person from a skeptical viewpoint, with a high index of suspicion of malingering or, at minimum, a self-serving posture. This perspective is inconsistent with the traditional empathic-listener stance necessary to the development of a patient-therapist relationship. While the evaluator must always maintain an attitude of respect for the evaluee, corroboration of the data and confrontation of inconsistencies often play an important part in the forensic assessment.

An area of controversy among forensic consultants is whether the expert should function solely as an objective evaluator or as a member of an adversarial legal team. Does the expert remain impartial or become an advocate? While there is a spectrum of views on this issue, I believe that the consulting party, the legal system, and society are best served by professionals who give objective opinions. It would be generally agreed that striving for objectivity gives the retaining attorney a clear view of what the expert can or will say at trial, and provides an opportunity for assessing the likelihood of success. Striving for objectivity fulfills the ethical obligation of the forensic psychiatrist,[13] maintains integrity, and protects the honor of the profession. Objectivity does not, however, preclude the forensic consultant from assisting in the planning of strategy. Indeed, the objective opinion of the consultant may provide useful information to assist counsel to decide whether to pursue, settle, or drop a specific matter, or emphasize or downplay particular issues.

Arguments for the advocacy approach state that the legal system is based on adversarial presentations in which each party is expected to present its case in the best possible light. No one side is without flaws. If that were the case there would be no dispute. Each side has an opportunity to present its case as it sees fit. It is not an obligation of one side (or its expert) to gratuitously reveal its weaknesses to the other. Moreover, each side has an equal opportunity to use expert witnesses. "Only a foolhardy lawyer would determine tactical and evidentiary strategy in a case with psychiatric issues without the guidance and interpretation of psychiatrists."[14] Indeed, in criminal cases, the United States Supreme Court has held that the state must provide an expert psychiatrist where an indigent defendant is unable to pay for one.[15] In that decision, the Court referred to the appointed psychiatrist's role as a member of a defense team.

Each forensic consultant must decide to what degree his or her role will be that of objective scientist or advocate. The adversarial nature of the system, as well as our tendency to promote our own opinions and beliefs, makes it difficult to exclude all advocacy from our roles. The providing of objective evaluations in itself makes the consultant an important part of the advocacy team and assists greatly in preparing for litigation. Once involved in the litigation process, the consultant should be a vigorous advocate for his or her own conclusions. Still, caution must be exercised to ensure that this enthusiasm for one's own opinion does not transfer automatically to zealous support for the cause of the retaining party. This path leads to loss of integrity and credibility.

The retaining attorney may want to have a report prepared, or, in order to avoid disclosure, may not want to receive one. In either case the preparation of a report is a useful exercise since the report gives the expert witness an opportunity to organize his or her thinking and review the validity of whatever conclusions have been reached. In cases where there is a long hiatus between the time of the clinical evaluation and the date of trial, a report can be an invaluable aid to memory and a means to reduce the time necessary for trial preparation. Reports may also provide reminders of issues and details which can be useful in future cases. They aid in an aggregation of experience.

The forensic psychiatric model just outlined provides a useful format for report writing. The legal question and the legal standard for addressing that issue should be carefully spelled out. Data should be kept separate from inferences, and facts should be separate from conclusions. A conclusory posture toward the legal issue, unsupported by clinical information, is to be avoided. In addition to clinical interviews, history, and mental status, the presentation of corroborative data is essential. A forensic formulation, in which the clinical data are applied to the legal standard, provides the logic through which the legal question is answered.

Pretrial Conference

The importance of a pretrial conference with the retaining attorney cannot be overstated. The expert should always insist on one. Attorney and witness must establish a dialogue which reviews the strengths and weaknesses of the case. There must be an opportunity to plan the attorney's direct examination of the expert, the exact questions which he intends to ask at the trial. Similarly, there should be an opportunity to anticipate the questions that will be asked during the opposing attorney's cross-examination. Actually role-playing these questions and answers gives the expert witness some facility with the processes, tactics, and opportunities of the courtroom. Role-playing prepares for pitfalls which may be encountered and frequently detects information gaps which can be filled before the expert takes the stand.

On the Witness Stand

Much of what follows has been gleaned from experience and advice from senior colleagues, attorneys, and judges, to whom I am exceedingly grateful. Some is common sense—perhaps the most valuable counsel of all.

APPEARANCE AND BEHAVIOR

Self-care will aid the expert witness who is about to give court testimony. It helps to pay attention to personal needs in anticipation of taking the witness stand. If possible, one should get a good night's sleep beforehand. Avoid last-minute, late-night cramming. Get to the courthouse early and familiarize yourself with the layout of the courtroom. Find the bathroom. Trying to testify while battling an expanding bladder is a doubly painful experience. Have a meal if need be. Why confront hypoglycemia as well as cross-examination? (Of course, no eating on the witness stand—this includes Lifesavers and so on.) While not feasible for the many people who depend on the energizing effect of caffeine to do intellectual work, avoidance of coffee and tea may be helpful, as caffeine may add to the existing nervousness.

Personal appearance is important. Surface may not outweigh substance, but jurors notice small things and form their biases accordingly. A clean shave or neatly trimmed beard, combed hair, and clean clothes add to a professional impression. Dress should be conservative, as though going to a funeral. It is best to look as middle-class as possible. Men should wear light-colored shirts, conservative neckties, and dark blue or gray suits, and never remove jackets in court. Jewelry should be avoided. Women should wear suits or business dresses. Skirts should be below the knees. Heels should be medium or low. Go for non-flamboyant, non-ostentatious "good taste."

Nonverbal behavior should be monitored for its effect on the jury. Nervous gestures, such as finger drumming, knuckle cracking, or fingernail biting, detract from a professional manner. A posture with arms folded tightly across the chest may be interpreted as defensive self-protectiveness. Do not cover your mouth or rub the bridge of your nose while speaking. Do not preen. Straightening the hair, brushing lint off clothes, and adjusting neckties are all associated with covering up. Certainly gestures may be used when appropriate. Counting on the fingers can help to accentuate main points, and pointing can add emphasis. (Do not overdo these.)

The experience of anxiety in court is universal and unavoidable. Psychiatrists in particular are not used to being on display as public figures. The consulting room is a very private place. It helps to remember that others have far more valid reasons to be nervous than you do. The principals in the courtroom drama, the plaintiff and defendant, and the attorneys have grave issues at stake. You and the judge, however, can rightfully remain calm. You are not on trial. Your life, your liberty, and your property are not at stake. You can rest assured, calm in the knowledge that you have no vital interests that will be compromised by your attendance at court, other than your reputation as a forensic psychiatrist.

Entrance and exit behavior are important boundaries to your testimony. If you have looked at the courtroom ahead of time, you will know where you will sit, where the other participants will be placed, and where you will take the witness stand. When you are called to testify, walk confidently to the witness stand, where you will be sworn in. If you can, engage the judge at the outset with a "good morning" or "good afternoon, Your Honor." This will begin a contact, a subliminal dialogue, which may be useful further along in the proceedings. After being sworn in, look at the jury. It is helpful to make eye contact with them as individuals. They make the vital decisions, and you want your nonverbal behavior to align you with them to the extent possible. However, never wink or smirk at them.

After being dismissed from the witness stand, leave the courtroom in the same professional manner as when entering. Do not saunter out, do not chat with people, do not loosen a necktie, do not show "relief." These behaviors suggest that testimony, as well as the expert, was dressed up for the occasion.

Take minimal notes to the witness stand as aids to your memory. Clear with your attorney what notes you do take with you. The cross-examining attorney has a right to see your notes, and after examining them, may question you specifically about them. Know your case. Know why you hold the opinions that you do. The witness stand is no place to figure this out. Resolve your doubts and ambivalence when you are preparing your testimony, or in conference with your attorney before you take the stand. Ambivalence tends to show up in word choice, and attorneys can be quite perceptive in picking it up. Surprise is anathema.

QUALIFICATION

In order to establish the admissibility of expert testimony, the credentials of the expert witness must be spelled out. Education (college, medical school, specialty training) and work experience allow recognition by the court as an expert. In addition, medical licensure and board certification, academic and hospital appointments, as well as any honors received, should be brought out by the attorney. Relevant publications, particularly those pertaining to the issues at hand, are also noteworthy. The demonstration of these credentials is an important factor in supporting credibility.

Qualifications should be elicited by a dialogue, a short question-and-answer exchange between attorney and witness. The monologue in answer to a single general question, such as, "Doctor, tell us about your education and experience," is likely to produce a soporific effect on the jury. Occasionally the opposing attorney will stipulate to the qualifications of the expert. This should be avoided by your attorney as it deprives the jury of knowing the breadth of the expertise being offered.

It is best not to engage in a discussion of one's theoretical orientation—Freudian, eclectic, or other. This information merely confuses the jury. For the court's purposes, the expert testimony will be about objective data and the inferences made from it.

DIRECT EXAMINATION

This interchange is the most difficult and most important phase of testimony. Sensitivity to nuances of language is critical. Professional jargon and complex words are to be avoided. If a technical or scientific term is used, it is best to translate it immediately to the jury. You can convey scientific expertise even while speaking in familiar terms. Assume that the average juror has not completed high school, so keep it simple but do not appear to be "talking down" to the jurors. Where you can, use the words of the examinee to demonstrate your points.

Intensifiers such as "very" and "surely" should be avoided, as well as glitches such as "kind of" or "I guess." Crisp, well-turned phrases convey confidence. Words of hesitation such as "uhf, well" or "you know" convey doubt. Repeated use of such words as "sir" and "thank you" diminishes the authority of the expert. The use of absolutes such as "I never" or "I always" should be discouraged; they have a way of coming back to haunt the expert during cross-examination. The expert should not depreciate his own testimony with words such as "honestly," "in all candor," or "I'm doing the best I can." Of course, the expert should not utter even the mildest profanity, obscenity, or racial or ethnic slur. In some areas of the United States even "hell" is blasphemy.

Attempt to anticipate the directions in which the questioning is going, and answer questions fully. The pretrial conference will help with this. Do not volunteer information beyond the answer to the question, as this may provide fodder for later cross-examination. Keep the data separate from the inferences, and proceed in a logical stepwise fashion toward your conclusions. Avoid speculation, conjecture, guessing. On the other hand, estimates, professional belief, and professional opinion are acceptable.

Pace is very important. Anxiety often tends to push a person into responding quickly. Resist this tendency. Listen carefully to each question and, if need be, pause before answering. Do not begin an answer before the attorney has finished asking the question. Objections by the opposing attorney will occur in the midst of testimony. Sometimes these are voiced simply to interrupt the pace of the expert's delivery. When an objection is made, stop talking. Do not attempt to talk over the objecting attorney. Wait until the judge has sustained or overruled the objection. Never speak when the judge is speaking. Listening carefully to the objection may provide clues about the direction that testimony should take.

CROSS-EXAMINATION

Remember when cross-examination begins that there is nothing personal in it. The opposing attorney is simply doing his or her job in the attempt to question, rebut, or disparage your testimony. The opposing attorney is paid to undermine your testimony, and may do so by attacking your education and experience,[16] the clinical evaluation you have performed, the ancillary information you have obtained, and the logic and reasoning by which you reached your conclusions. Even the validity of psychiatry as a profession is likely to be attacked. "The experienced cross-examiner has an armamentarium of tactics, including ad hominem attacks, argumentative questions, ploys calculated to 'shock' the witness, and other anxiety-inducing techniques that are intended to prompt negative demeanor, confusion and uncertainty in the witness."[17] Maintaining a dispassionate stance, with the calm assurance of your professional integrity, will protect against this assault.

The basic rule of self-preservation for witnesses going into this lion's den is always to be truthful and always courteous. The cross-examiner should be treated evenhandedly with the same respect shown to your own attorney. A sense of objectivity is communicated by presenting the same demeanor, even the same tone of voice, to both attorneys. Never argue or lose your temper. Do not use sarcasm or attempt to be witty. Humor is the prerogative of the attorneys and the judge.

A cardinal rule for responding to cross-examination is to pause and think before answering questions. Gutheil's "ten-second pause" acts as a shield against the buffeting of cross-examination.[18] If nothing else, it gives your attorney an opportunity to object. The cross-examining attorney will attempt to control the testimony by asking only questions to which he or she knows the answer. These are likely to be phrased in requests for yes or no answers. Questions should be answered briefly, and without volunteering additional information beyond the scope of the question. If you are finished with an answer, remain quiet and do not expand upon it. Do not add to your answer just because the examiner looks at you expectantly. If the examiner asks you if that is all you recollect, say "yes" if that is the case.

If you are interrupted while attempting to answer more fully, indicate that you had not finished with your response to the question. If you cannot answer the question in the form in which it has been put, you may say so. If you do not know the answer, acknowledge it. You are not expected to be omniscient, and showing that you know the limits of your expertise helps counteract an appearance of arrogance.

Do not attempt to answer questions you do not understand. It is the attorney's job to formulate intelligible questions, and not your job to educate him or to suggest good questions. Do not explain to the examiner that the question is incomprehensible because he has misunderstood terms of art in the profession. Do not help the examiner by asking questions, such as, "What do you mean by that?" If the attorney appears confused, do not try to clarify his confusion. You are not treating him.

Beware of compound questions and questions with double negatives. If a question is too complex to be held in your mind, it is too complex and ambiguous to answer. Think about the unstated assumptions within questions. If a question misstates your prior testimony, say so. Do not accept the attorney's characterization of time, distances, personalities, or events. Rephrase the question into a sentence of your own, using your own words.

Try to anticipate where you are being led, but do not expect to testify without having points scored against you. This is inevitable. There are two sides to every case. Your own attorney can seek to "rehabilitate" your testimony by clarifying these points on redirect examination. Do not allow the attorney to put words in your mouth. Pay particular attention to the introductory clauses preceding the essence of the question. Leading questions may be preceded by statements which are either half true or contain facts which you do not know to be true. Do not let the examiner put you in the position of adopting the half-truths or unknown facts, on which he will then base further questions. You may openly disagree with the implicit statements contained in these questions.

Be prepared to be questioned about your fee arrangements. Anticipate that you will be asked how much you have been paid "for your testimony." Make clear that you are paid solely for your time, not for your opinion.

Before going to court you should have carefully reviewed transcripts of any of your prior deposition testimony in the case. The cross-examiner will attempt to use deposition material to point out inconsistencies in your testimony. Be aware that the attorney is likely to have read transcripts of your testimony in prior similar cases, as well as any pertinent publications which you have written. These may be quoted out of context in order to attempt to show inconsistent testimony or opinions. In answering these challenges, you may need to explain the different contexts in which you made seemingly contradictory statements.

If challenged by the attorney's quoting material from an allegedly authoritative article or book which seems to contradict your testimony, there are several possible responses. One is to refuse to acknowledge the authoritative nature of the text. Medicine is an empirical science and, as such, does not have absolute authorities. If you know of flaws in the research or methodology of the publication, you can say so. In some jurisdictions, if you have not relied on the text you do not have to be confronted by it in court. Always ask to see the context of any quotation from a document, even your own writing. Also check the quotation. It may be misstated.

The courtroom is the judge's territory, and permission must be requested before moving in it. If you use lecture aids such as slides or blackboard, request the judge's permission before leaving the witness stand. The judge, who may seem intimidatingly powerful, can be also an ally and protective figure. You may ask the judge to have the court stenographer read back a question, or ask the judge for a moment of reflection. If uncertain about procedure, such as whether material which may be privileged should be divulged in open court, ask the judge for guidance. If the cross-examiner is genuinely harassing or badgering you and if your attorney has not objected, you may appeal to the judge for relief, though this approach must be used sparingly, and the judge may be reluctant to grant relief if your own attorney has not objected.

/ / /

Why would anyone deliberately suffer the slings and arrows of the courtroom? The forensic psychiatrist must endure constant chipping away at his narcissism. Constant criticism is to be anticipated, not only from the public but from colleagues as well. Yet work as an expert witness is an opportunity for the psychiatrist to apply clinical expertise in a different and exciting setting. Courtroom drama can be extremely stimulating. It is intellectually satisfying to work at this interface, translating concepts back and forth between the languages of law and psychiatry. The role provides a chance to move outside the consulting room and to encounter psychopathology not otherwise seen in routine practice. Most of all, acting as an expert witness is an unparalleled teaching opportunity. One can bring concepts of clinical psychiatry to a jury composed of people who have never before contemplated mental health issues. This educator role can provide immense professional satisfaction, plus the satisfaction of having served justice. Finally, there is a positive ethical benefit to society from having the legal system enriched by the complex insights and compassionate understanding of psychiatrists.

Notes

The author wishes to acknowledge the invaluable help of Ronald Schouten, M.D., J.D., in the preparation of this chapter.

1. A. A. Stone, *Law, Psychiatry, and Morality* (Washington: American Psychiatric Press, 1984).

2. T. G. Gutheil and M. J. Mills, "Legal Conceptualizations, Legal Fictions and the Manipulation of Reality: Conflict between Models of Decision Making in Psychiatry and Law," *Bulletin of the American Academy of Psychiatry and the Law* 10 (1982): 17–27.

3. P. J. Resnick, "Perceptions of Psychiatric Testimony: A Historical Perspective on the Hysterical Invective," *Bulletin of the American Academy of Psychiatry and the Law* 14 (1986): 203–219.

4. American Academy of Psychiatry and the Law, *Ethical Guidelines for the Practice of Forensic Psychiatry,* 1991.

5. R. Rosner, "A Conceptual Model for Forensic Psychiatry," in *Principles and Practice of Forensic Psychiatry,* ed. R. Rosner (New York: Chapman and Hall, 1994).

6. P. J. Resnick, "Guidelines for Courtroom Testimony," in *Principles and Practice of Forensic Psychiatry,* ed. Rosner.

7. J. R. Rappeport, "Effective Courtroom Testimony," *Psychiatric Quarterly* 63 (1992): 303–317.

8. S. Boyarsky, "Practical Measures to Reduce Medical Expert Witness Bias," *Journal of Forensic Sciences* 34 (1989): 1259–1265.

9. E. Tanay, "The Expert Witness as Teacher," *Bulletin of the American Academy of Psychiatry and the Law* 8 (1980): 401–411.

10. D. H. Schetky and E. M. Colbach, "Countertransference on the Witness Stand: A Flight from the Self?" *Bulletin of the American Academy of Psychiatry and the Law* 10 (1982): 115–121.

11. L. H. Strasburger, T. G. Gutheil, and A. Brodsky, "On Wearing Two Hats: Role Conflict in Serving Both as Psychotherapist and Expert Witness," *American Journal of Psychiatry* 154 (1997): 448–456. Group for the Advancement

of Psychiatry, *The Mental Health Professional and the Legal System* (Washington: American Psychiatric Press, 1991).

12. L. H. Strasburger, "Crudely without Any Finesse . . . The Defendant Hears His Psychiatric Evaluation," *Bulletin of the American Academy of Psychiatry and the Law* 15 (1987): 229–233.

13. American Academy of Psychiatry and the Law, *Ethical Guidelines for the Practice of Forensic Psychiatry.*

14. *U.S. ex rel. Edney v. Smith,* 425 F. Supp. 1038, 1047 (E.D.N.Y. 1976), aff'd without opinion 556 F.2d 556 (2d Cir.) cert. denied, 431 U.S. 958 (1977).

15. *Ake v. Oklahoma,* 470 U.S. 68 105 S.Ct. 1087 (1985).

16. W. F. Rowe, "Challenging the Expert Witness," *Criminal Justice* 7 (1992): 28–56.

17. R. L. Goldstein, "Psychiatrists in the Hot Seat: Discrediting Doctors by Impeachment of Their Credibility," *Bulletin of the American Academy of Psychiatry and the Law* 16 (1988): 225–234.

18. T. G. Gutheil, personal communication.

20

Narrative Truth, Historical Truth, and Forensic Truth

Alan W. Scheflin, J.D., L.L.M.

In the good old days, meaning the entire twentieth century up to the late 1980s, the number of malpractice lawsuits filed and won against psychiatrists, psychologists, and mental health professionals for non-somatic treatments was exceedingly small. In the small number of cases actually won by patients, relatively low dollar amounts were paid in damages. Whereas the average neurosurgeon expected to be sued once for every two years of practice, the average American psychiatrist was sued once for every 50 to 100 years of practice (Cohen, 1979). In general, although suits against other professionals were on the rise (one out of every four lawyers in California is sued for malpractice, according to its State Bar statistics), mental health professionals remained relatively unscathed by claims of professional negligence.

Unfortunately, these numbers are changing dramatically. The once-sacred couch or therapy room is now routinely violated by lawyers and litigants. Part of the reason may be that the heavily litigious climate in this country has caused a shift in the assessment of conduct away from the moral grounds of individual responsibility and toward the economic grounds of financially solvent institutional carriers. Risk-spreading has replaced individual accountability. Lawyers have further diminished the concept of personal responsibility by succeeding with a variety of imaginative, fanciful, and often unbelievable "excuse" defenses (Dershowitz, 1994; Scheflin, 1995). The current court-crazy climate, with its unending search for deep pockets, has led litigators to psychiatric malpractice insurers.

Back in those good old days, what a therapist did in the therapy room remained private. The wall that separated that room from the outside world was solid enough to keep confidences in and lawyers out (Lipkin, 1989; Simon, 1992; Appelbaum and Gutheil, 1991). Several legal developments, however, have rendered that wall porous, and recent events may have dissolved it almost entirely.

One of the most visible, and controversial, legal developments that has forged a connection between the therapy room and the outside world is the well-known *Tarasoff* decision (1976) requiring warnings to third parties threatened with violence by therapy patients (Simon, 1990). However, before the *Tarasoff* court imposed this judicially created duty regarding dangerous patients, several legal developments had already penetrated the sanctity of patient-therapist relationships. First, the courts had decided that duties were owed to third parties who were physically endangered by the negligence of the therapist. Thus, the psychiatrist's failure to inform the patient that a drug could cause drowsiness could be the basis of a lawsuit filed by a pedestrian who was injured when the patient fell asleep at the wheel. Second, courts had already protected patients from (1) improper conduct, such as sexual contact (Schoener et al., 1989); (2) experimental treatments involving physical contact with the patient, such as "sluggo" therapy (*Rains v. Superior Court [Center Foundation]*, 1984; *Center Foundation v. Chicago Insurance Company*, 1991), "direct analysis" (*Hammer v. Rosen*, 1960), and "Z-therapy" (*Abraham v. Zaslow*, 1975); and (3) highly controversial intrusive somatic treatments, such as ECT (Abrams, 1992) or psychosurgery (Scheflin and Opton, 1978; Shuman, 1977).

Perhaps the most important legal development for current concerns, however, is that legislatures had already required therapists to inform state authorities about any cases of suspected child abuse (Kalichman, 1993). These mandatory reporting laws were first enacted in the 1960s after a century of medical history demonstrated that physicians routinely examined and observed children who had been severely battered and yet those physicians had remained silent about the atrocities of which they had clear evidence (Behlmer, 1982). The publication of Kempe and colleagues' seminal paper on child abuse (1962) is credited with coining the term "battered-child syndrome" and with inspiring the mandatory reporting legislation now existing in every state. Not surprisingly, these mandatory reporting statutes extended from physicians to encompass all mental health professionals, as well as teachers and child care personnel (Everstine and Everstine, 1986). For the last thirty years mental health professionals have been legally required, under penalty of criminal prosecution and civil liability, to take an active role in the protection of children from molestation and abuse.

While the statutes have been credited with bringing the problem of child abuse to public attention and with providing effective help for battered children, they have not been without their critics. Some commentators have likened the mandatory reporting system to the Salem witch trials (Gardner, 1991), while others have observed that the child protective system serves an essential function despite its serious flaws (Myers, 1994; Alexander, 1993), some of which raise substantial difficulties concerning the continuation of the therapy (Levine, Doueck et al., 1995). At the heart of the attacks are two major issues: Are children telling the truth about being abused? And should mental health professionals become investigators, detectives, or police before reporting abuse to state authorities?

What Is Truth?

Ever since Pontius Pilate asked the question "What is truth?" two thousand years ago, the answer has become increasingly elusive. This has occurred, in part, because the concept of "truth" has undergone dramatic historical change (Schmitt, 1995; Campbell, 1992), especially in this "postmodern" age (Anderson, 1995). For psychiatrists, in the good old days, the answer was clear—in therapy, truth was what the patient believed (Frank and Frank, 1991). As Gravitz (1994) has noted, "in psychotherapy, more important than what actually occurred to a patient is what the patient believed occurred." Gutheil has cogently observed that "if a patient in therapy says something, assume it is true—i.e., that it captures some fundamental (but perhaps metaphoric or symbolic) truth about that person; but do not delude yourself that it is real, i.e., veridical, or that you know whether or not it actually happened just that way" (Gutheil, 1992). Outside the therapy room, however, a different truth has prevailed.

In recent years it has become popular to notice and highlight this difference between narrative truth and historical truth. The psychiatrist Donald P. Spence (1982, 1987, 1994a, 1994b), has articulated this distinction with eloquence. According to Spence, narrative truth is necessary and sufficient in therapy, but it is not adequate in courts of law. Thus, when an adult woman claims in therapy that she now remembers that she was molested as a child, the therapy may proceed with the assumption that the patient is correct, even if no such event ever occurred. The therapist's concern is not with the actual occurrence of the alleged incidents, but rather with its meaning for the patient's life story. If the patient is to testify in court, however, judges and juries are not interested in narrative truth. They require historical truth. Whether the acts of molesting actually occurred makes all the difference in a criminal or civil case, not whether the patient believes they occurred.

Common sense and careful observation inform us that there is a real distinction between the stories that patients tell their therapists, including the stories that therapists construct to aid patients, and historical truth, which is defined as events that actually happened in the real world. Stories in therapy may often be one-sided, exaggerated, distorted, misperceived, misremembered, or even wholly fictitious. On the other hand, many events that happen in the real world can be proven, measured, verified, and quantified, as is now required by the United States Supreme Court (*Daubert,* 1993) as a precondition for the admissibility of expert testimony. And so this dichotomy between narrative truth and historical truth captures a significant ideological point.

Nevertheless, in this chapter I want to suggest that there is little that is more malignant to the practice of therapy than making this distinction without careful consideration of its consequences. The distinction between narrative truth and historical truth can be a dangerous one, and it is wrong in its description of therapy, wrong in its understanding of historical truth, and wrong in its equation of historical truth with forensic truth. In short, I reject Spence's position that only narrative truth occurs or matters in therapy, and I reject his claim that only historical truth occurs or matters in courts of law. The consequences of these errors for professional risk management and for legal regulation of mental health professionals have already been most unfortunate.

Narrative Truth in the Therapy Room

An excellent illustration of the naive description of narrative truth may be found in Piper's (1993) discussion of sodium amytal's poor performance as a "truth serum." He notes that the drug's role as an aid to memory should be severely questioned because of the well-known capacity of subjects to lie, distort, fantasize, imagine, and respond to suggestion. But he conveniently ignores the most crucial fact—that people lie, distort, fantasize, imagine, and respond to suggestion *without* amytal and, indeed, as an ordinary part of their daily lives.

Sodium amytal may not be a truth serum, but then, nothing is: not even ordinary memory. Yet both memory and sodium amytal are capable of revealing truths that are independently verifiable. Piper's error is parallel to the error made by others (Perry et al., 1996; Karlin and Orne, 1996) when they criticize hypnosis on the grounds that its use with memory does not reveal only truth. It is *memory* that is fundamentally inaccurate. Improperly used hypnosis can cause further contamination, as can undue suggestion and leading questions (Scheflin, 1996, 1997b). Any retrieval technique, if used improperly, can contaminate memory. It does not follow, however, and it is not true, that hypnosis inevitably causes memory distortion (Brown et al., 1997). If used according to carefully constructed newly developed guidelines (American Society of Clinical Hypnosis, 1995; McConkey and Sheehan, 1995), hypnosis may be of exceptional assistance in the retrieval of accurate and hitherto inaccessible memories.

Piper, Orne et al., and others maintain a fallacious and harmful dual standard. On the one hand, they adopt the Loftus model of an inevitably malleable memory (Loftus and Ketcham, 1994); on the other hand, they then insist that any memory or psychotherapeutic technique be capable of producing truth. Yet, under their own model, historical truth is obviously unknowable from memory alone. The narrative approach, also called the "reconstruction of reality" approach, has generally been accepted by researchers studying memory (Brown et al., 1997), autobiographical memory (Ross, 1991), and the writing of history (Berkhofer, 1995).

Early researchers discovered that human senses are fallible (Munsterberg, 1908) and human memory malleable (Bartlett, 1932). It is from the work of these pioneers that Spence essentially has built his case. The logical conclusion of this reconstructionist position is that objective truth is inevitably unknowable. If our senses are untrustworthy, and our memory unreliable, then the past must always be known to us in a distorted fashion.

What happens in a therapy session? The patient selects and censors information, which is conveyed to the therapist. That information itself is based on inaccurate perceptions and incomplete or erroneous recollections. The therapist may then reconstruct "narratives" to explain the information presented (Freedman and Combs, 1996). The patient then constructs narratives to evaluate what the therapist is saying. The therapist's feedback responses to the patient further alter the patient's perceptions, and thus alter the information given to the therapist in response (Pearce, 1996). The final product is, by necessity, a shared construct which may be far removed from historical truth. In summarizing this point, Wesson (1985) has succinctly stated the inevitable progression of the slippage from reality to narrative: "From what 'really happened' to what the subject or patient remembers is one transformation; from what he remembers to what he articulates is another; from what he says to what the analyst hears is another; and from what the analyst hears to what she concludes is still another."

It therefore follows, under this model, that historical truth makes no appearance in the therapy room because patient and therapist have already gone through at least four layers of narration building a reconstructed reality. If therapy can only be narrative truth, and cannot be historical truth, what happens in the therapy session happens not for purposes of historic validation but rather for purposes of enabling patients to become more functional.

The theory of social reconstruction of reality has recently become popular. Its application to psychotherapy has been mixed. Some authors have leveled substantial attacks that psychotherapy is not scientific (Fancher, 1995) and others have gone further and argued it is based exclusively on myth (Dawes, 1994). Not surprisingly, these attacks have come at a time when mental health professionals are spending more time in court appearing as experts on an increasing number of issues (Felsenthal, 1995), a practice the anti-psychotherapy authors deplore. Other reconstructionists and historians have urged the reshaping of psychotherapy into more relativistic segments stressing flexibility over scientific validity (Cushman, 1995; Hale, 1995).

Given the initial premises of the reconstructionist position, psychotherapy is not "scientific" because the past is historically unknowable, at least without independent physical corroboration. It would therefore follow under this view that, if courts are wedded to historical truth, psychotherapy has no scientific role to play. While this point might make no difference if therapy stayed in the therapy room, it makes an important difference when the therapy reaches the courts.

Historical Truth versus Forensic Truth

Anyone who believes that courts of law are wedded to historical truth has not spent much time before judges and juries. While it is undoubtedly accurate to say that truth does serve a function in courts of law, other values, such as justice, fairness, mercy, and the preservation of individual rights, in fact have a more primary role. Indeed, one of the finer modern debates in law began with a lament and challenge by Judge Marvin Frankel (1975) that "our adversary system rates truth too low among the values that institutions of justice are meant to serve" (p. 1031) and the response by Professor Monroe H. Freedman (1975b) arguing that the Constitution protects the virtue of individual autonomy and also other rights and other values, despite historical truth.

We may test the hypothesis that courts of law insist on historical truth by examining a simple ethical question posed to all law students (Freedman, 1966, 1990). Suppose a lawyer is cross-examining a witness who the lawyer fully believes is telling the truth. The testimony of the witness is damaging to the lawyer's case. May the attorney use the cross-examination to attempt to persuade the jury that the witness is mistaken or lying? In short, may a completely truthful witness be cross-examined with the goal of convincing the jury of an untruth?

Legal commentators generally agree that this tactic, of making the historical truth appear to be untrue, not only is ethically permissible, it may even be mandatory. Chief Justice Warren Burger (1966) took a bigger step when he proposed that even prosecutors had the ethical right to distort the truth by impeaching the credibility of truthful witnesses. Wolfram (1986), however, in his textbook *Modern Legal Ethics,* cites cases suggesting Burger's view may be too extreme, and therefore unethical.

In *United States v. Wade* (1967), the United States Supreme Court, by a bare majority, held that the constitution mandates the presence of a lawyer at a police lineup. Justices White, Harlan, and Stewart disagreed that a *per se* rule requiring the presence of lawyers was necessary, as, for example, in cases where the witness knows or is closely related to the suspect, or in cases where the witness has spent a great deal of time with or had a very clear observation of the suspect. These justices acknowledged the relativity of perception and memory by noting:

> The premise for the Court's rule is not the general unreliability of eyewitness identifications nor the difficulties inherent in observation, recall, and recognition. The Court assumes a narrower evil as the basis for its rule—improper police suggestion which contributes to erroneous identifications. The Court apparently believes that improper police procedures are so widespread that a broad prophylactic rule must be laid down, requiring the presence of counsel at all pretrial identifications, in order to detect recurring instances of police misconduct. I do not share this pervasive distrust of all official investigations. (p. 251)

> I share the Court's view that the criminal trial, at the very least, should aim at truthful factfinding, including accurate eyewitness identifications. I doubt, however, on the basis of our present information, that the tragic mistakes which have occurred in criminal trials are as much the product of improper police conduct as they are the consequence of the difficulties inherent in eyewitness testimony and in resolving evidentiary conflicts by court or jury. (p. 254)

/ / /

While acknowledging that the criminal trial should *aim* at truth, White, Harlan, and Stewart also note that the search for historical truth is not the mandate of defense lawyers:

> Law enforcement officers have the obligation to convict the guilty and to make sure they do not convict the innocent. They must be dedicated to making the criminal trial a procedure for the ascertainment of the true facts surrounding the commission of the crime . . . But defense counsel has no comparable obligation to ascertain or present the truth. Our system assigns him a different mission . . . Defense counsel need present nothing, even if he knows what the truth is . . . If he can confuse a witness, even a truthful one, or make him appear at a disadvantage, unsure or indecisive, that will be his normal course. Our interest in not convicting the innocent permits counsel to put the State to its proof, to put the State's case in the worst possible light, regardless of what he thinks or knows to be the truth. Undoubtedly there are some limits which defense counsel must observe but more often than not, defense counsel will cross-examine a prosecution witness, and impeach him if he can, even if he thinks the witness is telling the truth, just as he will attempt to destroy a witness who he thinks is lying. In this respect, as part of our modified adversary system and as part of the duty imposed on the most honorable defense counsel, we countenance or require conduct which in many instances has little, if any, relation to the search for truth. (pp. 256–258)

The justices then quoted from several popular books on trial technique, all of which provided hints and techniques on twisting, distorting, or hiding the truth. The essence of this advocacy is captured in the following passage from Anthony Berkeley's (1929) classic murder mystery *The Poisoned Chocolates Case:*

> Facts were very dear to Sir Charles . . . There was no one at the bar who could so convincingly distort an honest but awkward fact into carrying an entirely different interpretation from that which any ordinary person (counsel for the prosecution, for instance) would have put upon it. He could take that fact, look it boldly in the face, twist it round, read a message from the back of its neck, turn it inside out and detect auguries in its entrails, dance triumphantly on its corpse, pulverize it completely, remold it if necessary into an utterly different shape, and finally, if the fact still had the temerity to retain any vestige of its primary aspect, bellow at it in the most terrifying manner. If that failed he was quite prepared to weep at it in open court. (pp. 55–56)

Suppose a defendant in a criminal case confesses to his attorney that he committed the robbery with which he is charged. The defendant does not want to testify, but he wants his attorney to allow his two friends to swear that the defendant was with them at 8:00 P.M., the time the victim claims the robbery occurred. The friends are telling the truth, but the victim is mistaken in believing that the robbery occurred at 8:00 P.M. rather than at 6:00 P.M., which is the actual time. May the attorney place into evidence truthful witnesses to persuade the jury of a falsity (his client's innocence)? In answering in the affirmative, a Michigan State Bar Opinion (1987) notes that "it is not the obligation of defense counsel to correct inaccurate evidence introduced by the prosecution or to ignore truthful evidence that could exculpate his client."

An old Tennessee case holds that a counsel who can summon up tears at will has a professional duty to do so on behalf of the client (*Ferguson v. Moore*, 1897). It is no wonder that an Illinois judge once instructed a jury that there were "tricks to all trades and the legal profession is the trade of all tricks" (*Forest Preserve Dist. of Cook County v. Mike*, 1954).

The adversary system is a search for one type of truth, but not historical truth. It is a search for forensic truth, by which what actually happened in the real world is discovered through filters that either prevent certain factual evidence from being admitted (statutes of limitation, for example) or permit other evidence, often deceptive in nature, to be introduced. The rules of evidence and the rules of procedure tightly control what the judge and jury may hear.

Several recent commentators have observed that forensic truth is far from equivalent to historical truth because the goals of the two are quite different (Angell, 1996; Jones, 1994). These authors emphasize the subjective, storytelling nature of forensic testimony, and the partiality of the witnesses, even experts, who tell those stories. The psychiatrist Bernard L. Diamond (1959) has questioned the possibility that an expert can ever be neutral, and not an advocate, in the forensic arena. Reidinger (1996) has commented on the differences between scientific truth and forensic truth by noting that neither conforms to historical truth:

Science is about uncertainty, probability, convergence; it's a peer-driven conversation—largely consensual—of tentative theories, imperfect proofs, criticisms and revisions. Even a well-established scientific theory—such as evolution—a fact, for scientists—remains incomplete and subject to revision according to the discovery of new evidence.

Law, to the contrary, is about settling arguments *now;* it's an adversarial enterprise whose real goal is not truth so much as victory and closure with justice. (p. 59)

At bottom there is a philosophical schism between science and law that neither Daubert nor any other decision can perfectly bridge.

Science will always be an uneasy guest in the courtroom, an intellectual discipline in which such terms as "proof" and "evidence" mean something different from what they mean to lawyers.

A bit of scientific evidence is like a piece of a puzzle slowly being put together. Some bits might not belong at all, and there will always be missing pieces, but eventually the picture becomes clear enough to support a general consensus about what it is and what it means.

Legal evidence, on the other hand, will be weighed on the scales of argument for credibility and persuasiveness, until the scale finally tips to one side or the other. Lawyers assemble evidence in an attempt to win—a notion foreign to the scientific method. (p. 62)

Further recognition of the differences between historical truth and forensic truth may be found in the United States Supreme Court's groundbreaking decision in *Daubert v. Merrell Dow Pharmaceuticals, Inc.* (1993), which is now the law in all federal courts and more than half of the state courts. *Daubert* involved the proper test for the admission into evidence of "scientific" expert opinion. Plaintiffs, claiming to have suffered birth defects because of their mothers' ingestion of a drug manufactured by the defendant, argued that courts should not exclude any scientific evidence because the scientific method requires that all viewpoints be available to be evaluated and tested. As the Court phrased plaintiffs' argument, rejecting expert-opinion evidence "will sanction a stifling and repressive scientific orthodoxy and will be inimical to the search for truth" (p. 596). The Court rejected this argument, primarily because the forensic proceedings are not a search for ultimate truth:

It is true that open debate is an essential part of both legal and scientific analyses. Yet there are important differences between the quest for truth in the courtroom and the quest for truth in the laboratory. Scientific conclusions are subject to perpetual revision. Law, on the other hand, must resolve disputes finally and quickly. The scientific project is advanced by broad and wide-ranging consideration of a multitude of hypotheses, for those that are incorrect will eventually be shown to be so, and that in itself is an advance. Conjectures that are probably wrong are of little use, however, in the project of reaching a quick, final, and binding legal judgment—often of great consequence—about a particular set of events in the past. We recognize that in practice, a gatekeeping role for the judge, no matter how flexible, inevitably on occasion will prevent the jury from learning of authentic insights and innovations. That, nevertheless, is the balance that is struck by Rules of Evidence designed not for the exhaustive search for cosmic understanding but for the particularized resolution of legal disputes. (pp. 596–597)

Ironically, there is much that narrative truth and forensic truth have in common. Both are types of truth that are shaped by technique to serve a variety of social purposes. Furthermore, the latest ideological movement in legal analysis has adopted the narrative perspective and now views forensic truth in the same manner that therapists view narrative truth. In essence, forensic truth is the choice among competing courtroom narratives. Not surprisingly, the concept of forensic truth has recently been shaped by the same forces that created the analysis of narrative truth.

As noted by Rieke and Stutman (1990), the idea that courts are engaged in the search for historical truth is based upon an assumption that "the legal process offers a reliable method for putting an accurate picture of an event in the mind of the judge or jury" (p. 46). Given the fallibility of the senses, the malleability of memory, and the suggestive tricks and storytelling skills of lawyers, this assumption has not withstood empirical testing, thereby leading Rieke and Stutman to describe the judicial process as "a narrative creative conception." Other scholars have agreed (Bennett and Feldman, 1981; Marshall, 1966; Cohen, 1950). A symposium at Yale Law School on this topic was reproduced as a groundbreaking book, *Law's Stories: Narrative and Rhetoric in the Law* (Brooks and Gewirtz, 1996).

The relativity of truth in therapeutic and forensic settings has certain implications for mental health professionals who leave the therapy room and enter the courtroom (Hoencamp, 1995). In particular, the claim that therapists should be responsible for historical truth has dangerous consequences, two of which I will single out for discussion. The first problem facing clinicians in court is their potential civil liability if they are historically inaccurate. This "liability for historical falsity" has recently become a real threat to therapists. The second problem, "testifying as to historical truth," punishes therapists if they do try to be historically accurate. Thus, therapists in court face a "damned if you do, damned if you don't" attitude brought about by a simplistic understanding of issues of narrative truth versus historical truth.

Liability for Historical Falsity

If everything discussed in a therapy session is narrative truth, then the mandatory reporting laws demand of therapists something they clearly are incapable of doing—spotting actual child abuse accurately in every case. Yet every state has mandatory reporting laws in reference to child abuse, many in reference to elder abuse, and many in other situations that may have a somatic base, such as gunshot wounds or unconsciousness.

The mandatory reporting laws are the ideal place to examine this distinction between narrative truth and historical truth because, until recently, the mandated reporters have generally enjoyed an absolute immunity for their reporting. This immunity makes a good deal of sense. In 1963, perhaps the first mandatory reporting law was passed in the country by the California legislature. The California Department of Justice discovered in 1978 that despite the existence of the mandatory reporting law, and despite the fact that the failure to report carried criminal penalties, only about 10 percent of all sexual abuse cases known to mental health professionals were actually being reported (*Krikorian v. Barry*, 1987). To correct this problem, and to encourage increased reporting of suspected child abuse, the California legislature passed a tougher law and applied absolute immunity to mandated reporters.

The legislators believed, and recent California courts have reconfirmed (*Stecks v. Young*, 1995), that the only truly effective method to prevent child abuse and protect abused children is to mandate that people who take care of children in a professional role or capacity report their suspicions of child abuse to the state. If the legislature mandated reporting, and then held therapists liable when the reports were proven false, therapists would have to become detectives (Hoorwitz, 1992). Indeed, they would have to become detectives who solved every crime, and did so correctly. Years of experience with Good Samaritan laws and with mandatory reporting laws demonstrate that the only way to obtain sufficient reporting is by providing reporters with absolute immunity. If reporting meant the threat of a civil lawsuit, who would report?

In recent years, the sanctity of the absolute immunity has come under attack, thereby making clinicians in some way responsible for historical truth. In *Stecks v. Young* (1995), a California Court of Appeals decision raised the threat of therapists being sued by nonpatients for reports that later turn out mistaken or unprovable. The facts of the case are quite simple. A twenty-nine-year-old woman in therapy reported that her parents had sexually molested her when she was a child. She also reported that her parents engaged in things called "brainwashing, human and animal sacrifice, and satanic worship." Because the daughter, who was diagnosed both as schizophrenic and as suffering from multiple personality disorder, was not living in her parents' household, the threat of continued molestation of her did not exist. However, she told the therapist that she was fearful about her niece and nephew, especially because her parents would be taking care of them during an upcoming high satanic ceremony in which the nephew might be sacrificed.

What should the therapist do in this situation? After hearing this story from her patient, the therapist dutifully reported the disclosures to the state authorities for their investigation. Next the outraged parents came along and sued the therapist, claiming to have been wrongfully accused of these heinous things. The court in *Stecks* did, in fact, hold that the absolute immunity in California's statute barred the parents from bringing a lawsuit against the therapist. But, in the concluding two paragraphs of the court's opinion, the judges warned that the case "professes the outer limits of immunity." There are, however, no outer limits of immunity in the California statute; the immunity is absolute. Nevertheless, the *Stecks* court has now urged the legislature to reexamine absolute immunity. And on what basis? According to the court:

> Typically, mandated reporters base their reports upon personal interviews with or observations of the alleged victim or abuser or upon information derived from other professionals treating or investigating the alleged abuse. By contrast, here the mandated reporter allegedly trusted the accusations of a purportedly schizophrenic patient, who had no personal knowledge that the children were being abused, and conveyed those accusations to the authorities.
>
> In circumstances where the mandated reporter is not drawing upon personal professional assessments of the victim or abuser or is not relying upon other trained professionals who have made such assessments, we submit that the application of absolute immunity warrants further reflection by the Legislature. Where such reports turn out to be false, the Legislature may deem it appropriate to apply qualified immunity and to permit recovery where the wrongfully accused person can establish that the report was known to be false or made in reckless disregard of the truth. However, absent a change in the statute, the trial court properly sustained the demurrer without leave to amend.

Interestingly, some reports of the *Stecks* case have erroneously stated that the "outer limits" were reached because of the factual claims of brainwashing, satanic abuse, and animal sacrifice. The court, however, says nothing about those allegations and does not appear to be concerned about the factual existence of these claims. The judges are quite clear that the therapist's failure to have done additional investigative work, to have questioned either the nephew or the niece, to have obtained an opinion from another mental health professional, or to have questioned the alleged abusers, was the sole basis of its concern about absolute immunity. Of course, had the therapist followed the court's advice, confidentiality would have been violated. Furthermore, nothing in the statute requires or mentions that therapists must either investigate accusations or get second opinions.

If the legislature does heed the court's request and eliminate absolute immunity, therapists will be put in the dangerous situation of having to guess correctly whether what a patient reports is historically valid. Therapists will need to demonstrate that they have conducted a sufficient investigation before notifying the state to conduct its own sufficient investigation. Nowhere does the *Stecks* court raise the issue of how the therapist should explain to the patient the fact that the therapist is investigating the patient's claims to see if they are true, or is consulting with other specialists to see whether the patient should be believed. The absolute immunity protection preserves the integrity of the therapeutic relationship from such destructive influences.

Of course, mandatory reporting itself may be destructive to the therapeutic relationship. But in the hierarchy of social values, every state has expressed a preference for the protection of children over the preservation of confidentiality and therapeutic loyalty. Lowe (1996) has recently observed that this preference for protecting children now even surpasses preserving the family unit. Lawmakers are in agreement that without such mandatory reporting there would be no effective means to remove children from abusive situations.

It is the function of the therapist to do therapy; it is the function of the state to investigate. Mixing up these roles is not advisable. In fact, the failure of the therapist to keep these roles separate may lead to the loss of the reporting immunity. In *Wilkinson v. Balsam* (1995), a husband filed divorce proceedings against his wife and requested custody of their young children. Shortly thereafter, the wife began therapy with a psychiatrist and told him she believed that her husband might have been sexually abusing their children. The psychiatrist saw the children for one session and concluded that the husband was indeed molesting them. Meanwhile, a doctor who examined the children found no evidence of abuse, and the wife's mother telephoned the psychiatrist to report that the wife was abusing the children. The psychiatrist, after telling the mother not to report her concerns to state authorities, continued to counsel the children as sex abuse victims and called state authorities to verify that the report against the husband which the wife filed was true. To make matters worse, when the state authorities interviewed the children they used highly suggestive techniques and ignored the statements from the children that they were "making it up" to please their mother. The psychiatrist received additional information from others that the wife was a child molester, but he ignored the information. After being arrested and suffering other losses, the husband sued the psychiatrist and the state authorities.

The federal district court judge found that the psychiatrist had assumed multiple conflicting roles of being an advocate as well as a therapist. The court noted that the psychiatrist had made up his mind from the beginning and had failed to conduct a reasonable, neutral inquiry before telling state authorities, the wife, and others that the husband was a molester. The psychiatrist's claim of absolute immunity was rejected on the grounds that the statute required that the report be made "in good faith," a condition not present due to the psychiatrist's obvious bias and dual conflicting roles. Furthermore, the immunity only extended to filing the report, not to giving his opinion to the wife, the police, and others.

The *Wilkinson* case is instructional on two points. First, it suggests that therapists must be most careful in selecting their roles. Once the therapy relationship begins, the advocacy relationship must be avoided. It would be interesting to have the court's view on whether the therapist who seeks independent verification of patient accusations against others necessarily slips into the advocate's role, thereby tainting both relationships. Second, the immunity granted by statutes does not extend beyond filing the necessary reports. It is, therefore, quite limited in its scope, perhaps because this limitation precisely fits the contours of the therapy relationship. Because a wider immunity might serve to induce therapists to become detectives, it has wisely been rejected.

While *Wilkinson* concentrated on the "in good faith" language in the immunity statute, a far broader, and more dangerous, analysis was developed by a lower court and judge in New York in *Caryl S. v. Child and Adolescent Treatment Services* (1994), an action against an adolescent treatment service. In this case, a five-year-old child, after visiting her paternal grandparents, told her mother that the grandmother had inserted a stick into her vagina and that it had caused her vagina to bleed. The mother took the child for a medical examination. The medical examination failed to confirm any lacerations. The mother then took the child to a treatment facility where, during the course of two years of treatment, the therapist came to the conclusion that the child was telling the truth and that there was molesting by the paternal grandmother. In a custody battle during the parents' divorce proceedings it was requested that the paternal grand-parents not be given any visitation rights and have no access to the child. And the therapist so testified.

The grandparents now claim that the therapist was negligent in reaching the diagnosis supporting the patient. The first line of defense in these third-party (nonpatient) cases has to do with the absence of any duty owed to the accused molester who is not in a therapeutic relationship with the therapist. The general rule of law has been that therapists owe duties to nonpatients in only two situations: (1) where a *Tarasoff* duty exists to warn a third party threatened by a dangerous patient, and (2) where physical harm to the third party is foreseeable, as, for example, when drivers and pedestrians are at risk because a psychiatrist prescribed a medication that causes drowsiness, but failed to tell the patient not to drive.

It is only within the last few years that courts have been willing to consider third-party liability suits in these abuse cases and in false-memory cases. Slovenko (1995a) applauds this potential liability as a means of redressing false accusations of childhood sexual abuse. He argues that the ordinary rules of negligence and foreseeability can be read to state that the therapist owes a duty to third parties. Bowman and Mertz (1996), on the other hand, in the most extensive review of the subject in print, detail why such third-party liability would be devastating to the mental health community. Appelbaum and Zoltek-Jick (1996) also have cautioned against new third-party duty rules, and have expressed grave concern about the adverse impact of such rules on all aspects of the practice of therapy. Brown, Scheflin, and Hammond (1997) warn that third-party liability rules have never been applied when the third party is in an antagonistic, or nonbeneficiary, relationship with the therapist's patient or the lawyer's client. They cite the ethical rules demanding loyalty to the patient in fiduciary relationships, and the conflict-of-interest rules that prohibit dual loyalties, as evidence that imposing third-party liability would destroy the ethical foundation of the mental health profession.

The judge in *Caryl S.* extended the identical foreseeability analysis used in physical harm cases to this case of emotional distress, an extension almost universally rejected by other courts. Thus, the treating therapist was held to owe a duty to the accused grandparents. The judge also held that New York's mandatory reporting law did not provide for absolute immunity, and so third parties may sue for "negligent misdiagnosis."

In this setting, "negligent misdiagnosis" means that the therapist is historically wrong, as proven by the courtroom narrative. But the failure to prove that the abusive events did occur does not itself prove that the events did not occur. It just proves that the evidence was insufficient. As a consequence, any time a report is filed in New York, a lawsuit is a distinct possibility.

Of particular interest in the *Caryl S.* opinion is the judge's reliance on two cases from other states in support of her conclusion that the law is moving to permit third-party lawsuits against therapists in emotional-distress cases. An examination of these two cases reveals, however, that the first is irrelevant and the second has been overruled to hold exactly the opposite of what the judge cited it to hold. The first case, *Montoya v. Bebensee* (1988) is irrelevant because it involved a *nonlicensed* therapist who acted outside the boundaries of law and who did much more than merely report abuse; and the second case, *W.C.W. v. Bird* (1992), has been overruled by the Texas Supreme Court in an emphatic opinion holding that therapists, as a matter of law, may not be sued by third parties. An attempt to dismiss the case on this point was rejected in *Caryl* (1997).

Perhaps the worst decision was reached by a judge and jury in a Pennsylvania case, *Althaus v. Cohen* (1994). A nineteen-year-old daughter went to a psychiatrist after having made accusations to the police of being molested by her parents. The psychiatrist listened to her story and conducted therapy. This was not a mandatory-reporting case because the daughter had already reported the molesting to the state officials. The therapist testified that some of what the daughter-patient told her was clearly unbelievable, and therefore not true. According to an Associated Press report (1994), "Some of the girl's claims were discounted immediately. She claimed her grandmother flew about on a broom, she was tortured with a medieval thumbscrew device, she bore three children who were killed, and she was raped in view of diners in a crowded restaurant." The daughter recanted and joined her parents in a lawsuit against the psychiatrist for treating the daughter as if the stories she told were true.

But the psychiatrist did not believe these things to be true, and she did not conduct therapy as if they were true. Furthermore, as Dr. Thomas Gutheil (1995) has noted, she "did not say that she was treating her patient as if the abuse was true. She said she was treating [the] symptoms she was showing and whatever cause there might be and I think that is a rather important notion. You treat symptoms; you don't treat causes in the usual sense of the word."

The jury held in favor of the parents and the daughter, and voted 10–2 to award the parents and daughter $272,000. But what did the psychiatrist do wrong? Perhaps it was that she failed to say to the patient "That's a lot of nonsense. I don't believe you." Had she said this, of course, she might have destroyed any trust in her that the patient had developed.

Althaus has been cited by Slovenko (1995b) as an illustration of why therapists, who are seekers of narrative truth in the therapy room, should be forced to become detectives answerable in the courtroom to a standard of historical truth. While this prospect is frightening enough, it is not quite accurate. The doctor in this case did not believe her patient and did not implant memories in her. The patient had already filed charges against her parents before she came to therapy, so real detectives had concluded that the abuse story, though not all of the details, was historically true. Furthermore, the psychiatrist did not accept the full story her client told her, and she did not encourage the client to sue her parents or take any outside action against them. If she were to act as a detective, what should she have done? What would have changed in the therapy? Indeed, the ultimate fear, and irony, of *Althaus* is expressed by Gutheil (1995): "What was so interesting was that the claim was that the doctor should have been a detective. But in this particular case it becomes fairly clear by the documents that it was the detectives who had planted the false memories in their repeated interviews of patients. So in a funny way, the doctor is told that, for not being a detective, the actual detectives are implanting the false memory, and the doctor is [then] blamed for implanting the false memory. It was a perfect triangle."

In *Althaus,* it appears that the therapist was successfully sued by the patient who joined with her family claiming that it was wrong for the therapy to be conducted according to the narrative developed by the patient, rather than the alleged historical truth which the therapist should have known by completely disbelieving her patient and totally ignoring her claims and expressed needs.

The idea that therapists should be detectives has become a popular refrain for advocates of "false memory syndrome." In general, they point to what they consider an epidemic of "recovered memory" therapists who are breaking up thousands of families by implanting false memories of childhood sexual abuse that supposedly happened decades earlier and only now is remembered. Moen (1995), an attorney defending families from allegedly false claims of sexual abuse, argues that therapists cannot hide behind the excuse of narrative truth when forensic issues are involved in the therapy. Moen, however, fails to present any discussion of how he expects therapists to be "detectives," and his brief paper does little more than suggest that therapists have to be held accountable for false accusations made by their patients. This suggestion, of course, would require strict liability. Therapists would have to hope that their patients would prevail in court, otherwise the therapists would be liable for failing to know historical truth. Slovenko (1995b) makes the same argument for accountability but also fails to articulate the nature of the detective role and its consequences to the therapy. Neither Moen nor Slovenko even hints at how their proposals would address the crucial issues that would necessarily arise if their demand that therapists also be detectives were implemented:

1. Should the patient be told that the therapist is conducting an investigation?
2. How does the therapist investigate without breaking the patient's confidentiality?
3. How thorough an investigation must be conducted? Should the therapist interview other family members, or go through old medical records, or check police files, and so on?
4. What should the therapist tell the patient about the investigation?
5. What should the therapist do if the therapist reasonably concludes that the patient is telling the truth?
6. What should the therapist do if the therapist reasonably concludes that the patient is not telling the truth?
7. What should the therapist do if the investigation fails to determine historical truth? Will the therapist be liable for, by hindsight, having made the wrong choice?
8. Should therapists receive training in investigation? Should graduate schools in the mental health professions offer mandatory courses in detective work?
9. How may therapists simultaneously meet their fiduciary duty of undivided loyalty to the client and their newly imposed reasonable-care duty to third parties who may be injured if the therapist is wrong about historical truth?
10. How can therapists avoid violating conflict of interest rules when they must mistrust the patient to the point of conducting an outside investigation, and they must be answerable to the very people the patient has come to therapy to discuss?

Testifying as to Truth

If it appears that the law is moving in a reckless and perilous direction when therapists are held liable for historical falsity, the law is no better when the issue concerns therapists testifying as to historical truth, as they would be required to do under the "therapists should be detectives" viewpoint.

Therapists are brought into court to express their opinions about historical truth, which may include the narratives discussed and developed in therapy. Many experts retreat into the more comfortable world of narrative truth by proclaiming that they do not work with historical truth at all. Yet these same mental health professionals then testify as if they had emerged from narrative truth into the bright light of historical truth. The law professor Marianne Wesson (1985), using the testimony given by mental health experts in the trial of Patty Hearst, has demonstrated this phenomenon with the instructive examples that follow.

THE "IT DOESN'T MATTER ANYWAY" PREMISE

Dr. Louis Jolyon West, in his testimony for the defense, described an event that led him to conclude that Patty Hearst had acted under duress, and therefore without criminal responsibility, while a captive of the Symbionese Liberation Army. Hearst, after her arrest, told a friend that when she was set free she would tell her story from "a revolutionary feminist perspective." Dr. West was asked during cross-examination to reconcile Patty's remarks to his conclusion that she had been acting under force when committing crimes with the SLA. West responded that Patty had told him that she made that statement only because Emily Harris, one of the more dangerous SLA members, was also in the room listening to her. West was then told that the prosecution could prove that no one else was present in the room at that time. He responded: "I'd find that fascinating; and, it would suggest to me that—and quite consistent with some of the other findings—that to her, Emily Harris was a constant presence as long as she was there." According to Wesson's analysis: "Dr. West, his factual premises discredited, retreated to the position that his conclusion was based on so many pieces of data that a blow to the truth value of any one piece of data could not affect his confidence in his opinion. Indeed, West demonstrated that he could cleverly reweave a new or contradictory fact into the fabric of his opinion so that it contributed to, rather than detracted from, the opinion's authority" (pp. 346–347).

Wesson also observes that a prosecution expert witness utilized the same ploy for "avoiding issues having to do with historical truth" (p. 347). Dr. Harry L. Kozol's opinion that Patty was acting out feelings of rebellion against her family was heavily influenced by a report that Patty had once lied about her mother's health in order to avoid taking a high school examination. As with Dr. West, the prosecution asked whether Dr. Kozol's opinion would change if it were proven that this incident never occurred. Kozol responded that his opinion would not change: "I am perfectly willing to believe it, but it doesn't change my opinion on the total picture, that is only one tiny item" (p. 347).

THE "I COULDN'T BE WRONG" PREMISE

An even more blatant attempt to circumvent the relativity of the narrative approach is found in the claim by experts that they could not be fooled, as if these experts had a pipeline to historical truth. Wesson provides an illustration in the testimony of Dr. Robert Jay Lifton, who based his opinion and testimony on Patty's own personal account of her captivity. When the prosecution provided evidence that the story Patty told was not historically correct, Dr. Lifton "suggested at first that it was not to be believed, and second that in any event it was quite consistent with his opinion, whether she was telling the truth or not."

> *Q:* . . . Doctor, did you hear the testimony in the courtroom that she told somebody to keep his expletive deleted head down?
> *A:* I either heard that testimony or read it.
> *Q:* And again is that consistent, in your theory, with your theory of terror and fear?
> *A:* Well, my impression was that she denied having said that and that that was quite uncertain as to whether she did say it.
> *Q:* Well, let's assume that she did say it . . .
> *A:* If she did say it, which I am not ready to assume, but if she did say it, it could be perfectly consistent with carrying out the role as well as she could of looking like a revolutionary bank robber. (pp. 347–348)

Lifton, at the end of his cross-examination, stated that it was not possible that he had been deceived by Patty.

Wesson notes that the very same doctors who claimed privileged access to historical truth also claimed that psychiatry provides no direct link to truth:

> Dr. West testified at one point, "I am not a detective. I am a psychiatrist." Dr. Martin Orne, a defense witness, agreed that he had testified in another trial that psychiatrists are not very good at "recognizing the truth." He elaborated that he could not testify with any degree of confidence as to whether "a specific event really happened." Dr. Orne did believe, though, that he could discern by the use of psychological tests whether an individual was truly afflicted with a pathological condition or was malingering. His distinction between historical truth and psychological truth seems quite useful. Unfortunately, it was left behind when Orne was asked on what factual premises he

based his opinion that Hearst had been under duress. He testified, "there were certain facts which were known and which I had from—particularly from the detailed history and compilation which Dr. West and Dr. Singer had made." In other words, Dr. Orne had to depend in the end on Patty Hearst's account.

Later in his testimony, Dr. Orne stated, "taking it all very carefully together, the weight of the data is unequivocally, [*sic*] in my view, that she was not simulating when I saw her. She was truthful with me." Hence his earlier careful distinction between his ability to detect malingering and his inability to detect falsehood seemed to have vanished even from Dr. Orne's own mind. By the end of his redirect testimony, Dr. Orne was asserting that he was confident that he had been working from an accurate history of Patricia Hearst's ordeal. (pp. 348–349)

THE "I'VE KNOWN IT ALL ALONG" PREMISE

Before Patty Hearst was captured, Dr. West wrote a letter to her parents in which he said:

Enclosed are a couple of reprints on the subject of so-called [brainwashing]. From them, you can see that considerable work from medical and psychiatric stand-viewpoint has been reported concerning the extent to which single-minded captors can profoundly influence individuals who come under their control. There's much that could be elaborated on the subject; but, at this time, I would make the following points: . . . there are historical precedents for special legal consideration if such a victim [*sic*] . . . In spite of the charges that have been filed against [Patricia], I believe powerful medical and legal arguments can be mobilized for her defense. (p. 350)

On cross-examination at the trial, West vehemently denied that the thoughts expressed in his letter had any influence on his examination of Patty and testimony on her behalf: "I approached the examination of this patient not only with my usual objectivity, but with excessive precautions against the fact that since I'm an expert on brainwashing and have been called by the Judge for this purpose, not to let myself be biased and to see things that I was looking for . . . I feel that this account, this case study of this patient, is as honorable and unbiased and scientific as any psychiatric case study that's ever been done" (p. 350).

Wesson observes that this triumph of scientific objectivity was undercut by Dr. West's own testimony. For example, in an illustration that violates all of the concerns of the false-memory movement, Dr. West testified that Patty suffered from "sleep deprivation." However, when he was asked whether Patty had ever claimed to be sleep-deprived, Dr. West astonishingly responded "She complained of practically nothing . . . I had to pry it out of her, all of it."

In violation of the rules of undue suggestion, Dr. West admitted that at the very outset of his examination he had informed Patty what her defense was to be, as follows: "To emphasize the involuntary and violent way in which you were dragged out of a relatively normal life with a forcible and terrifying sort of indoctrination that you got, and the tremendous pressure of threats in the beginning to make you subservient and compliant with the leadership of this group so that they would be able to keep control of you. I think myself that is the best explanation for what happened. I haven't heard anything to make me think otherwise. Doesn't that sound logical to you?" (pp. 350–351).

Dr. West's discovery that he was correct in his initial theory might be considered confirmatory bias because he was not neutral in his evaluation of Patty. Rather, he was her preannounced advocate with a blueprint on what he needed to discover from her in order to help her avoid criminal responsibility.

There is a close analogy between Dr. West's involvement with Patty Hearst and a well-known attorney's ethical dilemma presented in Robert Traver's brilliant book *Anatomy of a Murder* (1958) and the movie made of it in 1959. The dilemma begins when the attorney tells his client on their first meeting that before the client says anything he should know that the crime he is charged with has only a few defenses, which the attorney then explains in detail. After this preliminary discussion, the lawyer says, "now tell me your story." Monroe H. Freedman, in his excellent book *Lawyers' Ethics in an Adversary System* (1975a), observes that this practice is unethical because it conditions the client to distort the truth. Thus, the story the client tells the attorney will be a product of, and consistent with, the defense to be raised at trial. In this manner, the attorney's improper suggestions avoid the later ethical mandate of revealing to the court the client's intention to commit perjury. Under the American Bar Association Model Rules of Professional Conduct (1983), and the United States Supreme Court ruling in *Nix v. Whiteside* (1986), if the client told the truth to the attorney, and that truth was inconsistent with the defense, the client's intention to commit perjury must be revealed to the court. But if the client's story does not deviate from what he will say on the witness stand, there is no perjury known to the attorney. Thus narrative truth replaces historical truth in the avoidance of an ethical obligation.

Interestingly, Dr. West also testified that Patty's memory of her captivity was quite poor. Wesson aptly observes a link between West's testimony and the complaints of false-memory advocates about overzealous therapists:

> A situation more suited to the generation of a version of the historical truth that conforms to the examiner's expectations can hardly be imagined: a subject with little memory, an examiner who has already committed himself to a theory of the events, and an interviewing technique that consists of "prying" things out of the subject or suggesting them to her. Seen in this light, West's indignant claim that his opinion about Hearst is as "honorable and unbiased and scientific" as any case study ever done is reminiscent of Freud's assertion that his "Wolf-Man" study is entirely the product of his subject's memories, in which "no construction or stimulation by the physician played any part." (p. 351)

These illustrations of expert testimony bear witness to the conclusions drawn by Jones (1994) in her significant study of expert witnesses in the legal system. To those who claim that courts are engaged in the search for historical truth, Jones suggests that the opposite is in fact the case. She reports on how "lawyers use experts to construct stories" (p. 5) and on how experts dutifully play this role. The conclusion of this conspiracy is that "legality is constructed" (p. 13) and that "scientific and legal facts can be shown to be negotiated constructs" (p. 273) because: "determining what the facts say is a process of persuasion in both the legal and the scientific communities. Legal and scientific facts are not given; they are highly pre-fabricated. To look at how experts participate in the construction of facticity is to look at how they contribute to the apparent immutability of legal verdicts" (p. 5).

/ / /

It is too early to draw major conclusions about the interrelationship between narrative truth and historical truth. Nevertheless, it appears unconscionable for the legal system to whipsaw therapists, or others, between conflicting obligations. To claim that there is only narrative truth in the therapy room, but that if therapists do things we do not like we are going to hold them to a standard of historical truth, is logically and socially wrong. To ask therapists to become detectives is legally and ethically wrong. To make therapists choose between believing patients and believing third parties, and to expose them to extensive and costly liability whichever choice they make, is blatantly unfair.

The contentious distinction between narrative truth and historical truth in therapeutic and forensic settings must be eliminated because it is unworkable and contradictory in the ways discussed above. Perr (1975), in a remarkable paper entitled "Psychiatric Testimony and the Rashomon Phenomenon," explored the relative basis of truth in forensic settings, and the consequences for psychiatric testimony: "A number of years ago the Japanese motion picture, 'Rashomon,' focused on the interpretation of events as seen through the distorted eyes of the participants, whose perceptions were determined by their own needs or personalities. The Rashomon phenomenon applies to ordinary trial witnesses . . . all participants in the legal arena reflect some aspect of the Rashomon phenomenon" (p. 97).

Perr concluded that a legal judgment is not fact, nor truth, necessarily; rather it is a "measured evaluation based on probability." The attempt to know historical truth from the perspective of narrative truth is ultimately and always a search based on probabilities. Whether that search takes place in the therapy room or the courtroom makes no difference.

Once the pernicious idealistic distinction between historical truth and narrative truth is rejected, in its place may be substituted a role analysis that treats each separate therapeutic and forensic issue in light of the role mental health professionals ought to play, as a matter of policy, in our society. Under such a role analysis: (1) third-party liability would be eliminated because of the conflict of loyalty between patient and nonpatient that it would inevitably create; (2) mandatory reporting of suspected child abuse would retain absolute immunity for the reporter in order to protect children and guarantee sufficient obedience with the law; and (3) clinicians in and out of court would be encouraged to inform themselves fully on the scientific literature as well as the clinical literature in their fields.

Once such a role analysis is developed, we may move to apply it to some of the more intriguing questions yet to come, such as these: (1) By what standards should unorthodox and innovative therapies be measured? (2) May therapy be done without the informed consent of the patient? (3) May false memories be implanted for therapeutic purposes (Gravitz, 1994)? (4) May therapy be done outside the awareness of the patient (Scheflin, 1997a)?

References

Abraham v. Zaslow (1975). 1 Civil 33219, Cal. Ct. App., 1st Dist., Div. Three, Feb. 24.

Abrams, R. (1992). *Electroconvulsive Therapy.* 2nd ed. Oxford: Oxford University Press.

Alexander, G. (1993). "Big Mother: The State's Use of Mental Health Experts in Dependency Cases." *Pacific Law Journal* 24: 1465–96.

Althaus v. Cohen (1994). Case no. G.D. 92–20893, In the Court of Common Pleas, Allegheny County, Pa.

American Bar Association (1983), as amended through Feb. 1996. *Model Rules of Professional Conduct.* Chicago: American Bar Association.

American Society of Clinical Hypnosis (1995). *Clinical Hypnosis and Memory: Guidelines for Clinicians and for Forensic Hypnosis.* Des Plaines, Ill.: American Society of Clinical Hypnosis Press.

Anderson, W. T., ed. (1995). *The Truth about the Truth: De-confusing and Re-constructing the Postmodern World.* New York: A Jeremy P. Tarcher/Putnam Book.

Angell, M. (1996). *Science on Trial.* New York: Norton.

Appelbaum, P. S., and T. G. Gutheil (1991). *Clinical Handbook of Psychiatry and the Law.* 2nd ed. Baltimore: Williams and Wilkins.

Appelbaum, P. S., and R. Zoltek-Jick (1996). "Psychotherapists' Duties to Third Parties: *Ramona* and Beyond." *American Journal of Psychiatry* 153: 457–465.

Associated Press (1994). "Jury Sides with Family in Sexual-abuse Case." Dec. 18.

Bartlett, F. C. (1932). *Remembering: A Study in Experimental and Social Psychology.* Cambridge: Cambridge University Press.

Behlmer, G. K. (1982). *Child Abuse and Moral Reform in England, 1870–1908.* Stanford: Stanford University Press.

Bennett, W. L., and M. S. Feldman (1981). *Reconstructing Reality in the Courtroom.* New Brunswick, N.J.: Rutgers University Press.

Berkeley, A. (1929). *The Poisoned Chocolates Case.* London: W. Collins Sons.

Berkhofer, R. F., Jr. (1995). *Beyond the Great Story: History as Text and Discourse.* Cambridge, Mass.: Harvard University Press.

Bowman, C. G., and E. Mertz (1996). "A Dangerous Direction: Legal Intervention in Sexual Abuse Survivor Therapy." *Harvard Law Review* 109: 549–639.

Brooks, P., and P. Gewirtz, eds. (1996). *Law's Stories: Narrative and Rhetoric in the Law.* New Haven: Yale University Press.

Brown, D., A. W. Scheflin, and D. C. Hammond (1997). *Memory, Trauma Treatment and Law.* New York: Norton.

Burger, W. E. (1966). "Standards of Conduct for Prosecution and Defense Personnel: A Judge's Viewpoint." *American Criminal Law Quarterly* 5: 11–16.

Campbell, R. (1992). *Truth and Historicity.* Oxford: Oxford University Press.

Caryl S. v. Child and Adolescent Treatment Services, Inc. (1994). 161 Misc.2d 563, 614 N.Y.S.2d 661.

Center Foundation v. Chicago Insurance Company (1991). 227 Cal. App.3d 547, 278 Cal. Rptr. 13 (2nd Dist.).

Cohen, F. S. (1950). "Field Theory and Judicial Logic." *Yale Law Journal* 59: 238–272.

Cohen, R. J. (1979). *Malpractice: A Guide for Mental Health Professionals*. New York: Free Press.

Cushman, P. (1995). *Constructing the Self, Constructing America*. Reading, Mass.: Addison-Wesley.

Daubert v. Merrell Dow Pharmaceuticals, Inc. (1993). 509 U.S. 579, 113 S.Ct. 2786, 125 L.Ed.2d 469.

Dawes, R. M. (1994). *House of Cards: Psychology and Psychotherapy Built on Myth*. New York: Freeman.

Dershowitz, A. M. (1994). *The Abuse Excuse and Other Cop-outs, Sob Stories, and Evasions of Responsibility*. Boston: Little, Brown.

Diamond, B. L. (1959). "The Fallacy of the Impartial Expert." *Archives of Criminal Psychodynamics* 3: 221–236.

Everstine, L., and D. S. Everstine, eds. (1986). *Psychotherapy and the Law*. New York: Grune and Stratton.

Fancher, R. T. (1995). *Cultures of Healing: Correcting the Image of American Mental Health Care*. New York: Freeman.

Felsenthal, E. (1995). "Courts Hear Mental-health Experts in More Civil Cases." *Wall Street Journal*, Aug. 23, p. B1.

Ferguson v. Moore (1897). 39 S.W.341 (Tenn.).

Forest Preserve Dist. of Cook County v. Mike (1954). 3 Ill.2d 49, 119 N.E.2d 734.

Frank, J. D., and J. B. Frank (1991) *Persuasion and Healing: A Comparative Study of Psychotherapy*. 3rd ed. Baltimore: Johns Hopkins University Press.

Frankel, M. E. (1975). "The Search for Truth: An Umpireal View." *University of Pennsylvania Law Review* 123: 1031–59.

Freedman, J., and G. Combs (1996). *Narrative Therapy: The Social Reconstruction of Preferred Realities*. New York: Norton.

Freedman, M. H. (1966). "Professional Responsibility of the Criminal Defense Lawyer: The Three Hardest Questions." *Michigan Law Review* 64: 1469–84.

Freedman, M. H. (1975a). *Lawyers' Ethics in an Adversary System*. Indianapolis: Bobbs-Merrill.

Freedman, M. H. (1975b). "Judge Frankel's Search for Truth." *University of Pennsylvania Law Review* 123: 1060–66.

Freedman, M. H. (1990). *Understanding Lawyers' Ethics*. New York: Matthew Bender.

Gardner, R. A. (1991). *Sex Abuse Hysteria: Salem Witch Trials Revisited*. Creskill, N.J.: Creative Therapeutics.

Gravitz, M. A. (1994). "Memory Reconstruction by Hypnosis as a Therapeutic Technique." *Psychotherapy* 31: 687–691.

Gutheil, T. G. (1992). Letter, "Assessing Satanic Cult Abuse." *Psychiatric Times*, July, p. 9.

Gutheil, T. G. (1995). Personal communication, Nov. 17.

Hale, N. G., Jr. (1995). *The Rise and Crisis of Psychoanalysis in the United States: Freud and the Americans, 1917–1985.* Oxford: Oxford University Press.

Hammer v. Rosen (1960). 7 N.Y.2d 376, 165 N.E.2d 756, 198 N.Y.S.2d 65.

Hechler, D. (1988). *The Battle and the Backlash: The Child Sexual Abuse War.* Lexington, Mass.: Lexington Books.

Hoencamp, E. (1995). "Truth In- and Outside the Therapy Room: Some Theoretical and Practical Considerations." *Hypnos* 22 (Dec.): 198–203.

Hoorwitz, A. N. (1992). *The Clinical Detective: Techniques in the Evaluation of Sexual Abuse.* New York: Norton.

Jones, C. A. G. (1994). *Expert Witnesses: Science, Medicine, and the Practice of Law.* Oxford: Oxford University Press.

Kalichman, S. C. (1993). *Mandated Reporting of Suspected Child Abuse: Ethics, Law and Policy.* Washington: American Psychological Association.

Karlin, R. A., and M. T. Orne (1996). "Commentary on *Borawick v. Shay:* Hypnosis, Social Influence, Incestuous Child Abuse, and Satanic Ritual Abuse: The Iatrogenic Creation of Horrific Memories for the Remote Past." *Cultic Studies Journal* 13: 42–94.

Kempe, C. H., et al. (1962). "The Battered-Child Syndrome." *Journal of the American Medical Association* 181: 17–24.

Krikorian v. Barry (1987). 196 Cal. App.3d 1211, 242 Cal. Rptr. 312 (2nd Dist.).

Levine, M., H. J. Doueck, et al. (1995). *The Impact of Mandated Reporting on the Therapeutic Process: Picking Up the Pieces.* Thousand Oaks, Calif.: Sage.

Lipkin, R. (1989). "Intimacy and Confidentiality in Psychotherapeutic Relationships." *Theoretical Medicine* 10: 311–330.

Loftus, E., and K. Ketcham (1994). *The Myth of Repressed Memory: False Memories and Allegations of Sexual Abuse.* New York: St. Martin's.

Lowe, A. D. (1996). "New Laws Put Kids First: Reforms Stress Protection over Preserving Families." *American Bar Association Journal* 82 (May): 20–21.

Marshall, J. (1966). *Law and Psychology in Conflict.* Indianapolis: Bobbs-Merrill.

McConkey, K. M., and P. W. Sheehan (1995). *Hypnosis, Memory, and Behavior in Criminal Investigation.* New York: Guilford Press.

Michigan State Bar (1987). Opinion CI-1164.

Moen, S. P. (1995). "Consequences of the Therapist's Claim 'I'm Not a Detective,' " *Journal of Psychiatry and Law* 23: 477–484.

Montoya v. Bebensee (1988). 761 P.2d 285 (Ct. App. Colo.).

Munsterberg, H. (1908). *On the Witness Stand.* New York: Doubleday, Page.

Myers, J. E. B., ed. (1994). *The Backlash: Child Protection under Fire.* Newbury Park, Calif.: Sage.

Nix v. Whiteside (1986). 475 U.S. 157, 106 S.Ct. 988, 89 L.Ed.2d 123.

Pearce, S. S. (1996). *Flash of Insight: Metaphor and Narrative in Therapy.* Boston: Allyn and Bacon.

Perr, I. N. (1975). "Psychiatric Testimony and the Rashomon Phenomenon." *Bulletin of the American Academy of Psychiatry and the Law* 3: 83–98.

Perry, C., et al. (1996). "Rethinking Per Se Exclusions of Hypnotically Elicited Recall as Legal Testimony." *International Journal of Clinical and Experimental Hypnosis* 44: 66–80.

Piper, A., Jr. (1993). " 'Truth Serum' and 'Recovered Memories' of Sexual Abuse: A Review of the Evidence." *Journal of Psychiatry and the Law* 20: 447–471.

Rains v. Superior Court (Center Foundation) (1984). 150 Cal. App.3d 933, 198 Cal. Rptr. 249 (2nd Dist.).

Reidinger, P. (1996). "They Blinded Me with Science!" *American Bar Association Journal* 82 (Sept.): 58–62.

Rieke, R. D., and R. K. Stutman (1990). *Communication in Legal Advocacy.* Columbia: University of South Carolina Press.

Ross, B. M. (1991). *Remembering the Personal Past: Descriptions of Autobiographical Memory.* Oxford: Oxford University Press.

Scheflin, A. W. (1995). "Legal Commentary on the Diary." In H. Thornton, *Hung Jury: The Diary of a Menendez Juror.* Philadelphia: Temple University Press.

Scheflin, A. W. (1996). "Commentary on *Borawick v. Shay:* The Fate of Hypnotically Retrieved Memories." *Cultic Studies Journal* 13: 26–41.

Scheflin, A. W. (1997a). "Ethics and Hypnosis: Unorthodox or Innovative Therapies and the Legal Standard of Care." In W. J. Matthews and J. Edgette, eds., *Current Thinking and Research in Brief Therapy: Solutions, Strategies, Narratives.* New York: Brunner/Mazel.

Scheflin, A. W. (1997b). "False Memory and Buridan's Ass: A Response to Karlin and Orne, 'Hypnosis, Social Influence, Incestuous Child Abuse, and Satanic Ritual Abuse: The Iatrogenic Creation of Horrific Memories for the Remote Past." *Cultic Studies Journal* 13, no. 3.

Scheflin, A. W., and E. M. Opton Jr. (1978). *The Mind Manipulators.* London: Paddington Press.

Schmitt, F. F. (1995). *Truth: A Primer.* Boulder, Colo.: Westview Press.

Schoener, G. R., et al. (1989). *Psychotherapists' Sexual Involvement with Clients: Intervention and Prevention.* Minneapolis: Walk-In Counseling Center.

Shuman, S. I. (1977). *Psychosurgery and the Medical Control of Violence: Autonomy and Deviance.* Detroit: Wayne State University Press.

Simon, R. I., ed. (1990). *Review of Clinical Psychiatry and the Law,* vol. 1. Washington: American Psychiatric Press.

Simon, R. I. (1992). *Clinical Psychiatry and the Law.* 2nd ed. Washington: American Psychiatric Press.

Slovenko, R. (1995a). "The Duty of Therapists to Third Parties." *Journal of Psychiatry and Law* 23 (Fall): 383–410.

Slovenko, R. (1995b). " 'I'm Not a Detective' in 'Revival of Memory.' " Paper presented at a Conference on Law, Science and Society sponsored by the American Bar Association, Detroit, April 29.

Spence, D. P. (1982). *Narrative Truth and Historical Truth.* New York: Norton.

Spence, D. P. (1987). *The Freudian Metaphor*. New York: Norton.

Spence, D. P. (1994a). *The Rhetorical Voice of Psychoanalysis*. Cambridge, Mass.: Harvard University Press.

Spence, D. P. (1994b). "Narrative Truth and Putative Child Abuse." *International Journal of Clinical and Experimental Hypnosis* 42 (Oct.): 289–302.

Stecks v. Young (1995). 38 Cal. App.4th 365, 45 Cal. Rptr.2d 475 (4th Dist.), review denied Dec. 14, 1995.

Tarasoff v. Regents of University of California (1976). 17 Cal.3d 425, 551 P.2d 334, 131 Cal. Rptr. 14.

Traver, R. (1958). *Anatomy of a Murder*. New York: St. Martin's.

United States v. Wade (1967). 388 U.S. 218, 87 S.Ct. 1926, 18 L.Ed.2d 1149.

W.C.W. v. Bird (1992). 840 S.W.2d 50 840 S.W.2d 50 (Ct. App. Houston, 1st Dist., Tex.), rehearing denied Oct. 29, 1992.

W.C.W. v. Bird (1994). 868 S.W.2d 767 (Tex. Sup. Ct. 1994).

Wesson, M. (1985). "Historical Truth, Narrative Truth, and Expert Testimony." *Washington Law Review* 60: 331–354.

Wilkinson v. Balsam (1995). 885 F.Supp. 651 (D.Vermont).

Wolfram, C. W. (1986). *Modern Legal Ethics*. St. Paul: West Publishing.

21

The Perspective of the Plaintiff's Attorney

Clyde D. Bergstresser, J.D.

As psychiatrists and other mental health professionals, you want to practice your profession well and with dignity; you want to treat patients and help them live healthy productive lives. You are often dealing with patients in crises that are terrifying to them and their families. Our legal system requires you to predict things like dangerousness or suicidality that in many circumstances are not predictable. When you are wrong, as you are bound to be from time to time, the scientific foundation for your course of action is attacked if not ridiculed. Added to that, there are almost as many scornful jokes about psychiatrists as there are about lawyers. To many of you there is the perception that in recent years the legal system has invaded your shores. You want to know how to keep it away. Certainly, the last thing you want is to face a lawyer in a courtroom asking you difficult questions about what you did or failed to do.

How did we get to this place, and how can you protect yourself? These are the questions I frequently am asked to address from the perspective of a lawyer who has represented many patients in suits against mental health professionals. As you might suspect, there is no magic pill, no bunker you can lease or buy to insulate you from the effects of our legal system. Furthermore, it is not my opinion that the legal rights of patients are in conflict with good practice. In fact, I think that, viewed properly, there is a synergy between the two that encourages good practice.

There was a time when psychiatrists and other mental health professionals could practice without attention or interference from lawyers. That time has long since passed and is not likely to return. Lest anyone look back on that time too fondly, we must remember that a partial explanation for this inattention was collective fear and denial of all things related to "insanity." It was a time when mental patients were considered less than human, and therefore possessing and deserving of no rights. It was also a time when any woman who dared complain about a therapist's sexual exploitation quickly became revictimized and labeled a seducer who was the cause of the problem. Some subsequent therapists considered *her* to be in need of much therapy to determine why she wanted and permitted her own abuse to happen. For decades the psychotherapeutic community was aware of this problem and did nothing to bring attention to it or to stop it. Colleagues were not reported to licensing boards. Patients were discouraged from taking action. One must have some power to complain effectively.

A brief history of my involvement with the mental health system may address in part the question of how the legal system got so involved in your profession. It may also expose my bias.

I am an attorney who has been representing patients, including mental health patients, for over twenty years, primarily in the Commonwealth of Massachusetts. My start in mental health law began during my first year of practice in 1975, representing patients at Bridgewater State Hospital, a maximum-security facility intended for the "criminally insane." This facility was the venue for the filming of *Titicutt Follies,* the celebrated documentary by Frederick Wiseman exposing the subhuman conditions in which many of these patients existed. The Massachusetts legislature had recently enacted a statute, M.G.L., Ch.123, requiring the Commonwealth to satisfy stringent standards to continue the confinement of these patients under the strict security of a prison environment. Many of these patients who had served out their criminal sentences years before were receiving their first hearing since being hospitalized. In the interim, for some, decades had passed. This was the beginning of the era of deinstitutionalization.

The late 1970s was also the beginning of a wave of litigation by lawyers educated during the civil rights movement. They sought to demystify mental health law and to apply traditional notions of civil rights to mental patients. It was during this period that the seemingly contradictory notions of mental patients' rights to treatment and their simultaneous right to refuse treatment received recognition in federal and state courts throughout the country. My contribution to this body of law emerged from being one of the trial counsel (with Richard Cole and Robert Burdick) representing the plaintiffs in *Rogers v. Okin,* 478 F.Supp 1342 (D.Mass.1979); *Rogers v Okin,* 634 F.2d 650 (1st Cir. 1980); 738 F.2d 1 (1st Cir. 1984); 451 U.S. 906 (1972); 454 U.S. 936 (1981); 457 U.S. 291 (1982); *Rogers v.*

Commissioner, 390 Mass. 489 (1983). This class action was the first federal suit to successfully challenge the use of forced seclusion as a behavioral modification treatment modality and the use of antipsychotic medication within institutions without the informed consent of a competent patient in a nonemergency. As a result of this case, these rights were ultimately established in Massachusetts under both the Constitution of the United States and that of the Commonwealth. Court hearings are now routinely held in Massachusetts to determine the appropriateness of the involuntary use of antipsychotic medication, using a substituted judgment standard for incompetent patients.

Since that time I have represented many patients seeking damages in the prosecution and trial of tort actions. These include cases alleging malpractice, boundary violations including sexual exploitation, lack of informed consent, civil rights violations, wrongful death, and failure to warn, among others.

I have participated in many educational seminars and professional society meetings for mental health practitioners where the subject of risk management is addressed. In my opinion, far too often the lawyers involved in these occasions reinforce the myth that there is little correlation between the practitioner's negligence and the likelihood of civil liability. It may be the message you want to hear, but it borders on pandering. The reality is the opposite.

Given the widespread public relations effort in recent years by insurance companies, politicians, and political action committees, most jurors are predisposed to think that all malpractice cases are fabricated or exaggerated and that most plaintiffs' attorneys invent cases. Suits for damages by mental patients are still among the most difficult for patients to win. Many of the best malpractice lawyers will not even accept mental health cases because they know how difficult it is to prevail. It usually takes much more than just a breach of the standard of care. Rather, violations must be repeated or blatant. That is not to say that only meritorious cases are filed. Of course, civil suits are brought from time to time that have no merit. Usually these cases are filed by lawyers inexperienced in this field. It is rare that these cases ever make it to trial and rarer still that there would be a substantial verdict.

The best single way to avoid being successfully sued is to avoid being negligent; practice in accordance with the standard of care:

1. Do not accept responsibility where it is beyond or outside your area of expertise.
2. Seek consultation from your colleagues when treatment issues do extend

beyond your area of expertise; consult with a knowledgeable attorney
when complicated questions relating to a duty to warn arise.

3. Ensure that those allied professionals working under your license and/or
supervision are qualified for the tasks delegated to them and that they are
being professionally supervised.

4. Consider the risks your patients present to themselves and to others; perform an adequate and timely assessment where required.

5. Ensure that patients are being properly monitored when on medication.

6. Obtain consent from competent patients.

And the list goes on. It is the sum total of being a competent responsible
provider of health care.

What may be most useful for the practicing clinician concerned about
risk management is to address those departures from the standard of care
that frequently result in civil damage claims. There may be some comfort,
however, in briefly mentioning those areas of frequent complaint that
rarely if ever result in litigation. The most frequent calls a lawyer receives
are from patients complaining of bad therapy, wasted years, and wasted
money, all of which were not discovered until they finally got to their
present therapist. These are the kinds of cases we screen out over the phone
and are rarely filed by any lawyer, absent something extraordinarily bizarre
about the therapy. An example of what I mean by bizarre psychotherapy
would be a psychotherapist who, as a product of his own mental instability,
actively sought for many years to convince a patient that she was a multiple
personality, going so far as to make up names for these personalities, where
in fact the patient was not and never had been a multiple.

Next on the list of frequent calls are patients complaining of wrongful
hospitalization or commitment. Where the procedural requirements for
commitment have been satisfied, as they have been in virtually all of the
cases I have seen, no experienced lawyer will touch them. Even if there
have been procedural irregularities, where the patient was seriously mentally ill and in need of hospitalization, a patient will have an extremely hard
time finding a lawyer to pursue litigation. In this regard, the contingent
fee system really works to the advantage of mental health providers. Malpractice litigation is complicated, time consuming, and expensive, and very
few plaintiffs can front the costs. That means the attorney must invest not
only his time and the cost of his overhead but the costs of litigation. Any
lawyer litigating claims where there is little likelihood of a substantial recovery will soon be unable to pay his or her bills.

So what are the claims to be concerned about? Those where there is a real risk of a substantial recovery and those where the damages are the greatest. The risk is greatest where the patient is seriously abused, dead, or brain damaged or when someone else is dead or substantially injured or abused at the hands of the patient. For mental health professionals, at the top of the list must be suits arising out of suicide attempts (successful or resulting in substantial personal injury) where there is evidence of inadequate attention to diagnosis or treatment and/or a failure to protect the patient. Of course inpatients and outpatients with clinical depression or other forms of mental illness who can present serious risks of suicide form a large proportion of those patients seeking care. This makes it a risk most mental health clinicians will face frequently.

Of the malpractice cases I have handled arising out of suicide attempts, all but two settled before trial. Of the two that went to trial before juries, both resulted in plaintiffs' verdicts and substantial awards. This does not mean suicide cases are easy to win or are usually won. The opposite is true. It does mean that our firm is very selective about those we pursue. If a patient has a long history of mental illness and a long history of suicidal ideation with repeated attempts, we are very unlikely to file a complaint even in the presence of substantial departures from the standard of care. It is much too hard to overcome the presumption that the patient would have killed himself next week or next month even if prevention had been successful on the day in question.

Drawing on the cases I have handled and reinforced by my review of the literature, there are patterns of practice that emerge which increase the risk of error, inattention, and therefore tragedy. If you do not object to a lawyer commenting on clinical practice, I will list some of the areas of high risk that I have seen.

High on the list is the inappropriate reliance on "contracts for safety" to the exclusion of a competent mental health and suicide assessment by a practitioner qualified to perform the assessment and possessing sufficient information to make the assessment. Frequently, I have examined mental health professionals under oath after a suicide and asked them for the basis of their conclusion that a patient who had multiple risk factors for suicide did not require suicide precautions. All too often the mantra is that the patient "contracted" for safety and appeared sincere. I have seen contracts for safety relied upon by clinicians who never met the patient before and had no basis founded in experience for judging either the patient's "sincerity" or the patient's ability to maintain the contract in the presence of a history of impulsivity or even psychosis. Yet the contract was made and relied upon. I have seen contracts for safety relied upon by clinicians during the first day of a patient's admission to the hospital following a high-lethality suicide attempt, where the attempt was in breach of a then-existing "contract for safety."

In the absence of a therapeutic alliance, what does a contract for safety even mean? It certainly has no legal meaning. In addition, there are many reasons why patients enter into these contracts without ever intending to comply with them. Patients who have never been mentally ill before, patients who have never been in a mental hospital before, and patients with histories of personal and/or professional success and pride who find mental illness unacceptable may be motivated to present themselves as more in control than they are. Of course, the patient who really intends to kill himself is not likely to thwart his efforts by disclosing his intention and plan.

In the words of Douglas Jacobs, M.D., an acknowledged authority on suicide assessment and prevention: "We believe certain dangers may go unrecognized when using contracts. Clinicians widely believe that contracts prevent suicide, when in fact that has never been proven. Contracts can give staff a false sense of security when dealing with a suicidal patient . . . Do we ask our asthmatic patients not to breathe so hard or not to wheeze?"[1]

Where serious risk factors exist for suicidality, perhaps contracts for safety are most useful when a patient tells you he cannot agree that he will be safe. I often make the analogy to a mammogram in the presence of a palpable breast lump. If the mammogram confirms malignancy it must be acted upon, much like the patient who confirms he is not safe. If, however, a mammogram is negative, it cannot be relied upon to exclude malignancy in a lump since there is a false negative rate as high as 15 percent. Similarly, where the risk of error may be fatal, contracts for safety cannot substitute for a thorough history and evaluation, with appropriate precautions and vigilance.

Inadequate histories have been present in most of the cases we have pursued. A suicide assessment cannot be made without the pertinent information. You can be sure that during the course of litigation all of the historical risk factors that were known or should have been known at the time a suicide assessment was indicated will be thoroughly explored. Were the relevant questions asked? Were efforts made to speak with the family? I have seen circumstances where the spouse or parent was present at the time of admission, but nobody took the time to take a history from the closest family member which would have disclosed that the patient was withholding vital information relevant to a suicide assessment. This would be relevant not only to a determination of the risk factors but also to the question of the patient's ability to enter into a therapeutic alliance and be candid about feelings of suicidality. Was an effort made to contact the patient's most recent treater, who could be a valuable source of information for an assessment?

If none of these steps were taken and important information was not determined or known, a therapist lacks credibility in asserting that even if she or he had known that information, no further precautions would have been taken to prevent the suicide. Once you lose your credibility in front of a jury, you are in trouble.

There are several other issues that frequently arise in suicide cases. One area of inquiry is the competence, the level of training, and the supervision of the clinician performing the mental health assessment. All too often the least educated and least qualified clinician on an inpatient unit is delegated to perform the initial assessment. Where the initial assessment is inadequate, it often becomes a faulty foundation that is relied upon by the more qualified staff who evaluate the patient thereafter.

Know what you are signing and what it means to sign it. I have addressed senior psychiatric residents in some of our most prestigious training programs who have acknowledged that, despite never having performed an independent evaluation or assessment, they routinely sign off on plans changing levels of restriction and supervision or authorizing the placement or removal of restraints. Usually they are relying on the judgment of more experienced nursing staff who have been making these decisions for years. Of course, the reason they are being asked to sign these changes is that the nursing staff are not deemed to have sufficient education and training to be making the decision.

When and if disaster strikes, that same resident is going to look foolish explaining that it was policy to sign these orders without evaluating the patient. You can also be sure that this position will get no support from the unit chief and hospital administrators. I have examined a psychiatrist in a suicide case who explained that his signature on the patient's plan was just a matter of billing policy and did not require him to know anything about the patient or even to read and understand what he was signing. He acknowledged that a rubber stamp would have been adequate. I assure you, the jury was not pleased with his explanation.

Other questions to ask in assessing how your practices would hold up to scrutiny in the event of a disaster include the following. Does your hospital or clinic have protocols for suicide assessment and precautions, and are they being followed? Are the administrators who formulated policy aware of who is responsible for implementing it? Is anyone responsible for implementing policy or for reviewing compliance with established policy? When a suicide occurs in circumstances where a facility's own policies are being ignored, it is not an adequate defense to say that you were not even aware of the protocol for the removal of (for instance) robe belts, and the written policy did not comport with the standard of care in the community.

How is significant information relating to suicidality communicated to the staff responsible for establishing and implementing precautions? I have seen circumstances where emergency department staff obtained an appropriate suicide assessment, including pertinent history, which concluded that the patient could not contract for safety and required a locked inpatient unit. Even though the assessment was put in writing immediately, none of the information was communicated to the ward staff responsible for precautions, nor did the ward staff obtain a copy of the assessment. When the intake assessment was performed on the unit, significant history was not obtained and other history was distorted, resulting in inadequate precautions.

Another context in which litigation can arise following a suicide is premature discharge. I have seen this fueled by harried, overworked staff who are at their wits' end with a borderline patient who has pushed all their buttons and for whom they have been unable to find an alternate placement. However, appeasing the staff will appear a poor explanation for the patient who is suicidal at discharge and kills herself outside the hospital.

Potential liability can also arise where the premature discharge is insurance driven. Did the clinical staff do everything reasonably within their power to appeal an insurance-driven discharge? In this era of managed care and capitation agreements, clinicians and institutions with an economic incentive to provide less care will be the subject of increasing public scrutiny and discontent.

In my practice in recent years suicide cases are at least matched if not exceeded by complaints of boundary violations. We rarely pursue cases where the boundary violation did not include sexual intercourse. Of course the usual case involves a therapist having sexual relations with his or her patient. But we have had cases of sexual relations with a former patient and with the spouse of the patient. We have also pursued actions for loss of consortium by the husband where the patient is not at present complaining of the sexual contact by the therapist and may even be living with the therapist.

Depending on the profession, there are different rules relating to the issue of sexual relations with a former patient. The rules of the American Psychiatric Association were changed in July 1992 by a vote of 9 to 7.

The old rule—Section 2(1)—said: "Sexual involvement with one's former patients generally exploits emotions deriving from treatment and therefore almost always is unethical." The new rule reads: "the inherent inequality in the doctor-patient relationship may lead to exploitation of the patient. Sexual activity with a current or former patient is unethical." The wiggle room in the former rule of "almost always" was removed.

In 1992 the American Psychological Association passed a rule that reads: "Psychologists do not engage in sexual intimacies with a former therapy patient or client for at least two years after cessation or termination of professional services"—Section 4.07(a). The ethical code then lists seven factors to consider in determining whether even after two years sexual relations with a former patient would be an ethical violation.

Many psychotherapists find themselves in the role of subsequent treaters of patients with a history of sexual abuse by persons in positions of trust or authority. These could include prior therapists, pastors, teachers, parents or parent figures, and other relatives. A number of issues may arise during or after the treatment that you should consider in order to avoid an unintended disservice to your patient. Is there a duty to report the conduct to the relevant professional association or licensing board, with or without the permission of the patient? Should the patient be urged to report the conduct? Should the patient be urged to consult an attorney before the patient is clinically able to pursue civil litigation so that the right to sue is not lost in the interim by operation of a statute of limitations? Is it likely that your treatment records will be disclosed and you will be deposed or called as a witness in subsequent civil litigation and/or proceedings before a licensing or professional board? Should you agree to be an expert witness in any subsequent litigation, and if so what challenge should you expect on the grounds of bias?

Depending on the ethical rules of your profession, you may be under an explicit ethical obligation to report unethical conduct by other licensed professionals. You should of course become familiar with those rules. Whether the ethical rules require it or not, unless there are strong reasons not to report major boundary violations, it would be difficult to justify not advising your patient to make such a complaint. If, however, the patient is unwilling or not yet strong enough to consider filing such a complaint and does not give you permission to do so, the duty of confidentiality may supersede any duty to report. Patients whose trust has been abused in the past do not need to be revictimized by having their confidence betrayed by yet another therapist. You should consult with a knowledgeable attorney in your jurisdiction when this issue arises.

A subsequent treating therapist needs to be aware that there are statutes of limitations in all states requiring that personal injury litigation, including professionally abusive boundary violations, be filed within a limited period of time following the injury. Embarrassment, guilt, repression, denial, and other defenses interfere with a patient's ability to discuss the abusive conduct with anyone, much less consult an attorney. Therefore, a subsequent treating therapist is often the first person to learn of the conduct. Many jurisdictions, including Massachusetts, apply a doctrine referred to as the "discovery rule" to delay the running of the statute of limitations. For example, see *Riley v. Presnell*, 409 Mass. 239 (1991).

Pursuant to the discovery rule, if a patient, because of his defense mechanisms, is unable to understand that he suffered an injury as a result of boundary violations by a treater or parent, the statute may not yet have run out even if the offensive conduct occurred many years before. The subsequent treating therapist may be the most important witness on this subject. Once a patient brings a malpractice action of this type that puts her emotional harm at issue, in most circumstances she will be required to waive any patient/psychotherapist privilege as to the subsequent treater in order to pursue her claim for damages. The treater should be aware that the defense will scrutinize the process notes for any language that might be relevant to the patient's awareness which would trigger a running of the statute of limitations. Even your records generated during ongoing litigation will probably be discoverable by the defense.

If a subsequent treating therapist agrees to be an expert witness for his or her patient, the defense will challenge that therapist for having a bias. The defense will suggest that you will feel an obligation to testify only in ways that your patient will perceive as supportive or you will be risking the therapeutic alliance. I am not suggesting that this should preclude you from ever being an expert witness under those circumstances; I have used treaters for that purpose on occasion in my practice. But it must be done with an understanding of the hazards.

Another area of potential exposure relating to boundary violations is suits against employers. Are employers protected from tort exposure if they discharge a professional in their employ for having engaged in boundary violations without filing an ethical complaint with the relevant licensing board? What is your duty if a subsequent employer asks for a reference? What happens if you sit on your hands and others are victimized by the same therapist? How do you balance the duty to protect the public with your exposure for libel or slander or interference with contractual relations? These are difficult questions, and the answers will depend heavily on the facts of each case and the law and ethical rules in your jurisdiction and profession. In Massachusetts, I was a member of a legislative subcommittee that drafted model legislation to try to add some clarity and protection to this gray area, but as yet it has not been enacted.

The next broad category of psychotherapists' exposure to personal injury litigation arises when the patient under care negligently or intentionally causes injury to a third person. Generally the law does not impose a duty on an individual to exercise control over another to prevent her or him from causing harm to a third person. However, where a professional, particularly one licensed in the relevant community, has a special relationship with the person causing the injury, the law may create a duty to the society that granted him the license.

This area of the law raises a number of challenging and difficult questions. When do you have a "duty to warn" or a "duty to protect" a person whom your patient intends to harm or kill? Do you need the patient's permission? If your patient is an alcohol or drug abuser and you know or have good reason to believe he drives while intoxicated or high, do you have a duty to insist he have his license suspended? If he refuses, do you contact the police or the registry? If you do so, will you be exposed to a civil complaint for breach of confidentiality? What if your patient is taking psychoactive medication that you have prescribed and you have reason to believe she may abruptly terminate the medication, posing a risk of seizure while she is driving? What if your patient has a "recovered memory" of incest during your treatment and it later appears that this memory is tainted and false? Are you liable for damages to your patient *and* the now estranged family? These are some of the many questions that have come up at every conference I have attended because they arise out of common experiences within psychotherapy. There are no simple answers.

In the following discussion, any general principles or balancing tests that are raised are not intended as a substitute for consultation with a competent, knowledgeable attorney around a particular set of facts in a particular jurisdiction. Each analysis must be made with consideration of its potentially unique circumstances and the ethical standards, statutory law, and case law in your profession and your jurisdiction.

In the seminal case of *Tarasoff v. Regents of the University of California*, 551 P.2d 334 (1976), the California Supreme Court recognized and established a duty to warn a nonpatient of a risk of injury by a patient under the following circumstances:

> Once a therapist does in fact determine, or under applicable professional standards reasonably should have determined, that a patient poses a serious danger of violence to others, he bears a duty to exercise reasonable care to protect

the foreseeable victim of that danger. While the discharge of this duty of due care will necessarily vary with the facts of each case, in each instance the adequacy of the therapist's conduct must be measured against the traditional negligence standard of the rendition of reasonable care under the circumstances.

Many psychotherapists reacted with alarm to this newly articulated duty as lawsuits in their jurisdictions emerged to apply this doctrine. Throwing up their hands, psychotherapists would lament, How do I know what is foreseeable? Reaction from jurisdictions across the country has been varied. Some states followed *Tarasoff*'s lead, some jurisdictions limited the duty, and still others refused to establish this duty.[2] Several states enacted legislation to remove the mystery from foreseeability and to make it a much more difficult tort to pursue. For instance, the legislation passed in Massachusetts in 1989 (M.G.L., Ch 123 sec. 36B) creates a duty to act in specific situations. First, the statute creates a duty to take reasonable precautions to protect a third person where (1) the patient has actually communicated (2) to the licensed mental health professional worker (3) an explicit threat to kill or inflict serious bodily injury (4) to a reasonably identified victim (5) with the apparent intent and ability to carry out the threat. Second, the duty to take reasonable precautions is triggered by (1) a history of physical violence (2) known to the licensed mental health professional, (3) a reasonable basis to believe that there is a clear and present danger of (4) an attempt to kill or inflict serious bodily injury on (5) a reasonably identified victim.

The reasonable precautions that the Massachusetts statute contemplates include one or more of the following: (1) communicating the threat to the reasonably identified victim; (2) notifying the appropriate law enforcement agency; (3) arranging for voluntary hospitalization; (4) taking appropriate steps to initiate involuntary hospitalization (see M.G.L., Ch. 123, §1).

Determine the statutory requirements or common law duty as it exists in your state.

A frequent dilemma facing physicians and psychotherapists relates to the patient whose physical and or mental condition, or use of prescription or illicit drugs or alcohol creates a driving-related disability. Is there a duty to advise the patient to take action, a duty to report the noncompliant patient to the appropriate licensing or public health agencies or officials? Your jurisdiction may have laws or regulations that govern.[3]

Without attempting to assess the applicability of any one of these holdings to your jurisdiction, liability for injury to third parties or a duty to take reasonable action to protect third parties has been found under the following circumstances: where there has been a failure to warn a patient about a prescribed drug's driving-related side effects; a failure to warn a patient about the danger from abrupt cessation of a drug like Klonopin; a failure to warn the patient or his family about an impediment to driving stemming from a patient's medical or psychiatric condition.

A closely related question that is increasingly common is the duty of a health care provider to a nonpatient to warn of the risk of contracting a contagious disease such as HIV. In *Bradshaw v. Daniel*, 854 S.W.2d 865 (Tenn. 1993), a wrongful death action, the court found that a physician/patient relationship was unnecessary to impose a duty on the physician to warn the wife of a patient that he had Rocky Mountain spotted fever. However, the jurisdictions are not unanimous in imposing such a duty.[4]

Since the decision in *Ramona v. Isabella* (Cal. Super. Ct., May 13, 1994), cases are being filed by third-party family members alleging a loss of consortium and emotional harm allegedly resulting from negligently implanted false memories of sexual abuse. In *Ramona,* an adult patient, while undergoing therapy for bulimia, reportedly remembered for the first time having been repeatedly raped by her father between the ages of five and eight. Much of the remembering took place under sodium amytal, and the patient was assured that such memories could not be fabricated under this medication. A jury awarded $500,000 to the father.[5]

In recent years cases involving "false memory syndrome" have generated a cottage industry of competing experts. Zealots have emerged at both extremes. Of course, not all patients who exhibit behaviors that are consistent with those exhibited by sexually abused patients have been sexually abused. On the other hand, not all patients who have been sexually abused remember the abuse or its pertinent details at all times. Most competent professionals would agree that repression, denial, and dissociation do exist.[6] Of course, therapists must be careful not to do or say anything to contaminate the therapy provided to children and adults whose behavior is consistent with abuse. As with other areas of therapy, there is no substitute for experience, competence, and training.

The next wave of litigation will be carried by effects of managed care and capitation agreements linked to confidentiality agreements.[7] Increasingly, HMO and other managed care conglomerates squeeze patient care by providing primary care physicians with barely sufficient funds to cover overhead while creating large financial incentives for doctors to limit tests and referrals. In short, primary care physicians, the gatekeepers in these plans, stand to make significant financial rewards by not referring patients to potentially necessary specialists. The rewards to the executives of these conglomerates, arguably at the expense of patient care, are huge, with one executive reportedly receiving compensation of $20 million in a single year.

Not surprisingly, these managed care companies seek to insulate themselves from the predictable effects of these reverse incentives by contractually passing the malpractice risk to the doctors. Doctors are required to sign confidentiality agreements precluding disclosure of the financial incentives they have for withholding care. I doubt any judge would find such a confidentiality agreement enforceable when a patient who has been catastrophically injured because an MRI was not ordered or a neurological consult was skipped seeks disclosure of these financial incentives in the discovery phase of litigation. I also doubt that I have to describe the reaction a juror is likely to have to such a plan when (not if) these catastrophes occur.

We all must recognize that the amount of money available for health care per person is shrinking. The challenge for society and for the profession will be to establish checks and balances that encourage efficiency without compromising the quality of health care. We may all agree that relying on doctors to act against their economic self-interest without a serious counterbalance will invite intervention. In this era of "tort reform," the consuming public should also be very careful about defanging the civil justice system. A strong and effective bar of plaintiffs' lawyers may be the only ally of both the health care specialists and consumers in this battle. For those of you individually and through your professional associations paying your lobbyists to pass tort reform legislation that would make civil suits against health care providers economically unrewarding, remember the Chinese curse, "May all of your wishes come true."

I have some parting advice for the physician or health care provider who finds himself sued or about to be sued. Do not change or lose your records. Do not make "additions" or "corrections" to clarify what you meant. You would be amazed at how many people cannot resist the temptation to make sure that in hindsight the records say what was meant. When you get caught, your credibility will be destroyed, and it is very likely you will be caught. Copies of "lost" records have a habit of cropping up when you least expect it. Document experts are now very sophisticated in their ability to determine from writing patterns whether an entry was made all in one sitting, even from a copy. We have even had an understandably disgruntled divorced spouse of a defendant provide us with evidence of altered records. Of course *prior* to litigation or its threat, if records are inaccurate and it comes to your attention, you may make any addenda by dating the addition and making it clear that it is not contemporaneous.

My last piece of advice, both for your benefit and for the benefit of your patients, is to be well insured. In our system the only method of compensation for injury is a determination of fault. All human beings, even the best trained and the most careful, can be negligent. It can happen to you. It certainly can happen to me.

Notes

1. *RMF Forum* 14, no. 6, Dec. 1993.
2. See Michael L. Perlin, "Tarasoff and the Dilemma of the Dangerous Patient: New Directions for the 1990s," *Law and Psychology Review* 16 (1992): 29.
3. See "Liability of Physician for Injury to or Death of Third Party, Due to Failure to Disclose Driving Related Impediment," 43 ALR 4th 153.
4. See "Liability of Doctor or Other Health Practitioner to Third Party Contracting Contagious Disease from Doctor's Patient," 3 ALR 5th 370.
5. See "A Claim for Third Party Standing in Malpractice Cases Involving Repressed Memory Syndrome," *William and Mary Law Review* 37 (1995): 337.
6. See Barbara Pendelton Jones, "Repression: The Evolution of a Psychoanalytic Concept from the 1890s to the 1990s," *Journal of the American Psychoanalytic Association* 41, no. 1 (1993).
7. See "Extreme Risk: The New Corporate Proposition for Physicians," *New England Journal of Medicine,* Dec. 21, 1995: 1706–08.

22

Listen to Your Lawyer

David Gould, J.D.

In my more than twenty years of defending physicians and over one hundred medical malpractice trials, certain trends and historical perspectives have become quite apparent. In this chapter I will identify the most common sources of medical negligence claims and then discuss how to maximize the chances of a successful defense in the event of a malpractice action.

The most frequent source of medical claims is the patient who has had a bad result coupled with anger and/or hostility. In my experience, a negative result, although certainly a sufficient ground for commencing action in and of itself, is generally not independently a source of legal action. However, when a patient does not receive an adequate explanation for the negative result, a lawyer often becomes involved. It is common for a plaintiff sitting in a deposition to state that she tried many times to contact the physician for an explanation of an adverse outcome but either could not get in touch with the physician or was given a brief, curt, and unsatisfactory response. Many times I have come away from the deposition thinking that a little humanity, compassion, and, most important, time, could have avoided the entire problem.

This is not to say that "professional" plaintiffs may not crop up occasionally. But it has been my experience that greed alone is not the motivation for many such cases. Certain categories of cases that contain a common thread are worth discussing at this point, since we are attempting to identify areas that present a risk for the clinician. The most common types of cases involving mental health clinicians concern suicide, boundary violations, and the duty to warn.

These types of cases, like almost all medical negligence cases, are won or lost by what is contained, or not contained, in the medical record. It has been my experience that mental health notes, particularly in the outpatient setting, are, more often than not, deficient. Particularly in suicide cases, documentation of the clinician's thought process concerning suicidality, the need for preventive measures, and discussions with the patient is the most effective risk-prevention technique. Inadequate notes leave the clinician at the mercy of a plaintiff's attorney, especially when he is asked years later to recall an event that is poorly documented, if at all.

Similarly, boundary violation cases often reveal an appalling lack of notetaking. In such cases, the more thorough the documentation of what transpired at each therapy session, the better the chances of a successful defense. When notes are minimal or even lacking, the clinician is most vulnerable. In these types of cases, the allegation is that, in essence, there was never any therapy occurring at any session. A lack of documentation generally supports that assumption, while thorough notetaking as to what happened at each session strengthens the clinician's defense.

The type of documentation is important as well. Medical negligence trials often focus on the use of certain words in a record and how they are interpreted. Terms such as "confused" without further explanation should never appear in a record, since this general, vague term carries varying connotations and meanings to different people. Similarly, "depressed" can mean different things in different contexts and to different people. It is always preferable to set forth objective descriptions than to use imprecise, general terminology. Avoid using terms that carry negative connotations that do not accurately describe the clinical picture. Shorthand descriptions do not offer protection for the clinician who is called upon to interpret a note years later. Since memory fades with time, the more descriptive and complete the note, the easier it will be for the clinician to reasonably interpret it.

Similarly, in documenting informed consent discussions, avoid shorthand expressions such as "risks and benefits explained to the patient, she understands and consents." This note, of a type seen in many records, is quite useless since it does not detail the substance of the discussion. It is important to take the time to document the scope of the discussion using specific examples such as "I informed the patient that the common side effects of the medication are nausea, diarrhea, etc." It is important to write an objective and substantive note from which you will be able to draw reasonable inferences at some time in the future.

It is becoming increasingly common for physicians to hold a "post-mortem" when a negative event, such as a suicide, occurs. Such retrospective analysis of negative events may be discoverable by an adverse party in the event of litigation. Most, if not all, states have statutes which protect peer review from discovery. If such post-mortems are done under the purview of peer review, they will, in most states, be protected. If, however, there are routine conferences where such events are discussed and notes are made, these may be discoverable.

I have discouraged retrospective analysis where notes are made in the record of such meetings and conferences. I certainly do encourage peer review and learning from unexpected situations, but in the interest of risk management such analysis should be done in a privileged, confidential setting in order to ensure frank discussions and education without the fear of medico-legal implications.

Although it may seem obvious that one should avoid gratuitous comments about the care and treatment rendered by another practitioner, experience leads me to conclude that practitioners often cannot resist the temptation to criticize one another's performance. It is impossible to guess how many cases are started by a comment such as "Who did that to you?" More often than not, these comments are made by young, overzealous, and naive house staff in a large teaching facility. As soon as the patient leaves the facility, he calls a malpractice lawyer. Many cases could be prevented by the simple avoidance of gratuitous comments.

One additional area that bears comment here is the decision of whether to send a bill after an adverse event. Litigation can be precipitated when a widow receives a bill from a physician shortly after her husband has unexpectedly died. Although no one quarrels with the general proposition that practitioners are entitled to be compensated for their services, there are instances when it is worth thinking long and hard before sending a bill after an adverse event. One case that comes to mind involved a pediatric surgeon who was to do an elective circumcision on a seven-year-old boy, but who delegated the task to a first-year resident who had never done a circumcision before and who performed a terribly mutilating procedure unsupervised by a senior attending. Further, the parents were never informed that the original surgeon wasn't there, and then he sent the family to collection to pay his bill. Needless to say, after the family retained a lawyer to represent them in the collection matter, a malpractice lawyer was consulted, a lawsuit filed, and eventually a large settlement was agreed upon. The lessons of this case are obvious.

Practitioners, given their years of training, always have a desire to be helpful, be it to a patient, or, often to their own detriment, to attorneys representing patients. Since attorneys are trained as advocates for their clients, there may be occasions where an attorney representing a patient contacts a practitioner to talk about a particular course of treatment or even to give a pretrial deposition. The danger here is that the attorney may have an interest in engaging the clinician in discussion to determine whether there is a basis for a malpractice action against him or her. It is always wise, in the case of even the slightest doubt, to contact your malpractice insurer or risk manager before you speak to an attorney or appear unrepresented at a deposition. The insurer will evaluate the risk and exposure to you and, if it is determined that the assignment of counsel is appropriate, an attorney will be assigned to represent your interests. I am familiar with at least six cases in which, after appearing unrepresented at a deposition and giving damaging testimony, the physician has been added as a defendant.

Trends for the Coming Years

Recent years have seen a tremendous increase in the number of claims of alleged sexual abuse and harassment. There is no reason to believe that the frequency of these claims will lessen, since the basis of these suits is really one individual's story against another's. The difficulty in assessing these suits is that there is no "smoking gun" on the majority of the claims. The most effective way to defend such a suit is through complete and careful treatment records. Since the patient is alleging that there was no meaningful treatment, the more the clinician can point to records made contemporaneously with the alleged claims of abuse, the stronger his position will be. Of course, the reverse is also true. The more meager, or even absent, the record, the more precarious the position of the clinician.

As we attempt to predict future trends, the great unknown is the effect of managed care on the clinician's decisionmaking. The ultimate question is whether the clinician or the managed care provider or both will be responsible for the decision not to offer a procedure or test to a patient. The corollary question is whether a defense that an insurer or third-party payor refused permission for a procedure or test will be accepted by a lay jury when the clinician is sued for failure to order or perform that procedure or test. The clinician is held to the standard of care of the average practitioner in his specialty. When he recommends a test to his patient that is subsequently refused by the payor, the duty of the clinician is to inform the patient of the refusal and to then discuss the options with the patient. Those options include accepting the refusal and having the patient pay for the test or procedure himself. Discussions of options should be fully documented in the medical record.

A second area of concern in the upcoming years will be how capitated reimbursement plans will affect malpractice litigation. There are already a number of cases, with the list growing monthly, alleging that a clinician's judgment as to whether or not to order a test or procedure was clouded by the effect ordering it would have on the clinician's own financial interest. In other words, the allegation is that the clinician is in direct conflict of interest with the patient when the clinician's financial rewards are in question. The skillful plaintiff's attorney will attempt to argue that when the clinician's interests are in conflict with those of the patient, those of the clinician will always win. It is a virtual certainty that these types of claims are going to proliferate in the next several years. The defense to them is openness, communication with the patient, and adequate documentation of thoughts, impressions, and opinions.

Working with and Listening to Your Lawyer

There is very little that is more threatening to a clinician than involvement in a malpractice action. It is, however, possible to minimize the trauma by utilizing the steps and techniques discussed below. I have found that the initial discomfort among medical professionals at the commencement of a suit results largely from a fear of the unknown. Those becoming involved in the judicial system for the first time have a much more difficult time coping than do those who have had previous exposure to the courts in some form.

With the first flurry of activity, including receipt of a summons and complaint, correspondence from an insurer, and perhaps communication with a defense attorney, there comes a feeling of helplessness and, often, hopelessness. The process will be triggered by receipt of the summons and complaint, which you will forward to your insurer. It is at this point that perhaps the single most important decision in the entire case is made. That is, choice of defense counsel. All insurers have a list of approved defense counsel. It is a good idea to ask colleagues and peers whether they have been in a similar situation and, if so, whether they were pleased or displeased with their counsel. Since your defense lawyer will be an integral part of your life over several years of stress and anxiety, a known quantity is far preferable to putting your professional life in the hands of an attorney about whom you know nothing. Insurers will honor your request to have a particular approved attorney act as your defense counsel. Make that request prudently.

There is no substitute for your own active involvement in the process. Your attorney will control the tenor and pace of the litigation. However, you can exert a very strong influence over the proceedings by becoming an active partner with your attorney.

As mentioned above, the initial apprehension when confronted by litigation arises from fear of the unknown. Perhaps the most important task you can perform is to educate yourself about the system and the process. The more you know about what is going to happen, the better able you will be to deal with it. The process of education begins with the first contact from the insurer. Don't ever hesitate to ask the claims representative about the claims process, how your claim will be handled, or any other facets of the litigation from the claims-handling perspective. It is imperative that you cooperate fully with the claims representative, since he or she will be working quite closely with your attorney to prepare and coordinate your defense. The willingness to ask questions will go a long way toward helping you understand the legal system and survive in it.

Shortly after you forward the initial suit papers to your insurer, you should be hearing from your attorney. The initial communication is generally in writing but may be over the telephone. This initial communication will be an introduction and should ask you to contact the attorney and arrange an appointment to meet and discuss the case. At the first meeting the attorney should explain the legal process and the timing of various events in the case. Just as you will rely on your attorney to educate you about the legal process, your attorney will rely on you to educate him about the medical issues in the case. It is, therefore, imperative to attend the first meeting fully prepared. How should you prepare? First and foremost, you should review your records and be prepared to explain, in detail, your treatment and why you did what you did. Preparation presumes that you will be willing to spend whatever time is necessary to educate yourself and also to educate your attorney about the medical controversies implicit in the case.

Preparation also presumes that you are willing to be an active participant in your own defense. Experience has taught me that not everyone is willing to put the same commitment into preparing a defense. Keep in mind that these cases are invariably won and lost long before you ever set foot in a courtroom. They are won and lost by the preparation that both you and your attorney put into the case.

Another area in which thoroughness and willingness to be an equal partner are exceedingly important is the choice of an expert to review the records and testify on your behalf. Often I ask my client to help select an appropriate expert to review the materials and, if supportive, to testify at trial. Although attorneys and insurers have ample supplies of experts who are ready and willing to review malpractice cases, there are many occasions when an expert with a particular area of expertise is needed. This is one situation in which a defendant who is willing to be an equal partner in the process can make the difference between winning and losing. By searching for an appropriate expert, the defendant can provide invaluable input into his own defense.

Participating in the defense may take significant time, something not everyone is willing to provide. I am often struck by the reluctance of some individuals to become involved in their own defense. They look at their case as an inconvenience that matters only to the insurer. Nothing can be further from the truth. In most jurisdictions, settlements and verdicts on behalf of a plaintiff carry reporting requirements to State Boards of Registration and also to the National Practitioner Data Bank. Settlements and adverse verdicts may carry potentially negative ramifications with regard to credentialing or participation in certain managed care plans, as well as to medical licenses in certain instances. It is, therefore, critically important to maximize one's chances of a successful defense. Willingness to make the commitment to do whatever is necessary goes a long way toward maximizing the chances of a successful defense. It may include searching the medical literature for helpful texts and articles or it may involve a point-by-point rebuttal of what the plaintiff's expert has to say in a letter or an affidavit to a medical tribunal.

Yet another area in which thoroughness and preparation may make the difference between winning and losing is in answers to interrogatories. Interrogatories are written questions posed by one side to the other asking for certain information. The most common interrogatory posed by a plaintiff's attorney to a defendant clinician asks for the details of treatment. Over the years, the most common failing of thorough preparation I have seen is in the preparation of answers to interrogatories. A skillful plaintiff's attorney can effectively use answers that are incomplete or contain inconsistencies to the detriment of the clinician at the time of trial. By their very nature, interrogatories asking for details of treatment must be answered by the defendant, since the attorney was not present during treatment and is not aware of the intricacies and the details of treatment. Therefore the burden is on the defendant to answer the interrogatory. It is critical for the clinician, when preparing draft answers to interrogatories, to be compulsive in providing complete details concerning a specific course of treatment.

In an attempt to shortcut what can be a time-consuming and often unpleasant task, some defendants say "please refer to my office record" or provide an incomplete summary of treatment. Remember: since answers to interrogatories are signed under oath, they are, in their written form, actual trial testimony. Incompleteness and inconsistencies can have a profound effect on how a trial jury perceives the clinician, since the skillful attorney can use inconsistencies between answers to interrogatories and trial testimony to undermine the credibility of the testimony.

Such shortcuts are a formula for disaster. As plaintiffs' attorneys are becoming more skillful and better prepared, it is necessary for both the defendant's attorney and the defendant to be prepared to meet the challenge. A commitment to thoroughness is the initial step in meeting the challenge.

Depositions are addressed in great detail in another chapter, but a word about them from my perspective as a defense attorney is in order. Depositions are the single most important part of the pretrial discovery process. As answers to interrogatories are trial testimony, so are answers given at depositions. Depositions play two very distinct roles as trial of a case approaches. First, they allow the opposing attorney to assess you and how effective a witness you will make at trial. They also allow the attorney to think about what techniques may be useful to undermine your performance at trial. However, depositions also give you a "dress rehearsal" and an opportunity to size up your adversary and make some initial assessments of his ability.

The second area and certainly the most important function of a deposition for the plaintiff's attorney is that it presents the one and only chance to get your story, under oath, on the record. Literally, what you say at your deposition is your trial testimony, since the presumption is that you will be consistent between what you say in the deposition and on the witness stand. If there are certain positions concerning your treatment that are going to be the foundation of your testimony, they must be established in conjunction with your attorney. The *only* way these positions can be formulated is by face-to-face, one-on-one meetings.

The first meeting to lay the groundwork for your testimony and for the foundation of your case should occur shortly after receipt of the initial suit papers. A more important meeting should take place after you receive notice that a deposition has been scheduled. Under most circumstances, it is not acceptable to schedule a deposition preparation conference on the same day as the deposition. Since the deposition is a critical stage in the preparation of the defense, you must give yourself adequate time to prepare, develop whatever position is going to bind you at time of trial, and ask questions about the deposition process. I usually recommend a meeting for preparation no more than three weeks before the deposition. I have found that time frame to be the most workable and to allow ample time to schedule further sessions if they are needed.

At the predeposition conference, your attorney should begin to direct your thinking in the direction in which trial strategy will head. He should also familiarize you with the deposition process and instruct you what materials will be necessary for you to review. Since each attorney has a unique personality and style and likes to ask certain types of questions, your attorney should familiarize you with the style of the attorney who will be questioning you. In most jurisdictions the malpractice bar is relatively small, so this should not be a difficult task. For example, one lawyer might tend to use medical texts in questioning of clinicians. Another might like to use questions such as, "Doctor, it would have been bad medical practice if you had done . . ." These are the subtleties about which an experienced defense lawyer will be able to educate you. It should never be acceptable to have such a meeting with a paralegal or an associate who is not going to be with you at the deposition or is not going to be trial counsel.

Your attorney should also be able to educate you about the tack that he believes his adversary will take at the deposition and eventually at trial. By the time the deposition is taken, both you and your attorney should have access to this information from a number of sources, including answers to interrogatories detailing the substance of expected expert testimony and/or letters and affidavits submitted to medical malpractice tribunals. Since plaintiff attorneys rely on their experts to direct them as to a perceived negligent act or to a weakness in the defendant's position, it is these areas that they will attempt to probe at the deposition. By working with your attorney at the predeposition conference, you should be able to understand exactly where the opposing attorney will be heading with his questioning. The surest way to achieve a victory for a plaintiff is for the defendant to admit negligence or to actively second-guess himself; knowing in advance where the attack will lead should allow you to anticipate that attack and effectively counter it.

It is also of great importance to allow enough time to ask questions about the process. The key is to go into the deposition feeling comfortable with your understanding of the process and confident in your ability to counter the substantive medical questioning. Remember that no matter how much the attorney has delved into the subject matter, he has not completed a residency training program in your specialty. Be confident that your knowledge is vastly superior to that of any attorney who will be questioning you at a deposition. The opposing attorney can only ask the question—it is your answer that can do you harm. If you are prepared and comfortable, the deposition should allow you to make your points. Always remember that the goal of the deposition is not to try to convince your opponent of the futility of his position. That will never happen! The goal is to leave the deposition and be able to say "I didn't lose my case." I say this because the deposition is a one-sided opportunity for the opposing attorney to question you. Your attorney will not ask you any questions at the deposition since there is nothing to be gained by clarifying the plaintiff's questioning.

I hope it is apparent that the purpose of predeposition preparation sessions is to make you as knowledgeable and comfortable about the process as it is possible to be. I have heard too many times that, once questioning begins, the opposing attorney attempts to make the clinician whose deposition is being taken feel inadequate and uncomfortable. The more relaxed, comfortable, and confident you are about the deposition, the easier it will be to cope with the process.

After the deposition and as expert reports are accumulated, the strategy for the trial should become quite clear. At trial preparation sessions, the defendant clinician and his attorney should fine-tune the strategy. They should set the tenor not only for the clinician's testimony but for that of expert witnesses as well. The experts must testify that the clinician acted in accordance with accepted practice, assuming a certain set of facts. The cornerstone of that testimony is the assumption that certain facts to which the clinician will testify are true. Those facts must be developed through the clinician's testimony by the questioning of his attorney.

During the trial preparation phase, at some time the clinician and his attorney should be able to go question by question and answer by answer through the clinician's direct testimony. This is important for two reasons. First, the clinician's own testimony will form the basis for his defense and for supportive expert testimony. Second, there should be no surprises once the clinician is on the witness stand. Thorough and careful preparation should eliminate the element of surprise.

It is during this preparation stage that the clinician should be of greatest assistance to his attorney in defining and dealing with any medical issues. I often look to my client to educate me on the salient medical issues and help me develop lines of cross-examination of the adverse expert witness. Many times I have found the expertise of my client to be the greatest asset

I possess. The educational function is also one area where the clinician may exert the greatest influence. In helping to develop strategy and in formulating areas of cross-examination of the adverse expert, the clinician becomes an equal partner in the process. Along those same lines, I will often offer the defendant the opportunity of attending meetings with his experts. Although most times the defendant does not attend such meetings, there are occasions where his presence may be quite helpful.

I recall one case where the major defense of a very difficult neurosurgical case with devastating injuries involved interpretation of pre-operative and post-operative CT scans and MRI studies by the defendant physician. Since it was impossible for me to interpret the films and give the defendant's precise interpretation and explanation of exactly why he interpreted them as he did, he and I had two meetings with the expert to go over every aspect of these studies. By the time the expert testified and was questioned extensively about these films, he was as prepared as the defendant to discuss them and interpret them in a completely consistent manner.

The defendant's degree of preparation and active involvement in the entire system increases as trial approaches. Since the average medical malpractice trial lasts from five to ten days, the amount of information that is conveyed to the jury can be staggering. For several reasons, I always insist that the defendant be present at the trial from beginning (jury selection) to end (when the jury goes out to deliberate). First, the defendant has a tremendous stake in the outcome of the trial and should be actively involved in the entire proceeding. Second, the defendant may be able to provide useful tips for cross-examining the plaintiff's expert while the expert is on the witness stand. Finally, the presence of the defendant in the courtroom has a strong psychological impact on the jury. It is imperative for the jury to see with their own eyes that the outcome of the trial is very meaningful and important to the defendant.

The defendant's behavior and demeanor on the witness stand also influence the jury. More and more courts are trying to lessen the impact lawyers have on the outcome of trials. It seems that trial judges are utilizing new and unique techniques to even out situations where one attorney is far more skillful than the other. These judicial techniques run the spectrum from lessening the rather rigid rules of evidence that attorneys labor under to allowing jurors to ask questions of witnesses, either orally or in writing. All of these maneuvers are designed to try to ensure that the facts will be more important than theatrics.

Although it is certainly true that having the facts on your side and being able to present them in a cogent manner is your best defense, it is important to keep in mind that medical malpractice cases are often determined not only on the facts but by how jurors perceive the defendant. Jurors unconsciously process their intuitive feelings about the defendant into their verdict. Since the impact of lawyering is becoming less of a factor in professional negligence cases and since, to a large degree, qualified experts on either side of an issue tend to cancel each other out, the determinant often comes down to the jurors' perception of whether the defendant gave or attempted to give reasonable care. The way the jurors perceive the demeanor, delivery, and personality of the defendant on the witness stand may go a long way in deciding the outcome of a case. If jurors perceive the defendant as the kind of physician they would want caring for them, they will never hurt the defendant. If, on the other hand, they perceive the defendant as uncaring, abrupt, or hostile, they will be much more likely to find in favor of an injured patient.

It is also quite important to project competence, sincerity, and professionalism. Be sure you are thoroughly familiar with the records and documents you will be referring to in your testimony. It is disconcerting to watch a witness fumble through pages of medical records in an attempt to find a particular entry. That kind of behavior on the witness stand detracts substantially from the jurors' collective impression of the witness. I hesitate to say that form can be as important as substance from the perception of the individual juror, but certainly form can be an important adjunct to substance.

Nothing can be as important as the facts, but in the event of a substantial conflict in the facts, jurors must have something to fall back upon when attempting to determine which version of the facts is more accurate. The most obvious example is when the patient says the defendant said one thing and the defendant says he told the patient something very different. If those conversations are documented, there is really not much of an issue. However, in many cases there is no documentation. Thereupon, the jurors are asked to use their individual and collective instincts in determining what they believe to be the truth. In essence, they must determine whether the clinician defendant is lying. Jurors are much more likely to believe the clinician's version of the facts when they find him to be caring, competent, and professional. It goes without saying that if jurors perceive the clinician to be sloppy, arrogant, and unprofessional they are much more likely to find against him.

Certain general principles are clear when we discuss the form of testifying. First, know the record and be able to turn to the entry you need to refer to without fumbling through the record. Second, know the chronology thoroughly so that you can recite your course of treatment by heart when you are asked questions. Third, harbor no hostility toward the plaintiff or the attorney who represents him. I realize that this is easier to say than to do. However, it is critical to turn the other cheek on the witness stand. You must understand that the jury will be confronted by an injured plaintiff who is seeking a remedy for his injuries.

Although there is inevitably going to be sympathy for that injured individual, in the vast majority of cases injuries alone will not result in a verdict for the plaintiff. Claims experience shows that over 75 percent of verdicts in medical malpractice cases are for the defendants. With few exceptions, cases are brought to trial because the defendant's insurer and his lawyers believe the case to be defendable. Large plaintiff's verdicts are almost always the result of something gone awry during the trial. That something is most often a profoundly negative performance by the defendant.

Several years ago a neurosurgeon was sued in a football-helmet-injury case. The case was very weak, in terms of both liability and ultimate damages, from the plaintiff's perspective. The defendant physician was notorious for his temper, a problem that led to his undoing. During the trial the plaintiff's attorney showed him a stack of records and questioned him at great length about a number of small points. This infuriated the neurosurgeon. After the questioning, the attorney gave him the records, then turned to walk back to the podium. The physician threw the records at the attorney in full view of the jury. The jury found for the plaintiff in the amount of one million dollars.

/ / /

Although litigation is a difficult experience for any professional, understanding the process will make it easier to survive. By preparing thoroughly, by using your common sense, and by cooperating with your attorney as an equal partner, you will help maximize the chances of a successful outcome.

23

A View from the Bench

Hon. Kermit V. Lipez

The Jury

We are all more comfortable in familiar settings. When I walk into a court-room I have no sense of foreboding. When I walk into a doctor's office I want to leave immediately. I understand your need for a survival guide in court, where the stakes are so high: reputation, self-respect, credibility, and money. Although you will come to court believing you are entitled to vindication, you must convince the jurors of that entitlement.

Exposure to judgment is always an unsettling experience. Exposure to the judgment of strangers is particularly unsettling. We subscribe in our system of justice to the know-nothing model of jurors. If prospective jurors know you personally or by reputation, if they know something about your discipline, if they have had an experience similar to the events at issue in the trial, or if they have some opinions about any issue in the trial, they will almost surely be excluded from participation. Although we tell jurors they can use their common sense in evaluating the credibility of witnesses, we do not want their prior knowledge influencing judgments that should result only from the trial process. The jury trial is both an educational exercise for the jurors and an appeal to their hearts. You must impress the jurors with your facts. You must also persuade them with your lik-ability.

I have talked to many jurors after they have completed their trials to thank them for their service and to answer any questions they have about the trial process. I often find them eager to explain and justify their deci-sion, even though I make it clear they do not have to justify anything to me. The depth of their concern about their performance always impresses me. Jurors almost always take their responsibilities seriously.

I have also been struck in these conversations by the frequency of expressions of like and dislike about witnesses. Jurors believe witnesses they like. They disbelieve witnesses they do not like. The prevalence of these expressions is not surprising. Likes and dislikes translate easily into judgments about character. With people we know well, we can discern their reliability or unreliability despite our feelings about them. The abundance of evidence drawn from life permits these discriminations. The compressed reconstruction of life in the courtroom does not. In that setting likes and dislikes become the ruling passions, and they affect every judgment that jurors make about witnesses.

Often a telling detail is at the heart of these judgments: inappropriate clothing, a failed attempt at humor, a nervous fidget, an annoying verbal habit. Although it may seem unfair that jurors attach such significance to these details, we make snap judgments routinely in our own lives on the basis of such details. Indeed, we all accept the importance of "first impressions," which are quick judgments on character and capability based on scant evidence. Since trials ration time, jurors must make these snap judgments about witnesses who offer competing versions of the truth. That is why a trial is such a nerve-racking experience for the participants. The stakes are high. Time is short. Judgment comes quickly. The performance cannot be redone. As a witness, you must get it right the first time.

The Jury Instruction

You will have a better chance of getting it right if you understand what judges tell juries in their jury instructions about the process of evaluating credibility. These instructions on the evaluation of credibility generally distinguish between "fact" witnesses and "expert" witnesses. Fact witnesses offer information about what happened. Expert witnesses offer opinions about what happened. If you are testifying at a trial where your patient is suing somebody other than yourself, and you are there to describe how you treated your patient, you are testifying as a fact witness. If you are offering an opinion about the quality of care provided by another doctor on behalf of one of the parties, you are testifying as an expert witness. If you are the defendant in a malpractice case, and you testify about what you did to a patient and why you did it, you are testifying formally as a fact witness. Inevitably, however, your explanation of the "why" of the treatment puts your expertise on the line, and the jury will surely use the instruction on expert witnesses in considering your testimony.

I used the following credibility instructions in Maine. Although the language will vary in other jurisdictions, these instructions are representative of what judges throughout the country tell jurors about the evaluation of witness credibility.

Fact Witness

Ladies and gentlemen of the jury, one of the most important things that you have to do in any case, and certainly in this case, is determine the credibility, meaning the believability, of the witnesses. You are going to do that in part by using your common sense, meaning whatever you have learned in your various life experiences, and also by using a series of tests to analyze the testimony. There are a number of tests that can be used, and I am not trying to limit you in any way, but I will suggest a few tests that you can use if you think they are appropriate in this case.

You can consider each witness's age, experience, and intelligence. You can consider the way in which the witness testified on the stand. Was the witness forthright or evasive? Did the witness's testimony make sense? You can consider how well the witness explained away any prior inconsistent statements if you first find as a fact that there were prior inconsistent statements. You can consider whether the witness's testimony was corroborated or contradicted by the testimony of other witnesses or by the exhibits. You can consider how well each witness remembered what took place during the time period in question. You can consider how good an opportunity a witness had to make the observations that were made. You can consider whether there has been any motive, or lack of motive, shown for any witness to exaggerate or lie. Finally, you can consider what interest, if any, each witness has in the outcome of this case.

Again, this is not a complete list of the tests you can use, but this is the type of process you should go through in determining how much credibility to assign to the testimony of each witness. Do you want to believe everything that a witness said? Do you want to believe nothing that a witness said? Or, for one reason or another, do you want to accept a portion of what a witness said and reject the remaining portion? That is your decision to make.

Expert Witness

Ordinarily, ladies and gentlemen of the jury, we do not permit witnesses to express opinions about issues before the jury. Their testimony is confined to the facts in dispute. We make an exception to that rule, however, for a special category of witness that we call an expert witness. An expert witness is simply an individual who, because of training, education, or experience, has acquired some expertise in an area relevant to an issue in the trial. If that expert, based on that education, training, or experience, can offer an opinion that might be helpful to the jury in deciding an issue before it, we permit the expert to offer such an opinion.

You should understand that an opinion of an expert witness is no better than the underlying facts which support it. If you should decide that the opinion of an expert witness is based upon a mistaken or incomplete set of facts, or if you should decide that the opinion of an expert witness is not based upon sufficient education or experience, or if you should conclude that the reasons given in support of the opinion are not sound, or not supported by the evidence in the case, you may disregard the opinion of that expert witness entirely. On the other hand, if you decide that the expert witness does have a sufficient set of facts, that she does have sufficient education and experience, and that the reasons given for her opinion are supported by the evidence, then you may want to give that expert testimony considerable weight. It is up to you. Basically, you determine the credibility of an expert the same as you do that of a lay person.

Although lawyers and judges debate how well jurors understand complex legal instructions, much of that debate focuses on the often complicated legal principles applicable to the case. I am sure that jurors fully understand and apply these simple instructions on the evaluation of witness credibility.

As you can see, jurors are first told to use their common sense, a reminder that the laws of probability and human nature are not suspended in the courtroom. Common sense should not pose any problem for you. Jurors must use their common sense to evaluate the extremes of behavior, when a witness tries to make the preposterous persuasive. If you are trying to do that, you should not be in court at all.

Some of the fact witness instruction focuses on a witness who has seen or experienced an event and must now report that event to the jury. The quality of the reporting depends on the accuracy of the witness's observation and memory. Jurors are told to consider how age, experience, intelligence, and vantage point affect that accuracy. Although you will probably not be reporting a startling event in your testimony, such as an accident or a crime, you will be reporting the details of a relationship with a patient and a course of treatment. The accuracy of that reporting is critical to your credibility. The jurors will assess your age, experience, and intelligence in evaluating that accuracy. If you are uncommonly young or old, you must demonstrate that age has not impaired your capacities. If you are inexperienced, you must show that your training and skills are a good substitute for experience. If you are unintelligent, you should not be a doctor.

Your motive to testify favorably for yourself, and your interest in the outcome of the trial, will be self-evident when you are a defendant. Your challenge in testifying is to make yourself credible despite that obvious bias. To that end, you must avoid the kind of inconsistent statements noted in the credibility instruction. They impair perceptions of your competence, integrity, or both. Knowing that the judge will tell the jurors to think about how you testified, you must focus on presentation in your preparations.

The credibility instruction for an expert witness focuses primarily on an evaluation of the substance of the expert's testimony. That emphasis is logical. The expert witness is not reporting an event. Accuracy of observation and memory are not usually at issue. The expert witness is reporting a finding or an opinion, based on an analysis of data. The reliability of the opinion depends on the quality and quantity of the data and the quality of the intelligence that analyzed the data. Thus the jurors are told to focus on the facts underlying the expert's opinion, and on the expert's education and experience.

The concluding sentence of the expert witness instruction, however, tells jurors that they should determine the credibility of an expert in the same way that they determine the credibility of a lay person (another way of referring to a fact witness). Initially, I thought that instruction odd, given the differing emphases of the two instructions. I now realize that the instruction makes sense for two reasons. First, both instructions remind jurors that truth may come in mixed bags. They can accept all, some, or none of the testimony of a fact witness or an expert witness. Second, the expert witness is not a talking machine. The expert is a person of varying age, experience, and intelligence, subject to bias and inconsistency, and blessed or burdened with a pleasing or offensive countenance. The jurors should be reminded that many of the tests they use in evaluating the testimony of a lay witness should also be used in evaluating the credibility of an expert witness.

This reminder has a particular significance for you when you are testifying as a defendant in a malpractice case. As I have suggested, your role as a defendant inevitably makes you both a fact witness and an expert in your own defense. Implicit in your description of what you did is the opinion, based on your education, training, and experience, that you did the right thing. The jury's evaluation of your performance as a witness will involve simultaneously an evaluation of your credentials and the basis for your decisions (the essentials of expert witness evaluation), and an evaluation of your demeanor, consistency, and motives (the essentials of fact witness evaluation).

Given this dual focus of the jury, you must be as sensitive to the manner of your presentation as you are to its substance. If you are impressive substantively but offensive personally because of arrogance, hostility, impatience, or disinterest, you will fail to persuade. The converse is also true. A vacuous charmer is also unpersuasive. My emphasis on appearances does not imply that style can mask substantive weakness. It cannot. I emphasize the importance of appearances only because so many professionals insist that reason should always prevail, thereby forgetting those professors whose flawless lectures were never heard because they spoke so poorly. If you are unwilling to accept the importance of appearances in the courtroom, if you insist that you should prevail simply because you are right, you are setting yourself up for failure. Why should reason alone dominate in the courtroom when it is only one factor among many outside of the courtroom? The courtroom is not apart from life. It is a part of life. We trust people we like. Jurors are no different.

With this reality in mind, I offer some thoughts about your appearance in the courtroom.

Appearing in Court

STATUS AND SUBJECT MATTER

You enter the courtroom with the benefit of your status. Doctors are among the most highly respected professionals. You are lucky you are not a lawyer on trial. Why this great respect for doctors? Some of the answers are obvious: credentials, education, and the sheer intelligence required by the work. At a more subtle level, I believe jurors accord great respect to doctors because they derive reassurance from that respect. Everyone in the jury box has entrusted his or her fate to a doctor at some point. As a doctor in the courtroom, you are the doctor everyone has had or will have. If you are discredited, the jurors will be insecure about the doctors in their own lives. They will feel better about their own care if your care withstands scrutiny.

You also will be discussing a subject that is sure to interest jurors. Everyone feels vulnerable to illness. Jurors can easily place themselves in stories about sickness, treatment, and recovery. They will be listening intently to your story because they feel some personal stake in what they are learning.

Moreover, the trial puts the jurors in the odd role of judging a professional who is almost always judging and appraising them. That oddity emphasizes to the jurors their weighty responsibility, and you will almost surely have their close attention.

There are times when the fascination of jurors with the testimony of a doctor is palpable. I have seen jurors literally lean forward in their seats, their eyes riveted on the doctor. They know this is a key moment in the trial. They do not want to miss a word. That is the response you want. That is an opportunity for persuasion you must not squander.

DEMEANOR

As you testify, look at the jurors and make eye contact. Jurors talk about the witness who could not look them in the eye. They subscribe to the old-fashioned notion that a person who cannot look them in the eye is trying to hide something. On the other hand, the eye contact should not be overdone. I have heard jurors complain that a witness was trying to intimidate them with intense eye contact. As always, moderation is the key.

Be animated. Your clear interest in your subject conveys a caring that is important to your credibility. If you have a chip on your shoulder about being in court, pocket it at the courthouse door. Any displays of resentment, weariness, or hostility will offend the jury and impair your credibility.

TESTIMONIAL AIDS

If you can illustrate your testimony with a testimonial aid, such as a model, picture, or chart, use it. Jurors have different learning styles. Some learn better visually than they do orally. They need to see it to understand. Although such depictions may be a difficult task for a psychiatrist, I have seen some depictions of the human mind that were unforgettable.

LANGUAGE

Explain your subject as simply and directly as possible. If you have to use a medical term, explain its meaning without prodding from counsel. If the lawyer has to goad you into an explanation, the jurors may conclude that you do not care much about them or the proceedings. Worse yet, they may perceive in your fondness for obscurity a distasteful elitism and an attempt to prevent them from understanding.

Even if you lapse into jargon and forget to explain, you can redeem yourself with patient explanations and self-deprecating humor about the guild mentality of your profession and its fondness for big, unpronounceable words with simple meanings. While apologizing for the pedantry of your colleagues (do not use that word!), you can emphasize with your explanations that you are there to make your knowledge and work as accessible to the jurors as possible.

CREDENTIALS

The courtroom is no place for modesty about your education and your professional accomplishments. If you are a graduate of prestigious schools and board certified, if you have won honors and published articles and books, if you teach and lecture, tell the jurors about it. These accomplishments enhance your credibility. Many doctors testify to their credentials with a reluctance that I can only explain as a misguided fear of immodesty. Testimony by extraction loses much of its dramatic effect. A straightforward, unbroken narrative of your accomplishments is much more impressive. If you omit anything, your attorney can ask you about the omission.

If immodesty is an issue for you, you should understand that, as a defendant, you are entitled to present your credentials to the jury to enhance your credibility. If you are testifying as an expert witness, the recitation of your credentials serves an essential evidentiary purpose. Under our rules of evidence, an expert witness must be qualified to express an opinion on the subject at issue. That qualification is established by your credentials. Usually there is no dispute about the qualification of an expert witness to offer an opinion. If there is such a dispute, however, the argument over your qualifications will take place out of the presence of the jury, with the judge deciding as a preliminary matter if you are qualified to express the opinion. The judge's decision that you are qualified to express an opinion does not preclude opposing counsel from attacking your credentials in the presence of the jury in an effort to impair your credibility.

In cases where there is no dispute about your qualifications to testify as an expert witness, opposing counsel may magnanimously offer to stipulate to your qualifications (that is, agree that you are qualified to testify), supposedly to save time. Beware of such magnanimity. As I have indicated, your credentials relate both to your right to offer an expert opinion (to be decided by the judge) and to your credibility (to be decided by the jury). A stipulation to your qualifications prevents the jury from learning about the details of your credentials, and thus may lessen your credibility. Knowing what is lost by the stipulation, any experienced attorney will reject the offer to stipulate to your qualifications.

If jurors are forced to choose between irreconcilable accounts of a medical event, their choice may well turn on which witness has the most impressive credentials. That is not an irrational basis for choice. In our own lives we frequently choose professionals on the basis of credentials. Those credentials represent the unspoken judgment of others that this professional is reliable. Jurors look for such reassurance in making choices.

PREPARATION

If you are the defendant in a malpractice case, or if you are testifying as an expert witness, you will undoubtedly be well prepared. In both of these situations you have a large stake in your performance. In a third scenario, where you are testifying on behalf of patients who are suing somebody else for damages, and there is not such a personal stake in performance, you may get sloppy.

I have been astonished by the woeful lack of preparation by doctors in these situations, including an inability to remember the patient's name. Although the doctor with a busy practice cannot remember the details of treatment of hundreds of patients, there is always time to review a patient's file before testifying. Some doctors testifying as fact witnesses appear to have reviewed the file while driving to the courthouse. As a result, we waste valuable time in the courtroom while the doctor searches through disorganized files for a document that will refresh the doctor's recollection, much to the annoyance of the judge and jury. Such displays discredit the doctor and disserve the patient.

Although your patient did not come to you because of your skills as a potential witness, your obligation to that patient extends to giving a fair account of your treatment in court if circumstances require it. Displays of poor preparation by the doctor testifying as a fact witness often reflect contempt for the litigation process and anger at having to participate in it. You are entitled to your feelings. You are not entitled to harm your patient's case by venting these feelings with a sloppy performance in the courtroom.

DEPOSITIONS

Trials are preceded by an extensive discovery process through which the contesting parties learn about the facts of their competing claims in excruciating detail. Depositions are an essential part of this discovery process. They are statements made by you under oath before a court reporter, often in your own office, in response to questions posed by the attorneys.

If you are the defendant in a malpractice case, you will have been deposed before trial. If you are an expert witness you will probably have been deposed. If you are a fact witness you may have been deposed. As a defendant or an expert witness you will surely review your deposition before trial because of the stake in performance I have mentioned. Regrettably, if you are only a fact witness, you may not bother with that review.

Such an omission is inexcusable. Attorneys will mine your deposition in the hope of catching you in an inconsistency between your trial testimony and your deposition testimony. As noted in the jury instruction on credibility, jurors are told specifically that they can consider prior inconsistent statements in evaluating the credibility of witnesses. Although inconsistencies can be found in other sources, such as in your records or in statements you made to others, an inconsistency between your deposition testimony and your trial testimony is particularly damaging because both statements are made under oath. Presented with such an inconsistency, the lawyer cross-examining you will savor this question: "Doctor, which statement is true? The one you gave in your deposition, or the one you have given here?" You do not want to face this dilemma. You may be able to avoid it if you take a little time before trial to review your deposition.

CROSS-EXAMINATION

Cross-examination will be the most grueling part of your experience in court. As you are peppered with questions that permit only yes or no answers, you will feel enormous frustration. Stifle it. The cross-examining attorney has the right to ask such questions. You must try to be responsive. If you become combative and angry, you will fulfill the hopes of the cross-examining attorney, who knows that jurors may see in your frustration a raw nerve or, better yet, a guilty conscience.

Cross-examination is not the final word. The attorney who has called you to the stand will have an opportunity to conduct a redirect examination in which you have an opportunity to elaborate on your yes and no answers. Knowing this, I have rarely intervened to help a doctor or any witnesses who turned to me during a rigorous cross-examination and complained that they could not answer a difficult question yes or no. Moreover, if the attorney who had called the witness did not object to the question, there was even less reason to intervene. For these reasons, I think it is generally a bad idea for the doctor unhappy with cross-examination to initiate a plea to the judge for help.

There is, arguably, a more subtle way for you to deal with cross-examination questions that you feel unfairly demand yes or no answers. Instead of turning to the judge for help, you can simply say to the cross-examining attorney that the question as posed is unfair and you cannot answer it yes or no. The cross-examining attorney then must choose between backing away from the question and asking the judge to remind you of your obligation to answer a question that you have just told the jury is unfair. Although there may be some minimal risk for the cross-examining attorney in demanding that you answer such questions, much of that risk is dissipated when the judge accedes to the attorney's request and directs you to answer the question as asked. I have therefore seldom seen an attorney back off from the question.

I frankly have little patience with these games played by unhappy witnesses. Attorneys are supposed to object to inappropriate questions, not witnesses. You should let your lawyer, or the lawyer on your side of the case, do the objecting.

LEARNED TREATISES

You may find yourself cross-examined with the use of a "learned treatise." Although this legal term of art evokes images of massive medical school textbooks filled with pages of impenetrable print, a learned treatise can include something as simple as a medical journal or a monograph. The attorney will give you the title of the publication and ask if you are familiar with it. This inquiry should not surprise you because the attorney using the publication for cross-examination had to disclose in a pretrial memorandum that she was going to use it for cross-examination. If there was no such disclosure, the treatise cannot be used.[1]

The attorney may ask you if you consider the work to be reliable authority. If you consider it to be so, you should acknowledge its reliability. There is nothing to be gained by denying it. Although the cross-examining attorney has to establish that the work is authoritative in order to use it for cross-examination, this authority can be established in other ways if you will not oblige through your own testimony. The attorney, in the presence of the jury, will then read to you some portion of the publication and ask if you agree with it.

Although this procedure sounds simple enough, something unusual and powerful is taking place. Judges tell jurors that the questions of an attorney are not evidence. In this instance, however, the material in the treatise, read to the jury as part of a question, is going to the jury as evidence that the jury can use to discredit you. You can be sure that this evidence will contradict or impeach your testimony. Otherwise, the attorney would not use it.

There is nothing wrong with this procedure, and nothing you can do about it, other than to be well prepared to respond with the assistance of your attorney. Again, you should remember that your attorney will have the opportunity on redirect examination to get you to comment on the treatise material.

THE HIRED GUN

If you testify as an expert witness, you can expect cross-examination insinuating that your opinion has been purchased. This insinuation will be particularly potent if you testify frequently as an expert witness. The professional expert brings significant liabilities to the trial process. Through the discovery process in any case in which you have been designated as an expert witness, you may have to reveal the following: (1) the percentage of your work that involves serving as an expert witness; (2) the percentage of your work devoted to patients; (3) the amount of income that you receive from serving as an expert witness; (4) your hourly fee (which is almost sure to shock the jurors); (5) the amount you will be paid for your work in this case; (6) the percentage of time that you testify for either the plaintiff or the defendant in malpractice cases.

You will then be asked questions about this information at trial. If the picture that emerges from your answers is one of a professional witness who rarely sees a patient, almost always testifies for plaintiffs or defendants, and earns a ton of money doing it, including a goodly portion from this case, you will almost surely be a discredited expert witness. Jurors think doctors should see patients. If you have given up patients in favor of a lucrative career as an expert witness, jurors will view you as a hired gun entitled to none of the deference accorded real doctors in the courtroom.

THE BURDEN OF THE MENTAL HEALTH PROFESSIONAL

I believe that jurors are more wary of the mental health disciplines than they are of other medical specialties. Although they have probably had experiences with family physicians and internists, or orthopedists and cardiologists, jurors are less likely to have experienced a mental health professional. This phenomenon reflects a disinclination among the populace to seek help for mental problems because prejudices about such problems persist. These prejudices include skepticism about the reality of mental problems, and the suspicion that sympathetic doctors cannot discern false reporting. Despite the testing tools available to you, mental phenomena are difficult to measure. You cannot provide the objective measurements that are often reassuring to jurors.

If you are testifying as a fact witness or an expert, expressions of excessive sympathy for a patient or a party are always a bad idea. You must persuade with facts, not emotion. Seeing such emotions, the jurors will question your professional objectivity. If you are a mental health professional, these expressions of sympathy can be particularly damaging to credibility. They will deepen the concern for patient manipulation.

As a mental health professional, you also have the burden of being able to explain too much about human conduct. At times, psychological explanations of behavior seem too facile and convenient. To skeptical jurors, the ability to explain almost everything in terms of mental illness means that you are explaining nothing. For that reason, expert testimony that certain symptoms reflect a certain experience, such as child sexual abuse or rape, is usually not permitted in criminal cases to prove that experience. The symptoms are simply too consistent with too many types of experience. Although a diagnosis of sexual abuse accommodation syndrome or rape trauma syndrome may offer useful insights for treating patients, these diagnoses are too inexact to provide reliable evidence of a criminal act.[2]

Psychological testing also reflects the difficulty of transferring techniques so useful in the clinical setting to the courtroom. I have seen psychological testing used in many settings: competency hearings, personal injury cases, suppression hearings (when there is an issue about what a defendant understood in waiving the right to be silent), and in criminal trials when the state of mind of the defendant is at issue. Psychologists have difficulty conveying to jurors the meaning of test results, in part because translating a number into a comprehensible diagnosis is so difficult.

Obviously, such tests are appealing because they produce numbers, scales, and rankings. They seem to offer hard data in a soft science. Such certainty, however, usually disappears when cross-examination begins. Any variation by the examiner from a testing protocol can be fatal. There are always studies in the literature that read test results differently or that challenge the reliability of the test. I have rarely seen a case where I thought psychological testing advanced the cause of the party presenting it.

There is the added complication that you are often in court to explain and minimize the most outrageous human conduct. If you are testifying on behalf of the defendant in a criminal case who has committed violent acts, you are facing jurors who are powerfully motivated to punish. Although they may listen respectfully to your explanations, they will resist a suggestion that the explanation excuses anything.

You should not react to these problems by trying to oversell your subject or your science. Instead, a frank acknowledgment of the limits of your wisdom will impress the jury and ultimately make you more persuasive.

BEEPERS

In conclusion, I must acknowledge the limits of my own wisdom. There is no softer science than the study of the jury trial. Although I believe in my observations and advice, I offer none of it as gospel, except for this final admonition: turn off your beepers in the courtroom. I hate that sound. So do jurors. If you beep, we will conclude that you are rude, forgetful, careless, and self-important. Our minds will shut down. We will not hear another word you say. You will not survive our disdain. The courtroom is an unforgiving place.

Notes

1. I am reflecting the Maine practice with this statement; see M.R. Civ. P. 16(d)(3)(R). The practice may vary in other jurisdictions.
2. For other purposes, however, syndrome testimony can be useful in helping jurors understand the conduct of a woman or a child who has been abused and who, because of the abuse, acts in a way that seems inconsistent with the claim of abuse. For example, defense counsel in a child sexual abuse case often impeach a child witness by demonstrating a delay in reporting or recantation of the accusations, and then arguing that such delays or recantations are inconsistent with sexual abuse. There is ample clinical evidence that such behavior is not inconsistent with sexual abuse. Mental health professionals can help rebut this unfair inference by testifying about this clinical evidence.

Epilogue

Glen O. Gabbard, M.D.

The contributors to this book are, in the main, distinguished attorneys and eminent forensic psychiatrists. As a psychoanalyst and psychiatrist primarily identified with clinical work, and without forensic training, I am perhaps a strange bedfellow in this company of scholars. Nonetheless, as a teacher of psychiatric residents and a consultant to established colleagues, I have developed a particular perspective on the fear of litigation and its impact on clinical work. This fear is to some extent pervasive. Perhaps the best we can hope for is not to practice psychiatry without fear but to implement the specific preventive measures my fellow contributors have recommended and thereby contain and reduce our fear to manageable proportions.

I strongly endorse these steps, because the alternative is for clinicians to descend into paranoid anxiety that will both impair their clinical effectiveness and paradoxically increase their chances of being sued. In this chapter I will start with some observations about the psychology of physicians in general and psychiatrists in particular. I will then move to specific examples of the ways in which fear cripples the clinician's capacity to deliver competent and empathic treatment.

The Psychology of the Physician

Most applicants to medical school cite the wish to help people as a major reason for their career choice. Such altruistic motivations are admirable and have always constituted a pillar of the humane practice of medicine. Yet studies of the psychological characteristics of physicians (Gabbard,

1985; Gabbard and Menninger, 1988; Vaillant et al., 1972) suggest that, beneath the surface, a number of conflicts have found their expression in the pursuit of a medical career.

There is a broad consensus in the literature that compulsiveness is the hallmark of the physician's personality (Gabbard, 1985; Krakowski, 1982; Krell and Miles, 1976; Rhoads, 1977; Waring, 1974). In particular, a compulsive triad of doubt, guilt feelings, and an exaggerated sense of responsibility governs much of physicians' behavior. The adaptive aspect of these characteristics is that they contribute to diagnostic rigor. Physicians tend to be thorough. Most of us would prefer to have a compulsive physician caring for us if we were seriously ill. The maladaptive aspect is that physicians' lives may be constricted to the point where personal relationships are sacrificed to a single-minded pursuit of perfection at work. Indeed, while compulsiveness may be socially valuable, it is also personally expensive.

Self-doubt was a key characteristic that distinguished physicians from controls in a prospective study of men conducted by Vaillant and colleagues (1972). Their research also revealed that physicians who were front-line clinicians were more likely to have had emotionally impoverished childhoods than a control group of nonphysicians. Many physicians seem to feel that they did not receive the love they desired as a child, and they may work tirelessly with an unconscious fantasy that if they demonstrate enough self-sacrifice in their slavish devotion to their patients, they will finally achieve the approbation and admiration that they have long sought.

The second and third elements of the compulsive triad, guilt feelings and an exaggerated sense of responsibility, are intimately connected to self-doubt. Physicians are likely to blame themselves if a patient does poorly. They may become convinced that somehow they missed something that others would have noted, either in the diagnostic assessment or in the treatment planning. The tormenting self-blame characteristic of most physicians may reflect a response to a sense of helplessness and inadequacy. One reason for choosing medicine as a career may be a need to defend against a profound existential dread associated with feelings of impotence in the face of one's own death (Kasper, 1959; Krakowski, 1971). Physicians often harbor unconscious feelings of omnipotence in the form of exaggerated expectations. One of the great paradoxes of the physician is that those who feel most vulnerable to feelings of helplessness choose a profession that repeatedly reminds them of their impotence in the face of death and disease (Gabbard and Menninger, 1988).

Physicians' conflicts about their own aggression also enter into this pattern of compulsiveness. Because they have experienced their parents as lacking in the provision of adequate emotional nurturance, physicians often harbor resentment and rage at their parents. Strong, unfulfilled yearnings for dependency may coexist with this anger. Because both the dependent wishes and the rage are uncomfortable, the developing child may defend against them by reaction formation (that is, giving to others as a way of denying one's own neediness and anger). In fact, reaction formation was one of the chief defense mechanisms that differentiated physicians from controls in the study by Vaillant and colleagues. Through the selfless pursuit of helping others in a medical career, physicians may attempt to conquer their guilt for feeling angry at their parents (Gerber, 1983; Rhoads, 1977). Physicians may thus convince themselves that they have mastered their aggression by their altruistic daily behavior. As Karl Menninger (1957) noted, the practice of medicine affords "a unique opportunity to conceal conscious or unconscious sadism" (p. 101).

These factors all contribute to a fundamental insecurity in many physicians. They tend to be superego-ridden individuals with a desperate need to be needed. Long hours of overwork can be regarded as efforts to clear their consciences (Rhoads, 1977). In a study of 800 gifted men, Terman (1954) demonstrated that physicians as a group tend to feel inferior. Taking on more and more responsibility and exercising more and more self-denial are desperate measures to gain the approval they feel is so elusive. When physicians finally do receive praise and acclaim, they often find that they mistrust these expressions of gratitude and appreciation. Indeed, the physician's perfectionistic pursuit often seems to involve the hope for *relief* from relentless and tormenting superego demands rather than the experience of pleasure and a stable sense of self-esteem.

All of these characterological tendencies provide a fertile field for anxiety about malpractice litigation. Many physicians secretly lack self-confidence, no matter how many diplomas grace their office walls and no matter how impressive the respect of their colleagues. Daily reminders of fallibility haunt the physician. Hence nothing exposes the physician's fragile self-esteem so clearly as a malpractice suit. The thin veneer of self-confidence is pushed aside to reveal the underlying self-doubt and anxiety about self-worth and competence.

Some physicians live with a horror of being "found out." Their fundamental fraudulence will be laid bare. Their aggression will be unmasked. Their incompetence will be exposed. A lawsuit serves as a convenient nidus to externalize all of these internal fears because the threat of litigation may resonate so thoroughly with the physician's harsh superego. Even when colleagues are supportive, physicians who are sued may be convinced that they have been disgraced in the eyes of their colleagues. Many contemplate suicide as the only escape from the loss of face. In addition to realistic concerns, a malpractice suit often has the unconscious meaning of a transformation—the longed-for reward has become instead an accusation of incompetence. In the physician's heart, he or she may be convinced that the attack is well deserved.

Hypervigilance and Paranoia

If we understand that beneath the altruistic and well-intentioned motivations of the physician lurks a netherworld of anxieties, insecurities, and vulnerabilities, then we can appreciate why psychiatrists, like other physicians, dread the possibility of litigation. In a litigious era, psychiatrists may be so preoccupied with this fear that they begin practicing with a pervasive sense of hypervigilance. As one psychiatrist who had recently been sued put it, "With each new patient, the first question I ask myself is, 'Will this patient sue me?' " In this scenario the entire playing field of the doctor-patient relationship becomes radically shifted. Instead of seeing the patient as someone in need of help, the psychiatrist begins to see the patient as a persecutor. In this regard, the patient has become transformed into a part object rather than a whole person with a variety of conflicting feelings and motivations. A paranoid-schizoid ambiance is then jointly constructed by psychiatrist and patient as they proceed to scrutinize each other.

The concept of projective identification is a useful construct to understand communication between two individuals who are functioning in a paranoid-schizoid mode (Ogden, 1989). In this case, the psychiatrist projectively disavows an internal persecuting object (a more primitive version of the harsh superego), which is then placed in the patient where it can be controlled. Because of interpersonal pressure placed on the patient by the psychiatrist, the patient begins to identify (unconsciously) with the persecuting object that has been projected and begins to take on characteristics of that object. At the same time, the psychiatrist's hypervigilant behavior fosters a sense in the patient that he or she is being accused of something, so that in turn the patient begins to regard the psychiatrist as a potential persecutor. Hence the process can be characterized as akin to a situation where two mirrors reverberate with distorting reflections bouncing back and forth. A distorted image in one mirror leads to a slightly greater distortion in the opposite mirror and so on until the distortions have increased exponentially.

One of the damaging effects of these paranoid anxieties is that there is a self-fulfilling prophecy component to the process. In other words, if a patient is treated as a potential persecutor who may sue, the patient will genuinely begin to mistrust the psychiatrist and feel that the psychiatrist is not practicing with the patient's best interests in mind. The result may be an increase in the risk of litigation. In contemporary psychoanalytic thinking, the constructivist view of transference (Gill, 1994; Hoffman, 1983) has taught us that the patient's transference perceptions are partly based on the *real* behavior of the analyst. Accordingly, patients will develop paranoid transferences when psychiatrists behave toward them as though they are a threat. Moreover, part of this transference is that the psychiatrist is perceived as functioning in a self-preservative mode rather than an altruistic one. The patient has come in the role of a person needing help and finds that instead he or she is experienced as a potentially harmful person. This jarring realization subverts any semblance of a therapeutic alliance.

The mechanism described here paradoxically places the psychiatrist at increased risk for malpractice litigation. The commonplace wisdom that building a relationship of trust and a solid therapeutic alliance is the best prophylaxis against being sued continues to be a useful rule of thumb. The therapeutic alliance requires a sense of mutual collaboration of two partners in pursuit of a common goal. Mistrust on either side of the therapeutic dyad interferes with the formation of that alliance.

Fear of Boundary Violations

In recent years the psychiatric profession has come to a long overdue recognition that severe boundary violations, such as therapist-patient sex, can have a devastating impact on patients (Epstein, 1994; Gabbard, 1989; Gabbard and Lester, 1995; Gutheil, 1989; Gutheil and Gabbard, 1993; Simon, 1992). One of the unfortunate consequences of this heightened awareness in some quarters has been a countertransference rigidity that makes effective psychotherapy virtually impossible. Instead of regarding boundaries and the therapeutic frame as having an inherent flexibility, some psychiatrists have viewed them as encompassing a rigid set of absolute rules.

The therapeutic frame, and the professional boundaries that constitute the architecture of the frame, are not static constructs (Gabbard and Lester, 1995). They are best regarded as in a state of flux that varies with circumstances. Greenberg (1995) noted that there is an interactive matrix that serves to define the precise nature of the boundaries in each analytic dyad. Indeed, clinical experience suggests that we all shift flexibly with different patients based on our sense of the patient's needs. Hence we talk a little more with some patients, are a little more self-revealing with others, and somewhat more silent with still others. One reason that such flexibility is required is that varying degrees of "gratification" and "abstinence" have different meanings for different patients. Mitchell (1993), in advocating a flexible frame, made the following observation:

> It is apparent that one person's "firmness" is another's rigidity, and that one person's flexibility is another's "caving in." Both firmness and flexibility are important and should be among the considerations of any clinician struggling with these situations . . . The problem with the principle of standing firm is the assumption that it must mean to the patient what the analyst wants it to mean. Sometimes it does, and the patient feels encouraged by the analyst's ability to set limits, stand by his faith in the analytic process, resist allowing himself to be seduced into dangerous departures.
>
> However, while the analyst thinks she is standing firm, the patient may feel he is being brutalized in a very familiar fashion. Many patients are lost because they feel utterly abandoned or betrayed by analysts who think they are maintaining the purity of the analytic frame. The frame is preserved; the operation is a success; but the patient leaves, climbing off the operating table in the middle of the procedure. (p. 194)

This dilemma regarding the gratification-abstinence dialectic, often translated into flexibility versus rigidity, is particularly problematic with patients who suffer from borderline personality disorder. Many boundary violations that come to litigation involve such patients (Gabbard and Wilkinson, 1994; Gutheil, 1989). Setting "firm limits" on such patients may be a rationalization for an excessively rigid countertransference posture that grows out of a fear of the patient's intense object hunger. Therapists may make themselves emotionally unavailable to patients as a way of shoring up their own boundaries and assuring that they will not merge with the patient. As Lewin and Schulz (1992) observed, "The therapist presents the patient with a threat of loss in order to protect against what he sees as a dangerous invitation to fusion" (p. 80).

This posture of steely inaccessibility creates an impermeable membrane between patient and therapist. This very impenetrability creates formidable problems for the psychotherapy, because one of the fundamental paradoxes of the psychotherapeutic situation is that professional boundaries are maintained in order that both members of the dyad can cross the boundaries *psychologically* (Gabbard and Lester, 1995). A semipermeable membrane is necessary to facilitate empathy and projective identification.

In the psychotherapy of borderline patients, in particular, the therapist must be prepared to accept a variety of projections from the patient in order to make the treatment viable. A certain flexibility in the therapist's psychological penetrability is thus a requirement.

In the Menninger Treatment Interventions Project (Gabbard et al., 1994; Horwitz et al., 1996), we studied the impact of therapist interventions on the therapeutic alliance with borderline patients. One common technical error we observed in studying audiotaped transcripts of psychotherapy with borderline patients was the premature return of a "bad object projection." In other words, a therapist confronted with an intensely negative transference would attempt to "unload" the "bad object" by interpreting the projection and thus forcing it back down the patient's throat. The patient was unprepared to accept the projection and began to experience the therapist as a persecutor who could not be trusted. On the other hand, when a therapist could tolerate being cast in the role of "bad object," the patient ultimately could take the projection back on his or her own time schedule and could therefore use the therapist as an effective container of unacceptable aspects of the self.

Casement (1990) made the following observation: "Paradoxically, a part of the consistency that a patient needs from the analyst is that of *empathic responsiveness* to changing needs, which means the analyst sometimes is adaptive to the patient rather than remaining rigidly the same" (p. 333). He emphasized that there are important growth needs in borderline patients that must be acknowledged and facilitated through what is generally referred to as a holding environment. Partial transference gratifications are inevitable in the psychotherapy of borderline patients, and the therapist must be prepared to be "sucked in" to the patient's internal world to understand fully what the patient's experience is like. Countertransference enactments are now viewed as inevitable and potentially useful, if they can be discussed and understood (Gabbard, 1995; Jacobs, 1986; McLaughlin, 1991; Renik, 1993). Sometimes a therapist may feel that he or she has gone too far in the direction coerced by the patient, but the era of the "blank screen" therapist is over, and attempting to practice with the detachment of a surgeon may ultimately be riskier than becoming engaged at a psychological level with the patient's internal world.

Fear of Suicide

The impact of a patient's suicide on the treating psychiatrist may be devastating. Stress levels comparable to persons recovering from a parent's death are often experienced by psychiatrists after a patient has committed suicide

(Chemtob et al., 1988). The compulsive triad of self-doubt, guilt feelings, and exaggerated sense of responsibility is often activated by such events. Psychiatrists search their minds in the aftermath of suicide for what they might have missed. What subtle clue did the patient mention in the last interchange that suicide might be imminent? What errors of judgment were made in not hospitalizing the patient? And last but not least, will I be sued by the patient's family?

A vast discrepancy exists between the approach of a plaintiff's attorney and the clinical reality of suicide. While the plaintiff's attorney assumes that suicides are preventable and the psychiatrist must be at fault for not taking appropriate measures to prevent the suicide, the clinician knows that patients who truly want to kill themselves will ultimately do it regardless of psychiatric intervention. Clinicians also are aware that no one can predict which patient will commit suicide and which patient will only talk about it rather than act on it. In a study of 1,906 inpatients with affective disorders, Goldstein and colleagues (1991) used data on risk factors to attempt to develop a statistical model that would successfully predict suicide. Despite the best data available and a highly sophisticated computer model, the researchers failed to identify a single patient who committed suicide. They concluded that even when evaluating a high-risk group of inpatients, the prediction of suicide is not possible.

Nevertheless, psychiatrists berate themselves after a suicide and worry that their colleagues are viewing them as incompetent. Because of the narcissistic wound associated with a patient's suicide, many psychiatrists treat suicidal patients with round-the-clock observation by special nurses, physical restraints, and seclusion on inpatient units. The patient may never be given an opportunity to be alone long enough for suicide to be possible. However, intensive structure of this kind will not prevent suicides from ultimately occurring, and it may even give the patient the wrong message—that someone else, not the patient, is ultimately responsible for preventing suicide. In fact, Olin (1976) opined that if suicides never occur in a particular hospital, the treating staff are probably taking too much responsibility for the patients' behavior.

In outpatient settings as well as in hospital treatment, clinicians may unwittingly increase the chances of their patients' killing themselves if they are too fearful of that prospect. A number of observers (Gabbard, 1994; Hendin, 1982; Meissner, 1986; Richman and Eyman, 1990; Searles, 1979; Zee, 1972) have noted that when treaters fall prey to the illusion that they can actually save their patients from suicide, they may paradoxically be decreasing their chances of doing so. Much of this understanding grows out of the psychodynamics of the suicidal patient. A prominent psychological wish in the seriously suicidal patient is to have an unconditionally loving mother take care of every need (Richman and Eyman, 1990). Excessively fearful clinicians may attempt to gratify this fantasy by being available for phone calls at any time of the day or night and even during vacation periods. They may see their patient every day in the office and make a clear communication to the patient that they will become the unconditionally loving parent. Hendin (1982) has cautioned that this type of behavior exacerbates one of the most lethal features of some suicidal patients, which is their tendency to assign others the responsibility for their staying alive. Therapists who attempt to become the ever-present and unconditionally loving parent will find that this illusion is impossible to sustain, thus setting up the patient for a shattering disappointment that may increase the risk of suicide.

When clinicians are drawn into the role of savior, they are operating on the assumption that their provision of love and concern may somehow magically transform the patient's wish to commit suicide into a wish to live. Hendin has issued a cautionary statement regarding this assumption: "The patient's hidden agenda is an attempt to prove that nothing the therapist can do will be enough. The therapist's wish to see himself as the suicidal patient's savior may blind the therapist to the fact that the patient has cast him in the role of executioner" (pp. 171–172).

Suicidal patients remind us of our limitations. They can generate enormous hatred and anger in us that may coexist with the wish to rescue. Maltsberger and Buie (1974) warned that if clinicians cannot tolerate their own sadistic wishes toward such patients, they may be prone to act on countertransference feelings in a variety of ways, including forgetting to check on the patient, forgetting a patient's appointment, or subtly encouraging despair and hopelessness. When the countertransference hate is split off and disavowed, it may be projected onto the patient, who then must somehow manage the therapist's murderous wishes in addition to the preexisting suicidal impulses. When the therapist is using reaction formation to deny any sadistic wishes, Searles (1979) has described the following scenario:

> And the suicidal patient, who finds us so unable to be aware of the murderous feelings he fosters in us through his guilt- and anxiety-producing threats of suicide, feels increasingly constricted, perhaps indeed to the point of suicide, by the therapist, who, in reaction formation against his intensifying, unconscious wishes to kill the patient, hovers increasingly "protectively" about the latter, for whom he feels an omnipotent-based physicianly concern. Hence it is, paradoxically, the very physician most anxiously concerned to *keep the pa-*

tient alive who tends most vigorously, at an unconscious level, to drive him to what has come to seem the only autonomous act left to him—namely, suicide. (p. 74)

The fearful psychiatrist may discourage the patient from talking openly about fantasies of suicide and the meanings connected with those fantasies. The therapist may think that the goal is to get the patient to stop talking about suicide when in fact, that goal is more related to the therapist's needs than the patient's needs. Some patients may need to hang on to suicidality as a *thought* that does not actually lead to action because it provides them with an escape valve from an unbearable reality (Gabbard and Wilkinson, 1994; Lewin and Schulz, 1992). The therapist needs to empathize with the valuable psychological functions that suicidality may serve for the patient. Often the recognition of the adaptive aspect of suicide helps the patient feel understood and therefore less likely to act on the suicidal wishes. Nietzsche is alleged to have said, "The thought of suicide has saved many lives."

Many therapists have found that an open admission of their limits may be therapeutically useful. Henseler (1991) suggested that when a therapist acknowledges that he or she cannot stop a patient from committing suicide, there is often a calming effect. Such an acknowledgment may also lead to a greater collaboration in the psychotherapeutic task of understanding why the patient thinks that suicide is the only option.

/ / /

Much of my discussion has focused on dynamics in the psychotherapeutic setting. However, everything I have said applies equally to the psychiatrist prescribing medication for a patient. Pharmacotherapists who are terribly afraid of the harm they may do to patients and their subsequent vulnerability to lawsuit may deprive patients of much-needed treatment and expose them to the perils of *not* receiving adequate treatment. Many psychiatrists are afraid to prescribe clozapine, for example, because of an approximately 1 percent incidence of agranulocytosis in clozapine-treated patients. Nevertheless, considering the remarkable improvement seen in a substantial percentage of treatment-resistant schizophrenic patients who receive the drug, failure to prescribe clozapine out of fear may consign a patient to a virtual prison of psychotic torment, which may in turn lead to suicide, which occurs at a rate in schizophrenia second only to that of major depression (Roy, 1986). In fact, Meltzer and Okayli (1995) noted that clozapine treatment resulted in markedly less suicidality in a cohort of 88 neuroleptic-resistant patients treated with clozapine and prospectively evaluated for suicidality. The number of suicide attempts with a high probability of success decreased from five to zero. The researchers concluded that the overall morbidity and mortality of patients treated with clozapine may actually be less because the decreased risk of suicidality offsets the risk of agranulocytosis.

I have covered only a small sample of clinical situations where fear is the greatest obstacle to competent and sensitive clinical practice. The same principles can be applied to numerous other situations in a psychiatrist's practice. For example, the risk of suicide by refraining from the use of clozapine is analogous to the risk of suicide inherent in the psychotically depressed individual who may not receive electroconvulsive therapy when it is desperately needed.

In the practice of modern psychiatry, certainty is an elusive commodity. There is no risk-free clinical setting. Clearly the most sensible course is to build a solid therapeutic alliance in which the various treatment options are frankly discussed in terms of their benefits and risks for the patient. In the context of a good alliance, clinician and patient collaborate in assuming a shared risk while also hoping for an optimal outcome. In the final analysis, excessive fear in the clinician may be a much greater liability risk than adverse outcomes in the context of a good working relationship with the patient. However, by pursuing the instructions of the distinguished contributors to this book, the clinician will doubly benefit from a reduced risk of legal liability while enhancing patient care.

References

Casement, P. J. (1990). "The Meeting of the Needs in Psychoanalysis." *Psychoanalytic Inquiry* 10: 325–346.

Chemtob, C. M., et al. (1988). "Patients' Suicides: Frequency and Impact on Psychiatrists." *American Journal of Psychiatry* 145: 224–228.

Epstein, R. S. (1994). *Keeping Boundaries: Maintaining Safety and Integrity in the Psychotherapeutic Process*. Washington: American Psychiatric Press.

Gabbard, G. O. (1985). "The Role of Compulsiveness in the Normal Physician." *JAMA* 254, no. 20: 2926–29.

Gabbard, G. O. (1989). *Sexual Exploitation in Professional Relationships*. Washington: American Psychiatric Press.

Gabbard, G. O. (1994). *Psychodynamic Psychiatry in Clinical Practice: The DSM-IV Edition*. Washington: American Psychiatric Press.

Gabbard, G. O. (1995). "Countertransference: The Emerging Common Ground." *International Journal of Psychoanalysis* 76: 475–485.

Gabbard, G. O., et al. (1994). "Transference Interpretation in the Psychotherapy of Borderline Patients: A High-risk, High-gain Phenomenon." *Harvard Review of Psychiatry* 2: 59–69.

Gabbard, G. O., and E. P. Lester (1995). *Boundaries and Boundary Violations in Psychoanalysis*. New York: Basic Books.

Gabbard, G. O., and R. W. Menninger (1988). *Medical Marriages*. Washington: American Psychiatric Press.

Gabbard G. O., and S. M. Wilkinson (1994). *Management of Countertransference with Borderline Patients*. Washington: American Psychiatric Press.

Gerber, L. A. (1983). *Married to Their Careers: Career and Family Dilemmas in Doctors' Lives*. New York: Tavistock.

Gill, M. M. (1994). *Psychoanalysis in Transition: A Personal View*. Hillsdale, N.J.: Analytic Press.

Goldstein, R. B., et al. (1991). "The Prediction of Suicide: Sensitivity, Specificity, and Predictive Value of a Multimyriad Model Applied to Suicide among 1,906 Patients with Affective Disorders." *Archives of General Psychiatry* 48: 418–422.

Greenberg, J. R. (1995). "Psychoanalytic Technique and the Interactive Matrix." *Psychoanalytic Quarterly* 64: 1–22.

Gutheil, T. G. (1989). "Borderline Personality Disorder, Boundary Violations, and Patient-Therapist Sex: Medicolegal Pitfalls." *American Journal of Psychiatry* 146: 597–602.

Gutheil, T. G., and G. O. Gabbard (1993). "The Concept of Boundaries in Clinical Practice: Theoretical and Risk-management Dimensions." *American Journal of Psychiatry* 150: 188–196.

Hendin, H. (1982). "Psychotherapy and Suicide." In Hendin, *Suicide in America*. New York: Norton.

Henseler, H. (1991). "Narcissism as a Form of Relationship." In *Freud's "On Narcissism": An Introduction*, ed. J. Sandler, E. S. Person, and P. Fonagy. New Haven: Yale University Press.

Hoffman, I. Z. (1983). "The Patient as Interpreter of the Analyst's Experience." *Contemporary Psychoanalysis* 19: 389–422.

Horwitz, L., et al. (1996). *Borderline Personality Disorder: Tailoring the Psychotherapy to the Patient*. Washington: American Psychiatric Press.

Jacobs, T. J. (1986). "On Countertransference Enactments." *Journal of the American Psychoanalytic Association* 34: 289–307.

Kasper, A. (1959). "The Doctor and Death." In *The Meaning of Death*, ed. H. Feifel. New York: McGraw-Hill.

Krakowski, A. J. (1971). "Doctor-Doctor Relationship." *Psychosomatics* 12: 11–15.

Krakowski, A. J. (1982). "Stress and the Practice of Medicine: II. Stressors, Stresses, and Strains." *Psychotherapy and Psychosomatics* 38: 11–23.

Krell, R., and J. Miles (1976). "Marital Therapy of Couples in Which the Husband Is a Physician." *American Journal of Psychotherapy* 30: 267–275.

Lewin, R. A., and C. G. Schulz (1992). *Losing and Fusing: Borderline and Transitional Object and Self Relations.* Northvale, N.J.: Jason Aronson.

McLaughlin, J. T. (1991). "Clinical and Theoretical Aspects of Enactment." *Journal of the American Psychoanalytic Association* 39: 595–614.

Maltsberger, J. T., and D. H. Buie (1974). "Countertransference Hate in the Treatment of Suicidal Patients." *Archives of General Psychiatry* 30: 625–633.

Meissner, W. W. (1986). *Psychotherapy and the Paranoid Process.* Northvale, N.J.: Jason Aronson.

Meltzer, H. Y., and G. Okayli (1995). "Reduction of Suicidality during Clozapine Treatment of Neuroleptic-resistant Schizophrenia: Impact on Risk-Benefit Assessment." *American Journal of Psychiatry* 152: 183–190.

Menninger, K. A. (1957). "Psychological Factors in the Choice of Medicine as a Profession, Part II." *Bulletin of the Menninger Clinic* 21: 99–106.

Mitchell, S. A. (1993). *Hope and Dread in Psychoanalysis.* New York: Basic Books.

Ogden, T. H. (1989). *The Primitive Edge of Experience.* Northvale, N.J.: Jason Aronson.

Olin, H. S. (1976). "Psychotherapy of the Chronically Suicidal Patient." *American Journal of Psychotherapy* 30: 570–575.

Renik, O. (1993). "Analytic Interaction: Conceptualizing Technique in Light of the Analyst's Irreducible Subjectivity." *Psychoanalytic Quarterly* 62: 553–571.

Rhoads, J. (1977). "Overwork." *JAMA* 237: 2615–2618.

Richman, J., and J. R. Eyman (1990). "Psychotherapy of Suicide: Individual, Group, and Family Approaches." In *Understanding Suicide: The State of the Art,* ed. D. Lester. Philadelphia: Charles C. Thomas.

Roy, A. (1986). "Depression, Attempted Suicide and Suicide in Patients with Chronic Schizophrenia." *Psychiatric Clinics of North America* 9: 193–206.

Searles, H. F. (1979). "The 'Dedicated Physician' in the Field of Psychotherapy and Psychoanalysis." In Searles, *Countertransference and Related Subjects.* Madison, Conn.: International Universities Press.

Simon, R. I. (1992). "Treatment Boundary Violations: Clinical, Ethical, and Legal Considerations." *Bulletin of the American Academy of Psychiatry and the Law* 20: 269–288.

Terman, L. M. (1954). "Scientists and Non-scientists in a Group of 800 Gifted Men." *Psychological Monographs* 68: 1–44.

Vaillant, G. E., N. C. Sobowale, and C. McArthur (1972). "Some Psychological Vulnerabilities of Physicians." *New England Journal of Medicine* 287: 372–375.

Waring, E. M. (1974). "Psychiatric Illness in Physicians: A Review." *Comprehensive Psychiatry* 15: 519–530.

Zee, H. J. (1972). "Blindspots in Recognizing Serious Suicidal Intentions." *Bulletin of the Menninger Clinic* 36: 551–555.

///CONTRIBUTORS

PRUDENCE BAXTER, M.D.: Clinical Instructor in Psychiatry, Harvard Medical School; Director, Cambridge Court Clinic.

JAMES BECK, M.D., Ph.D.: Associate Professor of Psychiatry, Harvard Medical School; Associate Chairman, Department of Psychiatry, The Cambridge Hospital; author, *Confidentiality versus the Duty to Protect*.

CLYDE D. BERGSTRESSER, J.D.: Senior Partner, Bergstresser and Associates.

MARILYN BERNER, J.D., LICSW: Lecturer on Psychiatry, Harvard Medical School; Staff, Law and Psychiatry Services, Massachusetts General Hospital.

HON. JONATHAN BRANT: Lecturer in Psychiatry, Tufts University School of Medicine; Justice, Massachusetts District Court, Cambridge Division; author, *Law and Mental Health Professionals: Massachusetts*, 2nd ed.

RENEE TANKENOFF BRANT, M.D.: Assistant Clinical Professor of Psychiatry, Harvard Medical School; Supervisor and Lecturer, Children's Hospital, Boston.

TROYEN BRENNAN, M.D., J.D., MPH: Professor of Medicine, Harvard Medical School; Professor of Law and Public Health, Harvard School of Public Health; Division of General and Primary Medicine, Brigham and Women's Hospital, Boston.

ARCHIE BRODSKY, B.A.: Research Associate in Psychiatry (Law), Harvard Medical School, Program in Psychiatry and the Law, Massachusetts Mental Health Center.

HAROLD J. BURSZTAJN, M.D.: Associate Clinical Professor of Psychiatry, Harvard Medical School; Co-Director, Program in Psychiatry and the Law, Massachusetts Mental Health Center; coauthor, *Divided Staffs, Divided Selves: A Case Approach to Mental Health Ethics*, and *Medical Choices, Medical Chances: How Patients, Physicians, and Families Can Cope with Uncertainty*.

GLEN O. GABBARD, M.D.: Callaway Distinguished Professor of Psychoanalysis and Education, Menninger Clinic, Topeka, Kansas; Training and Supervising Analyst, Topeka Institute for Psychoanalysis; Clinical Professor of Psychiatry, University of Kansas School of Medicine; author or editor of twelve books, including *Boundaries and Boundary Violations in Psychoanalysis* and *Love and Hate in the Analytic Setting*.

DAVID GOULD, J.D.: Senior Partner, Ficksman and Conley.

THOMAS G. GUTHEIL, M.D.: Professor of Psychiatry, Harvard Medical School; Co-Director, Program in Psychiatry and the Law, Massachusetts Mental Health Center; coauthor, *The Clinical Handbook of*

Psychiatry and the Law; Divided Staffs, Divided Selves: A Case Approach to Mental Health Ethics; The Psychiatrist in Court: A Survival Guide; and *The Psychiatrist as Expert Witness.*

JAMES HILLIARD, J.D.: Lecturer on Law and Psychiatry, Department of Psychiatry, Harvard Medical School; General Counsel, Massachusetts Psychiatric Society; Partner, Conner and Hilliard.

LAWRENCE E. LIFSON, M.D.: Lecturer on Psychiatry, Harvard Medical School; Associate Clinical Professor of Psychiatry, Tufts University School of Medicine; Director, Continuing Education, Massachusetts Mental Health Center; faculty, Boston Psychoanalytic Institute; editor, *Understanding Therapeutic Action: Psychodynamic Concepts of Cure;* coeditor, *The Psychology of Investing* (forthcoming).

HON. KERMIT V. LIPEZ: Justice, Supreme Court of Maine.

PEGGY BERRY MARTIN, M.Ed., A.R.M.: Director of Education, Harvard Risk Management Foundation.

ALAN W. SCHEFLIN, J.D., L.L.M.: Professor of Law, Santa Clara University Law School; coauthor, *The Mind Manipulators; Trance on Trial;* and *Memory, Trauma Treatment, and the Law.*

ROBERT I. SIMON, M.D.: Clinical Professor of Psychiatry and Director, Program in Psychiatry and Law, Georgetown University School of Medicine; author, *Bad Men Do What Good Men Dream; Clinical Psychiatry and the Law* (now in its second edition); and *Concise Guide to Psychiatry and Law for Clinicians;* coauthor, *Psychiatric Malpractice: Cases and Comments for Clinicians;* editor, *Review of Clinical Psychiatry and the Law.*

LARRY H. STRASBURGER, M.D.: Associate Clinical Professor of Psychiatry, Harvard Medical School; Associate in the Program in Psychiatry and the Law, Massachusetts Mental Health Center.

RICHARD WARING, J.D.: Complaint Counsel, Massachusetts Board of Registration in Medicine.

///INDEX

Abandonment, 47, 147; referral viewed as, 49; termination of treatment viewed as, 216-217, 220; claim of, in malpractice litigation, 217, 218–220, 221, 237, 238, 239, 255–256, 257; legal concept of, 217–220

Abstinence, principle of, 197–198, 204

Abuse, 283. *See also* Child abuse/sexual abuse

Abusive patients, 242–243, 257

Access to patient records, 52, 75, 79, 83. *See also* Confidentiality

Accident law, 8

Acting out by therapists, 205–206, 212

Administrative costs, 17–18

Admissibility: of evidence/testimony, 262–264, 292; of expert testimony, 302, 308

Admitting privileges, 121

Adoption, 283

Advance directives, 41

Adversary system, 299, 304, 307–308

Adverse events: iatrogenic injury, 9–11; negligence as, 11; ratio of, to claims, 12, 13–14; medical costs of, 14–18; patient/physician relationship and, 92

Advertising by attorneys, 250–251

Advocacy, 239, 240; by expert witnesses, 289–290; in psychiatric practice, 313; role of therapist, 313

Affidavits, 234, 352

Aftercare, 130

Aggression of physicians, 372–373

Aiken v. Clary, 24, 25, 27

Althaus v. Cohen, 315–316

American Academy of Psychiatry and the Law, 274

American Bar Association Model Rules of Professional Conduct, 321

American College of Surgeons, 91

American Medical Association (AMA), 119, 128

American Psychiatric Association (APA), 105; Professional Liability Insurance Program, 117–118; position on duty to report impaired patients, 122–123; guidelines for psychiatric signatures, 147; code of ethics for boundary violations, 149, 336–337

Anonymity of therapists, 198, 208–209

Apology statutes, 260–261

Appeal rights, 48–49

Argus v. Scheppegrell, 120

Arrogance: of physician, 253, 258, 267; of witnesses, 355

Assault and battery: laws, 23, 24–25; by a patient, 66–67

Attorneys: consultation with expert witnesses, 286–290; referral by, 287; defense strategies, 299; distortion of the truth and, 305–307; consultation with, 339; as advocates, 347; working with, 348–356

Authorization to release information, 172

Autonomy of the patient, 199, 204, 205, 207, 245, 304

Battered child syndrome, 300–301. *See also* Child abuse/sexual abuse

Bean-Bayog, Margaret, 106

Bias, 321, 337

Billing practices. *See* Fees

Blue Cross/Blue Shield organizations, 58

Board of Registration in Medicine (Massachusetts), 91, 101, 103–104, 106

Borawick v. Shay, 263

Borderline patients, 376–377

Boston Psychoanalytic Institute, 106

Boundaries: setting and maintenance of, 92, 196–197, 200–201, 211; patient-physician, in psychotherapy, 106; exceptions, 195–196, 201–202; brief crossings of, 196; restitution of breached, 196, 200, 211; principles underlying, 197–200; therapeutic intervention and, 198–199, 206; crossings of, 200, 201–202; guidelines, 200–201

Boundary violations, 117, 118, 344; claim of, in malpractice litigation, 1, 96, 197, 200, 212, 338–339, 344, 345; in child and adolescent therapy, 85–86; in psychiatric practice, 117, 118; in supervisory arrangements, 149–151; ethics of, 195, 200, 212; progressive, 196, 201, 206–207, 210–212; effect on quality of care, 201; in times of crisis, 201–202, 206; involving prescription medications, 205; in managed care facilities, 206; money-driven, 209; prevention of, 211–212; physical contact, 300; sexual exploitation, 331; sexual relations with current patients, 331, 338; sexual relations with former patients, 336–337; documentation as risk-prevention strategy, 345; fear of, 375–377

Bradshaw v. Daniel, 341

Brainwashing, 320

Brandt v. Grubin, 219

Bridgewater State Hospital (Massachusetts), 330

Burger, Warren, 305

California Medical Association Insurance Feasibility study, 8, 10, 12

Canterbury v. Spence, 25–27, 34, 40, 129

Capitation agreements, 336, 341, 348. *See also* Malpractice insurance companies

Care: impact of lawsuits on, 2; continuity of, 70; effect of loss-prevention efforts on, 92–93, 98; value of claims data in improvement efforts, 93–94; appropriate, 130; effect of boundary violations on, 201

Caryl S. v. Child and Adolescent Treatment Services, 313–315

Causation judgment, 9

Cause of action in malpractice litigation, 218

Certification, 102–103, 135

Child abuse/sexual abuse, 72, 84; mandatory reporting of, 52, 72, 77; confidentiality issues and, 77, 80; claim of, in malpractice litigation, 80, 132–136, 263; liability issues, 84–85; recovered memories of, 117, 132–136, 263; truth about, 301–302, 309–317; false accusations of, 309–317, 323

Child and adolescent therapy: confidentiality issues, 72–73, 75–78; informed consent issues, 72, 73–74; parents' involvement in, 72, 73–74, 75; risk management, 72–80, 84–85, 86–87; role of therapist in legal proceedings, 73; documentation, 74–75; malpractice considerations, 80–82; role of therapist in, 80–82, 83–84; liability of therapist in high-conflict divorce, 82–84; trauma and sexual abuse liability issues, 84–85; juvenile delinquents and offenders, 85; boundary violations and, 85–86

Child Behavior Checklist, 262

Child protection statutes, 77

Children: informed consent to medical treatment and, 41–43; privacy rights of, 65; custody of, 73, 80, 83, 283, 312–314; prescription medications for, 127

Christy v. Saliterman, 122

Chronic illness, 16, 37–38, 242; competence issues and, 37–38

"Circle of confidentiality," 65

Civil litigation, 282–283, 342

Civil rights violations, 331

Claims data, 93–96

Class action suits, 330–331

Clinician in court: as defendant, 2, 8, 80, 81, 84; testimonial privilege and, 78–80; as consultant, 82; conflict-of-interest issues, 133–134; roles of, 133–134, 225–226; as plaintiff, 228; depositions, 231–234; trial procedures, 235–236. *See also* Expert witnesses; Fact witnesses; Testimony; Witnesses

Clinics, 91

Coddington v. Robertson, 218

Collaboration of caregivers, 96–98. *See also* Medical backup

Compensation for injuries, 8, 11, 12, 14–19, 252

Competence: issues in informed consent, 34–38; guardians/conservators and, 35, 37, 38; testimonial capacity, 35, 37; elements of, 36–37; chronic illness and, 37–38; involuntary commitment and, 39–41; documentation of, 55–58; issues in contracts against suicide, 178, 180; to terminate treatment, 210; to consent to treatment, 247; evaluations of, 283

Comprehensive Drug Abuse Prevention and Control Act, 190

Computer(s): documentation, 69–70; programs for medical decisionmaking, 147–148

Confidentiality, 81; conflict with the law, 2; documentation of treatment and, 50–53, 61–65, 69–70, 79–80; managed care liability and, 50–53, 238; waiver of right to, 51, 62, 221; as distinct from privilege, in patient records, 61–64; denied to insured patients, 63; exceptions to, 63, 76, 77–78, 85; circle of, 65; of computerized documentation, 69–70; in child and adolescent therapy, 75–76; mandatory reporting and, 77, 337; vs. duty to warn or protect, 77–78; issues in high-conflict divorce cases, 83; in claims data, 94; breach of, 156, 339; boundary violations and, 195, 202, 205; in treatment settings, 210; termination of treatment and, 221; expert witnesses and, 229; agreements, 341, 342

Confinement of mental patients, 330

Conflict of interest, 133–134, 348; in child and adolescent therapy, 81; expert witnesses and, 230; third-party liability and, 314

Consent. See Informed consent

Consultants/consultation, 136; patient identity and, 53; model of supervision, 141, 142–143; in supervisory arrangements, 146–148, 151; concerning boundary violations, 150, 211, 212; forensic psychiatric, 247–248; psychiatric, 281, 282–283; forensic, 283, 284, 286–290; ethical obligations of, 289–290

Consumer protection legislation, 63

Contract(s): actions, 45, 62; third-party, 45–46, 49–50, 53, 131; breach of, 62, 178; treatment, 76; therapeutic, 83–84; managed care, 135; medical backup, 144; fee agreements, 287; for forensic consultation, 288; confidentiality agreements, 341, 342. See also Suicide risk: contracts against suicide

Controlled Risk Insurance Company, 96, 99n9

Cooper, Jeffrey, 96

Costs: of patient injury, 14–18; health care, 16; of psychiatric malpractice, 17; containment vs. standards of care, 44, 46–48, 209, 220, 237

Countertransference, 86, 151, 201, 207, 211, 212, 375, 376; enactments, 377, 379

Court(s): decisions and directives, 2, 9; protective orders, 51, 77–78; orders to provide patient records, 51–52, 75, 79–80; testimonial privilege statutes, 78–80

Credibility. See Testimony: credibility of

Criminal litigation, 281, 285

Crisis situations, 211, 329; confidentiality issues and, 64–65; informed consent issues and, 74; boundary violations during, 201–202, 206

Custody of children, 73, 80, 83, 283, 312–314

Danzon, Patricia, 8, 11–13, 15

Data bank information about physicians, 112, 350

Daubert v. Merrell Dow Pharmaceuticals, Inc., 262, 263–264, 267, 278, 302, 308

Death. See Wrongful death

Decision trees, 54, 55, 270

"Deep pockets" principle, 140, 141, 299

Defensive medicine, 2, 18, 125, 254–255, 257

Defensive psychiatry, 126, 134, 182, 183

Deinstitutionalization, 330

Depositions, 231–234, 296, 344, 347, 365–366; as testimony, 351–352; predeposition conferences, 352–353; vs. trial testimony, 366

Diagnosis: compromised by sexual boundary violations, 202; misdiagnosis or failure to diagnose, 243, 260; negligent misdiagnosis, 314–315

Diamond, Bernard L., 307

Disability: adverse events and, 9–11, 16; distinguished from preexisting disease, 16, 17; claims, 283–284, 288

Disabled abuse, 52

Disciplinary action against physicians. See Licensing boards: disciplinary function

Disclosure: issues, 24, 25–27, 37; written agreement, 64; of sexual abuse, 84; of financial incentives for withholding care, 342

Discovery process, 52, 231, 338, 351, 365–366, 368

Divided treatment. *See* Medical backup

Divorce, 283; child and adolescent therapy and, 72–73, 75, 80; high-conflict, 80, 82–84

Documentation (general discussion), 134, 135, 136; of patient competence, 55–58; objectivity in, 66–67; changing entries, 67–68; computerized, 69–70; of drug prescriptions, 119, 125, 129, 190, 191–192; of prescription medications, 119, 125, 129, 190, 191–192; of boundary violations, 345; terminology, 345; of sexual abuse cases, 347

Documentation of treatment: "write smarter not longer" strategy, 54–60, 65–67; progress vs. process notes, 57–60, 61; use of forms, 59–60; for trial proceedings, 60–61, 68, 69, 290, 342–434; confidentiality issues, 61–65, 69–70; informed-consent issues, 63, 345; institutional incidence reports, 66; failure to keep notes, 68–70; as risk-prevention strategy, 74–75, 345, 347, 355; in managed care facilities, 244

Domestic violence, 72

Dooley v. Skodnek, 120

Drug: trials, 34; distribution laws, 110; manufacturers, 118; tolerance, 119, 121; abuse programs, 195

Drug Enforcement Agency (DEA), 110; prescription medication regulations, 187, 191–193

Drugs. *See* Prescription medications

Due process hearings, 52

Duty of care, 118, 132; for suicidal patients, 177, 179; boundary violations and, 197; fiduciary, 199–200; for incompetent patients, 219

Duty to protect, 52, 77–78, 85, 131, 338, 339–340; from violent patients, 202. *See also* Duty to warn

Duty to treat. *See* Duty to care

Duty to warn, 52, 77–78, 85, 131, 339–340; regarding violent patients, 202; third parties, 300, 314; of risk of con-

tracting a contagious disease, 341. *See also Tarasoff v. Regents of the University of California*

Edwards v. United States, 118

Eichhorn, John, 96

Elder abuse, 52, 310

Emancipated minor doctrine, 42, 74

Emergencies. *See* Crisis situations

Employee Retirement Income Security Act (ERISA), 132

Entitlement, 250, 251

Ethics: violations, 62; standards of conduct, 105–106; of physicians in managed care facilities, 239; expert witnesses and, 287; in law, 305, 321; in mental health professions, 314, 323, 337; of patients, 338–339. *See also* Boundaries

Evaluations: clinical, 81, 83, 84, 288–289; performance, 141; psychiatric, 171, 283; of expert witnesses, 263; of competence, 283

Experimental and research procedures, 300; informed consent and, 33–34, 41

Expert testimony, 2, 25, 27, 352; on standards of care, 48; on behalf of current patient, 288; admissibility of, 302, 308; scientific, 308

Expert witnesses, 269, 296–297, 350; clinicians as, 2, 25, 98, 118, 132; role of, 133–134, 228–229, 230, 281, 285, 358–362; as fact witnesses, 227, 229–231, 263, 358–359; treating physicians/therapists as, 229–231, 285, 338; conflict-of-interest issues, 230; evaluation of, 263; consultants as, 267, 281, 282–283; fees paid to, 274, 285, 287, 288, 295, 368; law-vs.-psychiatry considerations, 282; contexts of litigation and, 282–284; psychiatric evaluations provided by, 283; legal definitions used by, 284–286; defined, 285–286; effectiveness of, 285–286; consultation with attorney, 286–290; ethics and, 287; qualification of, 287, 292–293; as distinct from clinicians, 288; as advocates, 289–290; pretrial conference, 290–291; direct examination of, 293–294; cross-examination of, 294–296, 353–354, 368; distortion of the truth and, 322; bias of, 337, 361; jury instruction regard-

ing, 358, 359–360; deposition of, 365–366. *See also* Expert testimony; Fact witnesses
Exploitation Index, 211

Fact witnesses: treating physicians as, 2, 226–228, 262, 263, 265, 268–269, 358–359; expert witnesses as, 227, 229–231, 263, 358–359; psychiatric, 285; defined, 285–286; jury instruction regarding, 358–359, 360; role of, 358–362; deposition of, 365–366. *See also* Expert witnesses; Witnesses
Failure: to report, 310 (*see also* Mandatory reporting); to warn, 331; to protect, 333; to treat, 333
False-memory syndrome, 316, 320, 322, 323, 341. *See also* Child abuse/sexual abuse
Families: limited drug prescriptions for, 110–111; litigation-prone, 133, 242–243, 247; patient/physician relationship and, 135–136; guilt in, 248, 256
Federal Licensing Examination (FLEX), 103, 104
Federation of State Medical Boards, 102, 103, 112
Fees: billing guidelines for physicians, 107; contingency, 287, 332; billing sent after an adverse event, 346
Fifth Pathway Programs, 103–104
Fitrak v. United States, 120
Food and Drug Administration (FDA), 119, 126–128
Forced seclusion, 331
Forensic psychiatry, 177, 246, 270; consultations and evaluations, 81–82, 83, 283, 284, 286–290; model, 284–285, 290
Foreseeability: of suicide, 167–168, 171; of harm to third parties, 314, 339–341; and failure-to-warn litigation, 339–340
Fragmented care, 121
Frankel, Marvin, 304
Freedman, Monroe H., 304, 321
Fromm-Reichman, Freida, 211

Gestalt therapy, 201
Gier v. Educational Serv. Unit No 16, 263
Government regulation of medical practice. *See* Licensing boards
Grievance procedures, 49

Guardian ad litem, 38, 79, 83, 225–226. *See also* Competence: guardians/conservators and
Guilt: of clinician/physician, 245–246, 259–261, 372; of family, 248, 256; as basis for malpractice litigation, 252–253, 256; over patient suicide, 378
Gunshot/knife wounds, mandatory reporting of, 52, 310
Gutheil, Thomas, 65, 294, 301, 315

Harlan, John Marshall, 305–306
Harvard Law School, 8, 281
Harvard Medical Practice Study (New York hospitals), 8–9, 18–19; iatrogenic injuries and, 9–11; litigation records, 11–14; costs of patient injury, 14–18; negligence rates/claims ratio, 93, 256
Harvard Medical School, 8; Department of Continuing Education, 2–3; Program in Psychiatry and the Law, 256
Harvard School of Public Health, 8
Harvard teaching hospitals, 96
Hawker v. New York, 101–102, 111
Health care delivery, 91, 140
Health Care Quality Improvement Act, 112
Hearst, Patty, 318–322
Hilliard, James, 146
Hinckley, John, 281
HMOs, 91. *See also* Managed care facilities
Homeopathy, 105, 125
Hospitals: iatrogenic injuries, 8–11; liability insurance for, 90–91; risk-management programs, 97–98; premature release of patients from, 117, 118, 130–131, 161, 164–165, 336; psychiatric, 130–132, 168, 174; teaching, 141–142
Household production losses, 16, 17
Hypnosis, 263, 302–303
Hypochondria, 239–240

Iatrogenic injuries, 8–11; insurance coverage for, 90–91; prevention of, 94
Immunity: absolute, 310–312, 323; limited, 313
Impostors, medical, 104
Informed consent, 23, 40, 81, 83, 205, 323; intentional torts vs. negligence, 24–25; professional and materiality standards for, 25, 27, 28; disclosure issues

Informed consent (*continued*)
and, 25–27, 37; hypothetical scenarios, 27–30; voluntary, 30, 31–32, 33, 34, 35, 37; knowledge of assent, 30–31, 37; malpractice litigation and, 30–31, 38–39, 269, 270; "reasonable person" standard for, 30–31, 129; coercion and, 31–32, 33, 35; institutionalized populations and, 32–34; competence and, 34–38; chronic illness and, 37–38; involuntary commitment and, 39–41; exceptions, 40–41, 63; by proxy, 40–41; children and, 41–43, 72, 73–74; documentation of, 63, 345; prescription medications and, 127, 129–130, 331; failure to obtain, 130, 331; statutes, 130; of patient to divided treatment, 144, 145; by suicidal patients, 172; autonomy of patient and, 199, 205; boundary violations and, 205; pro forma, 244, 246, 255
Innovative treatments, 196
Insanity defense, 281
Insurance. *See* Malpractice insurance; Medical insurance
Intentional tort theory, 24–25
Interrogatories, 350–352
Interspousal abuse, 82
Involuntary commitment, 39–41, 78

Johnson v. Ward, 218–219
Joint Commission on Accreditation of Healthcare Organizations (JCAHO), 91
Judges, 296, 354
Jury, 357–358; in malpractice litigation, 331; impression of the defendant, 354–356; opinion of witnesses, 357–362; instructions to, 358–362, 366
Juvenile delinquency, 80, 85

Kaimowitz v. Department of Mental Health of Michigan, 33–34
Knapp v. Eppright, 219
Kozol, Harry L., 318–319

Law's Stories: Narrative and Rhetoric in the Law (Brooks and Gewirtz), 309
Lawsuits against practitioners. *See* Malpractice litigation
Law vs. psychiatry, 281–282
Lawyers. *See* Attorneys
Lawyer's Ethics in an Adversary System (Freedman), 321

Learned treatises, 367–368
Legal rights of patients, 329–330
Liability, 1–2; impact on patient care, 2; protection measures, 48–49; prevention, 69; vicarious, 143, 144; in termination of treatment, 217; civil, 300, 309, 310, 331, 337; for historical falsity, 309–310; third-party, 314, 322. *See also* Managed care liability
Liability in psychiatric practice. *See* Psychiatric practice
Liability insurance: for hospitals, 90–91. *See* Malpractice insurance
Libel, 338
Licenses, medical, 145–146, 187
Licensing boards, 101–102, 113, 284, 292; licensing function, 102–105; disciplinary function, 105–113; reporting of ethics violations to, 338–339
Lifton, Robert Jay, 319
Litigation: records, 11–14; against alleged child abusers, 135; reimbursement for, 140; claims-handling perspective, 349. *See also* Malpractice litigation
Loss prevention: efforts by malpractice insurance companies, 90, 91, 92–93, 97–98; effect on quality of care, 92–93, 98; techniques and issues, 94–95; guidelines, 96–97; educational approaches to, 97–98
Lozano, Paul, 106

Magic, patient's wish for, 257–259
Malpractice: prevention, 2, 8; tort law and, 7–9, 62; reform legislation, 12–13, 18; documenting clinical care and, 69; crisis (1973–1975), 90; sharing of claims information, 93–96
Malpractice, psychiatric, 17, 19, 31
Malpractice insurance, 8, 17, 89, 90–91, 343, 347; premiums, 2, 8, 19, 90, 96; intentional tort coverage, 25; contract actions not covered by, 45, 62; market, 89, 90; captive, 90, 91; claims rates, 90; commercial vs. self-insurance programs, 90–91; claims management, 92–93, 98; suicide-related claims, 96–97; required coverage, 105; APA-sponsored, 117–118; for supervisory relationships, 135, 140; "deep pocket" principle of, 140, 141, 299; for psychiatrists, 145, 299; sexual misconduct excluded from cover-

age, 217; capitation agreements, 337; denial of benefits, 347–348
Malpractice insurance companies: loss-prevention efforts, 90, 91, 92–93, 97–98
Malpractice law: reform, 12–13, 18
Malpractice litigation, 1–2, 8–9, 62, 331, 344; as deterrent, 11, 93; rates of, 11–14; exploratory suits, 14; no-fault alternative to, 18–19; informed-consent claims, 30–31, 38–39, 269, 270; recovered abuse memories and, 80, 132–136, 263; prevention, 93–96, 237, 256, 261; collaborative study of claims, 96; civil actions, 106, 309, 310; standard-of-care claims, 112, 119, 121; increase in number of claims, 117–118, 241, 299, 347; elements of, 118, 229; involving prescription medications, 118–119, 125, 126, 189–191, 300, 380–381; negligence claims, 132, 256, 265, 299, 355; premature-release-of-patients claims, 132; suicide of patients and, 166, 167, 168, 175, 177–179, 245, 333, 378; boundary-violation claims, 196, 197, 200, 212; sexual misconduct claims, 202, 212; abandonment and termination-of-treatment claims, 217, 218–220, 221, 255–256; statute of limitations for, 218; clinician as defendant, 228; physician-patient-family relationship and, 237–238, 246; managed care risk factors, 237–239; risk factors for, 237–239, 247–248; high-risk families and, 242–243; high-risk clinicians and, 243–246; injury-related claims, 250–251; media and social factors, 250–251; role of technology in, 251–252, 263; emotion-based, 252–257; physician as defendant, 263; third-party (nonpatient), 310–317; high-risk areas, 332–333; average length of trial, 354; preponderance of verdicts for the defendant, 356; fear of, 371, 373–374
Mammograms, 105
Managed care facilities: boundary violations in, 106; psychiatric practice in, 117, 118, 125–126; split-treatment arrangements in, 121; influence on treatment boundaries, 202; confidentiality issues and, 205, 341–342; financial (cost-containment) limitations in, 209,

220, 237, 341–342; restrictions on physicians and clinicians, 209, 220, 237, 244–246, 341–342, 347; termination of treatment, 220; discouragement of referrals from, 243, 244, 341–342; documentation of treatment in, 244; standards of care, 347–348
Managed care liability, 44, 92, 237, 247–248; third-party contracts, 45–46, 53; cause of action, 45–49, 53; indemnification clauses and, 49–50; confidentiality of records, 50–53, 238; premature release of patients, 130–132; recovered abuse memories and, 135; patient-physician-family relationship and, 237–238, 246; prevention, 238–239; denial of benefits and, 239, 247; litigation-prone patients and, 239–242, 243; litigation-prone families and, 242–243, 247; high-risk clinicians and, 243–246
Mandatory reporting, 52–53, 72–73, 77–78; immunity from lawsuits and, 310–313, 77, 322; of gunshot/knife wounds, 52, 310; of suspected child abuse, 52, 72, 77, 300–301, 309–317; failure to report, 77; of impaired physicians, 110; of impaired patients, to the DMV, 122–123, 339, 340–341; of prescriptions to drug-dependent patients, 192–193; effect on therapeutic alliance, 311–313; of intent to commit perjury, 321; of sexual exploitation by therapists, 330, 337; of foreseeable danger to third parties, 339–341; of settlements and verdicts, 350. See also Duty to protect; Duty to warn
Massachusetts General Hospital, 96
Massachusetts Medical Society, 106, 109
Massachusetts Psychiatric Society, 106
Mature minor doctrine, 42, 74
Media, 250–251, 281
Medicaid, 14
Medical backup: prescription medications and, 140; supervisory arrangements concerning, 143–148
Medical boards. See Licensing boards
Medical insurance, 63, 107, 111, 146–147, 239; billing practices and, 107, 111; denial of coverage, 131. See also Malpractice insurance
Medicare, 14

Memory science, 135; use of truth serum, 302, 341; use of hypnosis, 302–303; reconstruction of reality theory, 303–304. *See also* Child abuse/sexual abuse: recovered memories of

Menninger, Karl, 373

Menninger Treatment Intervention Project, 377

Mental disorders, 72; required reporting of, to DMV, 122–123; violence and, 153–165; suicide and, 167; medical-legal issues in treatment for, 283

Mental health care: balance of practice and legal requirements, 2; cost vs. standards of care, 44

Mental health law, 330

Methadone clinics, 192–193

Metzloff, Thomas, 8

Miller v. Greater Southeast Community Hospital, 218

Mills, Don Harper, 8

Modern Legal Ethics (Burger), 305

Monitoring standards, 96

Montoya v. Bebensee, 315

Moon v. United States, 119

Mulder v. Parke Davis and Co., 128

Multiple personality disorder (MPD), 210, 211

Narcissism, 250, 267; of clinician, 237, 244; of patient, 240–241; of expert witnesses, 296

Narcotic treatment programs, 192–193

National Association of Insurance Commissioners (NAIC), 12

National Board examination/certificates, 102–103

National Board of Medical Examiners (NBME), 103

National Practitioner Data Bank, 112, 350

Neglect through abandonment, 217

Negligence: tort litigation for, 9–11; death as result of, 10; rates, 11; vs. intentional torts, 24–25; expert testimony regarding, 25; law, 25; disclosure issues and, 25–27; patient's right to appeal in cases of, 49; adjudication of, 50; in prescribing medications, 118; of supervision, 143, 144; in care of suicidal patients, 169, 179; in psychotherapy, 197, 202; of substitute physician, 219; admission of, 245–246; and likelihood of civil liability, 331–332; third-party injuries and, 339

Negligent misdiagnosis, 314–315

Neutrality, duty of, 198–199, 204, 206

Nix v. Whiteside, 321

No-fault compensation, 12, 15–16, 17–19

No-harm contracts. *See* Suicide risk: contracts against suicide

Nondisclosure issues, 24

Nonmedical therapists, 140, 145

Nursing homes, 91

Objectivity, scientific, 320

Omer v. Edgren, 199

Orne, Martin, 319–322

Osteopathy, 105

Over-the-counter drugs, 119

Pain and suffering compensation, 15–16, 18

Parents: rights concerning child's treatment, 64–65; right to see child's medical records, 74–76, 79; custodial, 76; informed consent and, 83

Patient Care Assessment Regulations of the Board of Registration in Medicine (Massachusetts), 91

Patient-physician-family relationship: malpractice litigation and, 237–238, 246

Patient-physician relationship, 92–94, 118; autonomy of patient in, 2, 199, 204, 205, 207, 245; sexual, 105, 336–337; guidelines for psychotherapists, 106–107; financial, 107, 209; physical contact in, 107–108, 207–208; gift giving and, 108; self-disclosure by physician in, 108; social, 108–109; family members and, 109, 135–136; sexual, 118, 202–211; with suicidal patients, 121; boundary issues in, 149; baseline, 190; trust-based, 197, 199–200; rule of abstinence in, 197–198, 204; duty of neutrality in, 198–199, 204; verbal interaction in, 205–206; personal, 206–207; post-termination, 206–208; in managed care facilities, 244–245; long-term, 250; effect of expert testimony on, 288; effect of legal changes on, 299–300; fiduciary, 314; fear of litigation and, 374–375; inaccessibility of therapist in, 376–377. *See also* Therapeutic alliance

Patient records. *See* Confidentiality; Documentation
Patient's rights: to refuse treatment, 2, 23, 38–39, 330, 331; to appeal, 48–49; to refuse to testify, 61–62
Peer review, 346
Performance evaluations, 141
Perjury, 321
Per se rule, 305
Personal injury law, 8
Personal injury litigation, 339
Physical examinations, 189–190, 207
Physician abuse, 82
Physician Health Services (PHS) (Massachusetts), 109–110
Polypharmacy, 124–125
Prescription medications, 110–111, 117, 118–130, 189–191, 193, 244; liability areas, 117, 118–119, 190–191; exceeding recommended dosages, 118, 119–121; malpractice litigation involving, 118–119, 125, 126, 189–191, 380–381; monitoring, 119–120, 121–124; for suicidal patients, 120–121, 178, 245; nonadherence to, 121, 122; split treatment arrangements and, 121; side effects, 122, 124, 254; duty-to-warn (disclosure) issues, 122–123, 127, 129–130; addictive, 123, 205; polypharmacy, 124–125; inappropriate indications, 124–126; failure to prescribe, 125; package insert (PDR), 126, 128; off-label prescribing, 126–128; informed consent concerning, 127, 129–130; limited prescribing privileges for, 146; registration of physician and drug, 187, 192; dispensing without prescription, 187–189; for immediate family of physician, 191; self-prescribing of, by physicians, 191; for drug-dependent patients, 192–193; guidelines for dispensing, 193–194; boundary violations involving, 205; antipsychotic, 331
Prevention strategies for malpractice litigation, 18, 19, 93–96, 257, 261. *See also* Loss prevention; Risk management
Privacy rights, 62, 65
Privilege, 78, 81; as distinct from confidentiality in patient records, 61–64; patient/psychotherapist, 338. *See also* Testimonial privilege
Projective identification, 374

Pro se rule, 288
Psychiatric practice. *See* Patient-physician relationship; Therapeutic alliance
Psychiatric records, 50, 51–52
Psychiatry vs. the law, 281–282
Psychology: of the physician, 371–374; of the psychiatrist, 374–375
Psychosis. *See* Violent patients
Psychotherapy, 106–107, 108, 133, 332; negligence in, 197; reimbursement for, 238; historical truth and, 304

Ramona v. Isabella, 133, 341
Ramon v. Farr, 128
Rape trauma syndrome, 369
Raymond, Sherwin H., 111–112
Raymond v. Board of Registration in Medicine, 111–112
Reaction formation, 379
Reasonableness standard in assessing suicide risk, 167
Reasonable person standard, 30–31
Reconstruction-of-reality theory, 303–304
Recordkeeping. *See* Documentation
Recovered memories of childhood abuse. *See* Child abuse/sexual abuse
Referral: as abandonment, 49; assessment of patients from, 56; of high-risk cases, 81; of family members, 135; to narcotic treatment programs, 193; to avoid boundary violations, 212; termination of treatment and, 217, 218–219, 220–221, 255; confidentiality issues in, 221; discouraged in managed care facilities, 243, 244, 341–342; at termination of treatment, 255; by attorneys, 287; to specialists, 341–342
Refusal of treatment, 2, 23; informed consent and, 38–39, 331; by involuntarily committed patients, 39; legal rights of, 330
Regulation, 2, 136. *See also* Licensing boards
Resource allocation, 238–239
Risk management, 255, 331–332; clinical, 1–2, 3, 136; techniques, 65, 119; informed consent in child and adolescent therapy, 73–74; documentation as technique for, 74–75, 345, 347, 355; documentation of treatment as, 74–75, 345, 347, 355; confidentiality issues, 75–78; testimonial privilege and, 78–80; excep-

Risk management (*continued*)
tions to privilege, 80; malpractice issues, 80–82; in high-conflict divorce proceedings, 82–84; at hospitals and health facilities, 91, 97–98; prevention of medical injury, 94; actual care scenarios, 94–95; principles, 140, 257–259, 331–332; in medical backup arrangements, 145; in supervisory arrangements, 148–149, 151–152; in treatment of violent patients, 153–162; assessment of suicide risk as, 171; for managed care liability, 237, 247–248; forensic psychiatric consultation as, 247–248; emotion-based, 256–257; therapeutic alliance as, 257; apology for bad outcome as, 259–260; errors in judgments of the truth, 302. *See also* Loss prevention; Suicide risk
Risk Management Committee (Harvard hospitals), 96
Risk Management Foundation of the Harvard Medical Institutions, 2–3, 96; Suicide Risk Advisory Group, 96–97
Risk Management Standards, 91
Rogers v. Okin, 330–331
Rosner, Richard, 284
Rules of evidence, 354

Sarchett v. Blue Cross of California, 48–49
Self-determination, patient's right of, 2, 199, 204, 205, 207, 245
Self-disclosure: by therapist, 198, 208, 210
Settings for treatment, 209–210
Sex-biased therapy practice, 207
Sexual abuse, 82; of patients, 105–106; recovered memory of, 263, 339, 341; false allegations of, 309–317, 323, 339; patients with history of, 337; documentation, 347. *See also* Child abuse/sexual abuse
Sexual abuse accommodation syndrome, 369
Sexual exploitation: fiduciary patient-physician relationship and, 199–200; as boundary violation, 202–211, 212; of terminated patient, 206–208
Sharing of information: regarding claims, 93–96; consent of patient in medical backup arrangements, 145
Signature of physician, 146–147, 335
Slander, 133, 136, 338

Social Transformation of American Medicine (Starr), 101
Social welfare programs, 14–15
Somatic treatments/conditions, 300, 310
Specialists, 140; referral to, 243, 244
Special Purpose Examination, 103
Spence, Donald P., 301, 302, 303
Split-treatment arrangements. *See* Medical backup
St. Charles v. Kender, 45
Standard of care, 44, 45, 121, 331–332; duty to treat and, 46–48; redefinition of, 48; prescription medications and, 128, 194; for alleged victims of sexual abuse, 135; for suicidal patients, 168, 172, 182–183; minimum, 190; boundary violations and, 197; medical decisionmaking and, 238; in malpractice litigation, 282–283; departure from, 333; community, 336
Standard of proof, 282
Starr, Paul, 101
State-funded systems of care, 55
State medical boards. *See* Licensing boards
Statute of limitations, 218, 307, 337, 338
Stecks v. Young, 310–312
Stewart, Potter, 305–306
Stone, Alan, 281
Street drugs, 119
Subpoenas to access patient records, 52, 79
Substance abuse, 72; by physicians, 105, 109–111; treatment, 108, 208
Substandard care, 251; claim of, in malpractice litigation, 9–11, 12, 14, 48; discipline of physician and, 112
Substituted consent, 41–42. *See also* Informed consent
Substituted judgment, 39, 331
Substitute physician. *See* Medical backup; Referral
Suicidal patients, 106, 243; involuntary commitment of, 78; prescription medications for, 120–121, 178, 245; anxiety associated with treating, 166, 169, 177, 183, 377–381; in acute crises, 171, 175; under care of substitute physician, 219; psychodynamics of, 378–380
Suicide: pacts, 176; prevention, 334–336, 378; cases, 344–346
Suicide risk: contracts against suicide, 166, 174–175, 176–180, 181–183, 333–334, 336; assessment vs. prediction of,

166–167; risk-benefit analysis, 167, 168–169; reasonableness, foreseeability, and prediction, 167–168, 171; documentation of assessments of, 167–169, 172, 176; hospitalization or discharge of patient and, 168–169, 172, 182–183, 236; management of suicidal patients, 169, 172–173; indicators, 169–171; assessment methods, 171–174; therapeutic alliance and, 175–176, 181–182; clinical risk management and, 179–180; management, 179–180; assessment, 180, 183, 333–336; clinical vignette, 180–183; in managed care settings, 336; high-risk cases, 336–339; prediction model, 378

Suicide Risk Advisory Group (SRAG), 96–97

Supervision: of other therapists, 135; by psychiatrist, 140–141; consultation model of, 141, 142–143; oversight model of, 141–142; liability in relation to, 143; negligent, 143, 144; boundary issues in, 149–151

Supervisory arrangements, 135, 140, 143

Tarasoff v. Regents of the University of California, 2, 62, 131, 300, 314, 339–340

Technology, medical, 244, 251–252, 263

Termination of treatment: sexual exploitation of patient after, 206–208; feelings of loss and grief by the therapist, 208; billing practices and, 209; viewed as abandonment, 216–217, 220; referral of patient, 217, 218–219, 220–221, 255; by patient, 219; documentation of, 220, 221; guidelines, 220–221; confidentiality issues in, 221

Testamentary capacity, 35, 37

Testimonial capacity, 35, 37

Testimonial privilege, 61, 78–80

Testimony: forensic, 81–82, 83, 119, 132, 134; expert, 262, 263; reliable and relevant standards for, 263; principles of effective, 264–265, 271, 273, 276; witness attitudes and, 265–266, 267, 291–292, 362–367; content of, 274–277; recommendations for, 278–279; depositions as, 296, 351–352; of historical truth, 309, 317–322; credibility of, 342–343, 351, 354–355; interrogatories as, 351; testimonial aids, 363; terminology used in, 363–364. *See also* Expert

witnesses; Fact witnesses; Trial; Witnesses

Testing, psychological, 369

Therapeutic alliance: suicide risk and, 175–176, 181–182; contracts against suicide and, 176–177, 180; boundary maintenance in, 197; informed consent and, 205; advocacy-based, 240, 313; admission of clinician error and, 245–246, 257, 259–261; as risk management, 257, 259, 375; mandatory reporting requirements and, 311–313; absence of, 334; competence of patient to enter, 335; with borderline patients, 376–377. *See also* Patient-physician relationship

Therapeutic privilege, 40

Therapist shopping, 241–242

Third parties: protection of, 2, 77–78, 85, 202, 300, 314, 339–341; contracts with, 45–46, 49–50, 53, 131; malpractice litigation by, 310–317

Third-party payers of medical costs, 15, 16, 131; contractual liability of, 45–46, 53, 131, 314, 322; contracts containing indemnification clauses, 49–50; release of medical records to, 75, 238; denial of benefits by, 247–248. *See also* Malpractice insurance companies

Titicutt Follies, 330

Tort law: reform, 7, 15, 18, 342; compensation function of, 8, 11, 12, 14–15; negligence cases, 9–11; substandard care and, 9–11, 12, 14

Tort litigation, 338; deterrent effect of, 7, 9, 18; efficiency of, 12, 13–14; intentional torts vs. negligence, 24–25

Tort system, 252

Transcripts of depositions, 234

Transference, 201, 207, 211; during trial procedures, 236; paranoid, 375; gratifications, 377

Trauma, 80, 84–85, 240, 266

Treatment: review boards, 41; alliances, 54; teams, 65–66, 143; length of sessions, 210–211; uncertainty of, 259

Trial: administrative proceedings as alternative to, 283–284; strategies and techniques, 306, 351–352, 353; rules of evidence, 307, 309; rules of procedure, 307; documentation at, 338; preparation, 349–356, 365; pretrial discovery process, 351, 365–366, 368; average length of, 354

Trust, 337; as basis of patient-physician relationship, 197, 199–200, 205; betrayal of, 254–255, 257

Truth: about child abuse, 301–302, 309–317; historical (actual, provable), 301–302, 303–304, 309–317, 319–320; inside the therapy room, 301–304, 322; narrative (told and believed by patient), 301–304, 323; forensic, 302, 304–309, 322–323; narrative vs. historical, 302, 310, 321, 322–323; distortion of, 303, 305, 306, 322; memory and, 303; historical vs. forensic, 304–309; scientific, 307–308; testimony regarding, 309, 317–322; standard of, 316; psychiatry and, 319

Truth serum (sodium amytal), 302, 341

Underclaiming, 8

Undue suggestion, 321

United States Medical Licensing Examination (USMLE), 102

United States v. Moore, 190

United States v. Tran Trong Cuong, 189, 190

United States v. Wade, 305

Utilization review, 46–47, 131–132

Videotaped depositions, 232–233

Violent patients: negligent release of, from hospitals, 117, 118, 130–131, 161, 164–165; prescription medications for, 126–127; legal issues and, 153, 162; assessment of, for clinical risk, 153–161, 164; case study, 162–165; confidentiality vs. boundary violations, 202; assessment of, for litigation, 283

Wage losses from adverse events, 16, 17

Waiver: of testimonial privilege, 78–79; of confidentiality, 84, 221; of privileges, 338

W.C.W. v. Bird, 315

Wesson, Marianne, 318–319, 322

West, Louis Jolyon, 318, 319–322

White, Edward Douglass, 305–306

Wickline v. California, 46–47, 131, 132, 220

Wilkinson v. Balsam, 312–313

Wilson v. Blue Cross of Southern California et al., 131–132

Wiseman, Frederick, 330

Witnesses: alibi, 226; character and status, 226, 362–363; rebuttal of, 226; cross-examination of, 236, 271–277, 366–367; ethical standards for, 262, 272, 273, 276; role of, 264; attitudes and appearance of, 265–266, 267, 291–292, 362–367; direct examination of, 266–270; communication with attorney, 267–268; credentials of, 268, 364–365; fees paid to, 268; redirect examination of, 277; credibility of, 335, 358–362, 369; treating therapist as, 338; direct testimony by, 353. See also Clinician in court; Expert witnesses; Fact witnesses; Testimony

Workers' compensation, 17

Wrongful death, 10, 156, 217, 219, 331, 341

Wrongful hospitalization or commitment, 332

Yale Law School, 309

Younger, Irving, 272